Wills Eye Hospital

COLOR ATLAS & SYNOPSIS OF
Clinical Ophthalmology

Neuro-Ophthalmology

THIRD EDITION

EDITORS
Peter J. Savino, MD
Clinical Professor of Ophthalmology
University of California San Diego
Shiley Eye Institute
La Jolla, California

Helen V. Danesh-Meyer, MD, PhD, FRANZCO
Sir William and Lady Stevenson Professor of Ophthalmology
Department of Ophthalmology
University of Auckland, New Zealand

SERIES EDITOR
Christopher J. Rapuano, MD
Director and Attending Surgeon, Cornea Service
Co-Director, Refractive Surgery Department
Wills Eye Hospital
Professor of Ophthalmology
Sidney Kimmel Medical College at Thomas Jefferson University
Philadelphia, Pennsylvania

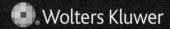
Wills Eye Hospital

COLOR ATLAS & SYNOPSIS OF
Clinical Ophthalmology

Neuro-
Ophthalmology

THIRD EDITION

Wolters Kluwer

Philadelphia • Baltimore • New York • London
Buenos Aires • Hong Kong • Sydney • Tokyo

Acquisitions Editor: Chris Teja
Editorial Coordinator: Lauren Pecarich
Manufacturing Coordinator: Beth Welsh
Marketing Manager: Rachel Mante Leung
Production Project Manager: Barton Dudlick
Design Coordinator: Stephen Druding
Production Services: S4Carlisle Publishing Services

Cover image courtesy of Dr. Harry Bradshaw.

Third Edition

9 8 7 6 5 4 3 2 1

Printed in China

Library of Congress Cataloging-in-Publication Data

ISBN-13: 978-1-4963-6689-4
ISBN-10: 1-4963-6689-1

Cataloging-in-Publication data available on request from the Publisher.

To Marie and Mike
Juliette and Emily

Contributors

Jurij R. Bilyk, MD, FACS
Professor of Ophthalmology
Department of Ophthalmology
Thomas Jefferson University Hospital
Philadelphia, Pennsylvania
Attending Surgeon
Skull Base Division
Neuro-Ophthalmology Service
Wills Eye Hospital
Philadelphia, Pennsylvania

Helen V. Danesh-Meyer, MD, PhD, FRANZCO
Sir William and Lady Stevenson Professor of
    Ophthalmology
Department of Ophthalmology
University of Auckland
Auckland, New Zealand

Adam E. Flanders, MD
Professor of Radiology & Rehabilitation Medicine
Department of Radiology/Neuroradiology
    Division
Thomas Jefferson University Hospital
Thomas Jefferson University
Philadelphia, Pennsylvania

Rahul M. Nikam, MBBS, DMRD, DNB
Fellow
Department of Radiology
Thomas Jefferson University
Philadelphia, Pennsylvania
Fellow
Department of Medical Imaging
Nemours Alfred I. duPont Hospital for Children
Wilmington, Delaware

Peter J. Savino, MD
Clinical Professor of Ophthalmology
University of California San Diego
Shiley Eye Institute
La Jolla, California

Kiran Shankar Talekar, MBBS, MD, DABR
Assistant Professor of Radiology
Radiology, Neuroradiology
Sidney Kimmel Medical Center
Thomas Jefferson University
Physician Faculty
Radiology and Neuroradiology
Thomas Jefferson University Hospital
Philadelphia, Pennsylvania

About the Series

The beauty of the atlas/synopsis concept is the powerful combination of illustrative photographs and a summary approach to the text. Ophthalmology is a very visual discipline that lends itself wonderfully to clinical photographs. Whereas the seven ophthalmic subspecialties in this series—Cornea, Retina, Glaucoma, Oculoplastics, Neuro-ophthalmology, Uveitis, and Pediatrics—employ varying levels of visual recognition, a relatively standard format for the text is used for all volumes.

The goal of the series is to provide an up-to-date clinical overview of the major areas of ophthalmology for students, residents, and practitioners in all the health care professions. The abundance of large, excellent-quality photographs (both in print and online) and concise, outline-form text will help achieve that objective.

Christopher J. Rapuano
Series Editor

Preface

We undertook the task of writing this atlas to be part of a larger work, that of the Wills Eye Hospital Multi-Specialty Atlas series. Being part of a larger work and the format in which it was produced required that we deal with certain limitations.

The book is an atlas and therefore cannot be encyclopedic; certain information had to be omitted. We chose to include those topics that are the most frequently encountered entities in neuro-ophthalmology. These are problems that the general ophthalmologist face on any given day in the office. We have tried to include the most clinically relevant material in each topic. We have purposely omitted the more exotic neuro-ophthalmologic syndromes.

Because this series is a smaller, soft-covered publication designed to be portable, certain limitations were imposed on the photographic array. We could not present some of the multiple series of eye movement disorders in more standard ways but hope that the way we have displayed them makes sense to the reader and is not confusing or obfuscating.

Some of the photographs may be smaller than we would ideally like, but in order to have a full exposition of the photographic variations of an entity (ocular motility, visual field, and neuroimaging), we chose to make them smaller and try to include them in one area, ideally on one page, so the reader would not be constantly flipping back and forth between text and photographs.

We hope that our compromises to the format have not sacrificed clarity and ease of reading and interpretation.

We include two invited chapters, one on basic MRI information for the general ophthalmologist, kindly written by Drs. Adam E. Flanders and Kiran S. Talekar, MD, from the Division of Neuro-Radiology at Thomas Jefferson University. Chapter 13 on orbital disorders with neuro-ophthalmologic implications is authored by Jurij R. Bilyk, MD, of the Oculoplastic Service at Wills Eye Hospital. He also authored the section on Traumatic Optic Neuropathy in Chapter 5. We express our gratitude to these authors for their willingness to contribute to the atlas and for their flexibility in tailoring their chapters to our format.

This atlas could not have come to completion without the involvement of Jack Scully of the Audio-Visual Department at Wills Eye Hospital. His expertise, tireless dedication to making the photographs in this book as good as they could be, and incredible good humor over many months in dealing with the authors is greatly appreciated. He literally had a role in the exposition of every single photograph in this atlas.

We hope that the work will be useful to residents in ophthalmology and will be helpful to the practicing ophthalmologist. If we have accomplished this, we have succeeded in our task.

Peter J. Savino
Helen V. Danesh-Meyer
Editors

Contents

Wills Eye Hospital

COLOR ATLAS & SYNOPSIS OF
Clinical Ophthalmology

Neuro-Ophthalmology

THIRD EDITION

Examination of the Afferent Visual System

INTRODUCTION

The purpose of the neuro-ophthalmic afferent examination is to detect visual abnormalities (acuity or visual field) and to determine if they are because of neuro-ophthalmic disorders. The neuro-ophthalmic examination should be preceded by a thorough history of the presenting complaint, a detailed past medical history, social history, ocular history, list of medications, and review of systems. The emphasis of the history should be listening to how the patient characterizes the visual symptoms, in particular, the time course of symptoms of visual loss, the laterality, and any associated symptoms. For example, it is crucial to discriminate between sudden visual loss and the sudden *awareness* of visual loss. Associated symptoms should also include systemic conditions that may be relevant. For example, in a patient with sudden visual loss over the age of 60 years, the patient should be asked about concomitant symptoms of giant cell arteritis. It is the responsibility of the clinician to explore these possible associations. The history should be followed by a comprehensive ophthalmologic assessment that may

identify non–neuro-ophthalmic causes for the visual disturbance (e.g., microhyphema as a cause of transient visual loss). Only the parts of the examination that are directly relevant to the neuro-ophthalmic examination will be discussed in this chapter.

VISUAL ACUITY

Patients can have decreased acuity from a variety of causes. The starting point of the neuro-ophthalmologic examination is to determine the *best-corrected* Snellen acuity in each eye separately. A variety of targets can be used to test visual acuity (VA) at distance (Fig. 1-1). Several methods may be used to determine if the VA can be improved and what is the likely cause of the poor vision.

- Refraction
- Pinhole: A series of pinholes measuring 2 to 2.5 mm are placed before each eye as its fellow is occluded (Fig. 1-2). Improvement in acuity with pinhole indicates a refractive or media (e.g., cataract) cause of decreased vision.
- Bright light near vision: An improved near acuity with appropriate reading glasses

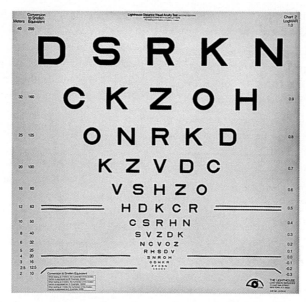

FIGURE 1-1. Bailey-Lovie visual acuity chart. The retro-illuminated Bailey–Lovie chart is placed at a distance of 4 m from the patient.

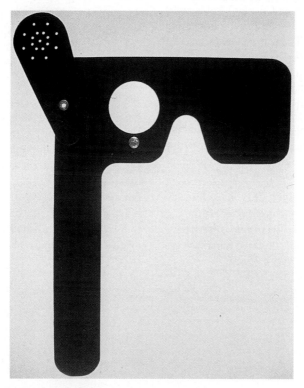

FIGURE 1-2. Pinhole occluder. Occluder with pinholes that can be rotated into position in lieu of performing a refraction.

and a bright light indicates that the cause of decreased vision is refractive or cataracts.

• Potential acuity devices: a variety of apparatus project images (Snellen optotypes or lines) directly on the retina, thus bypassing any refractive or media cause for decreased vision.

Improvement in VA to normal with any of these methods obviates the need to search for a neuro-ophthalmic cause of visual loss. Failure to improve the acuity, on the other hand, means further investigations for other causes, including neuro-ophthalmic diseases, are in order.

COLOR VISION

The purpose of color vision testing is to detect acquired unilateral or bilateral color loss, which occurs with optic neuropathies, disorders of the optic chiasm, and, more infrequently, some occipital disorders (see Chapter 7). Most optic neuropathies produce loss of color perception relative to VA, whereas in retinal or macular disease, the acuity may be poor but color vision is relatively preserved. Acquired dyschromatopsia is a useful clinical finding to support the presence of an optic nerve disorder.

It is important to remember to test each eye separately and to test color vision before testing pupils because the bright light can produce transient color desaturation. Color vision may be tested with the following:

• Ishihara pseudoisochromatic or Hardy–Rand–Rittler plates: The patient is asked to identify the numbers displayed using each eye

in turn (Fig. 1-3). This tests predominantly red–green color deficiencies. The number of correctly identified plates with each eye is recorded. The control plate can be read if the VA is better than 20/400. If the patient does not see the control plate, it is pointless testing the remainder of the plates. If the patient only sees the control plate, then this is recorded as "control only."

• Farnsworth panel D15: This panel has 15 caps with colors that are to be placed in order, starting with the closest hue to the reference cap, until all 15 are placed in sequence. A number on the back of each cap indicates its correct position in a normal sequence. This test identifies tritan (blue), deutan (green), and protan (red) color anomalies.

• Farnsworth Munsell 100 hue: This tests actually consists of 85 (not 100) caps in 4 boxes (Fig. 1-4) and is similar in concept to the D15 test. The 100-hue test can determine the severity as well as the axis of color anomaly. The Farnsworth Munsell 100 hue test most thoroughly assesses color vision, but because it is tedious and cumbersome, it is not usually performed as a first-line color vision test.

• Color comparison: At times, asking the patient to determine the amount of red in a test object (mydriatic bottle cap) with each eye to detect the percentage of red desaturation (e.g., OD 100%, OS 75%) will reveal subtle color anomalies (Fig. 1-5). Although this is a subjective test, it has been demonstrated to correlate strongly with the presence of a relative afferent pupillary defect (RAPD).

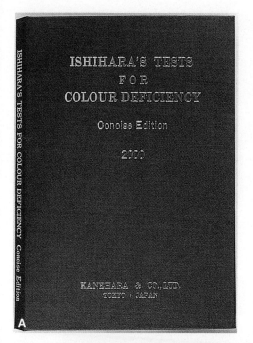

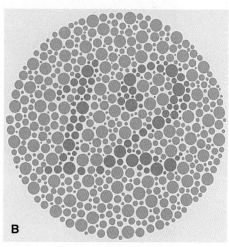

FIGURE 1-3. A. Ishihara pseudoisochromatic color-plate book. B. The first plate (12) is the control plate and is recognizable except with profound visual loss.

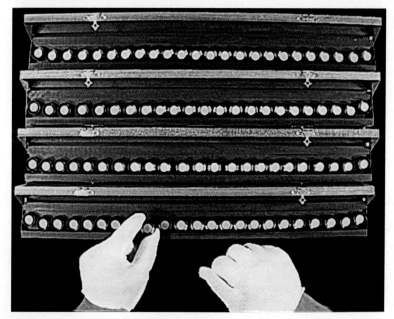

FIGURE 1-4. Farnsworth Munsell 100 hue color vision test. The patient uses gloves and under standard illumination is asked to arrange the caps in sequence with respect to the color reference cap in each box.

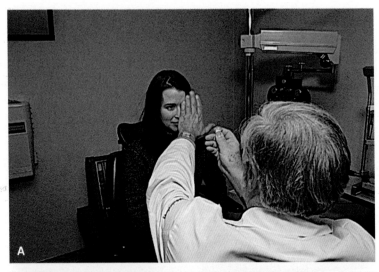

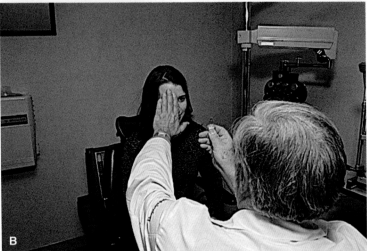

FIGURE 1-5. **Red desaturation test.** Color comparison between right eye (**A**) and left eye (**B**).

PUPILLARY TESTING

Pupillary testing should be performed on every patient. Several parameters should be assessed during pupil testing. These include the following:

- Size and regularity of pupils
- Presence of anisocoria (discussed in Chapter 12)

- Relative afferent pupillary defect (RAPD)
- Response to light (discussed in Chapter 12)
- Response to near (discussed in Chapter 12)

Relative Afferent Pupillary Testing

Testing for the presence of an RAPD should be performed on every patient. The presence of an RAPD indicates an optic neuropathy or severe retinal disease. Patients should be tested in the dark while they fixate in the distance. A bright light, either a halogen muscle light or indirect ophthalmoscope, is shone in each eye separately. The light illuminates each eye for the same amount of time (prolonged illumination of one eye may bleach the retina asymmetrically and produce an RAPD when none exists) and is swung between the eyes rapidly. In a unilateral or asymmetric optic neuropathy, the afferent input to the midbrain pupillomotor centers will be less than when the same light is presented to the unaffected eye. Therefore, weaker pupillary constriction occurs in *both* pupils when the affected eye is tested and more when the contralateral eye is tested. Hence, when the light swings to the normal pupil, both pupils constrict. Swinging back to the affected side causes relative dilatation of both pupils. It is important to remember that failure to constrict or a more rapid release of the constriction may indicate a very mild optic neuropathy. Finally, even though the examiner is looking at one pupil, it is important to remember that both pupils are changing equally and examining either pupil will result in the same interpretation of the test (**Fig. 1-6**).

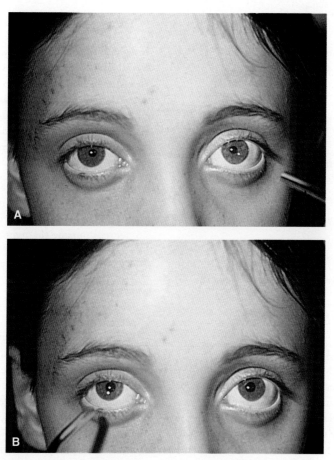

FIGURE 1-6. **Pupillary examination.** Both pupils constrict when the light is directed into the left eye (**A**), but they both dilate when it is swung to the right eye (**B**). Both constrict again when the light is swung back to the left eye (**C**).

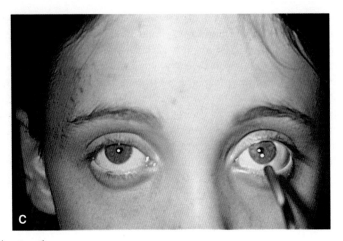

FIGURE 1-6. (*continued*)

The RAPD may be produced by

- anterior chamber or vitreous hemorrhages,
- large retinal detachments or macular lesions,
- unilateral or asymmetric optic nerve disorders,
- chiasmal compromise (as long as there is asymmetric visual loss),
- optic tract lesions.

The RAPD is *not* produced by

- cataract,
- refractive errors,
- lesions posterior to the lateral geniculate body,
- nonphysiologic visual loss.

AMSLER GRID

The Amsler grid consists of a central dot for fixation surrounded by a grid pattern. Each eye is examined separately. The patient is instructed to look only at the central dot and to report (or draw) any scotomas or other alterations of the grid. Defects may be due to neuro-ophthalmic or retinal disease. The presence of metamorphopsia (straight lines appear curved) is an indication of a retinal and not an optic nerve abnormality. We find it useful to use the red grid on the black page as the first test because patients with subtle optic neuropathies may have a normal white on black Amsler but an abnormal red on black Amsler (Fig. 1-7). If the red Amsler is normal, the white need not be tested.

The Amsler grid falls on the central area and encompasses 10 degrees around the fixation point. The optic disc, and thus the blind spot, is 5 degrees outside the temporal border of the grid.

CONTRAST SENSITIVITY

Snellen acuity is routinely tested in a high-contrast setting (black letters on a white background) (Fig. 1-8). Decreasing the contrast can expose visual defects that may otherwise go undetected. Patients with optic neuritis, for example, often have poor contrast sensitivity despite "normal" acuity and color vision. A variety of methods may be used to test contrast sensitivity. We do not test it on all patients but find it useful in patients with visual complaints but with an otherwise normal examination.

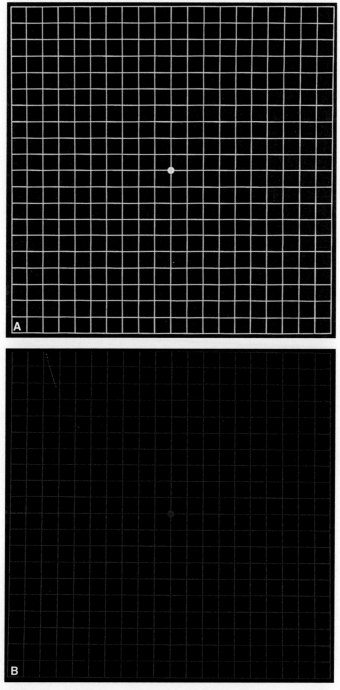

FIGURE 1-7. **Amsler grids.** A series of test plates can be used but the white (**A**) and red (**B**) squares on a black background are most useful.

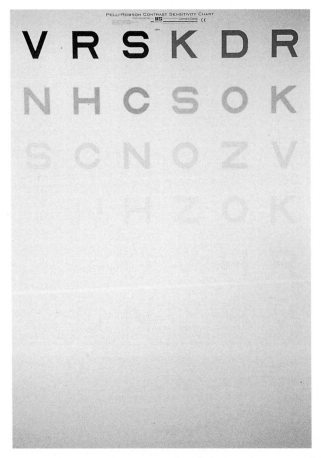

FIGURE 1-8. **Pelli-Robson contrast Sensitivity Chart.** The Pelli–Robson chart consists of 16 triplets of letters that gradually decrease in contrast. A normal response is correctly identifying 14 of the 16 triplets.

BRIGHTNESS COMPARISON

A simple comparison of brightness sensitivity between the two eyes is a sensitive test for unilateral optic neuropathy and has been shown to correlate strongly with the presence of an RAPD. A light (from a muscle light or indirect ophthalmoscope) is shone directly into each eye separately, and the patient is asked to fixate the light. The light source is held approximately 30 cm from the patient's eye and lined up to be in the center of the visual axis. Care must be taken to shine the light directly along the visual axis in both eyes because shining the light obliquely in one eye will influence the patient's response. The patient is then asked the following questions: (1) Is the light equal between the two eyes or is one brighter? If one is brighter, then the patient is asked, (2) if you give the value of 100 to the brighter light, what value would you give to the light when it is shone in the other eye? Alternatively, "If the light in the brighter eye is worth one dollar, how much is the light in the other eye worth?"

If the answer to question 1 was that the light in both eyes is equal, this makes optic neuropathy as the cause for the visual disturbance less likely.

PHOTOSTRESS RECOVERY TEST

This is a useful test to help differentiate between maculopathy and optic neuropathy. The principle underlying this test is that recovery of retinal sensitivity following exposure to a bright light is based on regeneration of visual pigments that were bleached during the exposure to light. A delay in this process occurs in diseases that affect the photoreceptors or the adjacent retinal pigment epithelium. It is independent of the neural pathway. The test is performed as follows on each eye independently.

1. Determine the best-corrected VA in each eye.
2. Patient looks directly into bright light source held at 2 to 3 cm for 10 seconds.
3. Record the time taken for the return of VA to within one line of the best-corrected acuity.

Most normal patients will have a recovery time of less than 30 seconds, and the recovery time between eyes is within 10 seconds. Macular disease, but not optic nerve disease, may cause a prolongation in the photostress recovery time. This is particularly useful for unilateral or subtle macular diseases.

OPHTHALMOSCOPY

Examination of the fundus is an essential part of the neuro-ophthalmic examination. This can be performed with direct or indirect ophthalmoscopy. We recommend assessment of the optic disc with a 60-, 78-, or 90-diopter hand-held lens that allows stereoscopic examination.

Other aspects of the neuro-ophthalmic examination are covered in other portions of the text.

- Visual fields (Chapter 2)
- Ocular motility (Chapter 7)

Visual Fields

INTRODUCTION

Testing visual fields is an integral part of the neuro-ophthalmologic examination in any patient with an afferent system problem. In fact, any patient who has decreased vision that cannot be explained on an ocular or refractive basis should have a visual field test.

PRINCIPLES THAT CONTRIBUTE TO VISUAL FIELD INTERPRETATION

Extent of the Normal Monocular Visual Field

- Nasally 60 degrees
- Superiorly 60 degrees
- Inferiorly 70 to 75 degrees
- Temporally 100 to 110 degrees

Retinal Nerve Fiber Anatomy

The basis of visual field defects is the anatomic structure of the retinal nerve fibers. The visual field and retina have an inverted and reverse relationship. Relative to fixation, the inferior visual field falls on the superior retina. The superior visual field falls on the inferior retina, the temporal visual field on the nasal retina, and the nasal visual field on the temporal retina.

Lesions of the optic nerve produce specific patterns of visual field defects within the central 30 degrees of the visual field because retinal nerve fibers enter the optic disc in a specific pattern.

- Arcuate nerve fiber bundles: The superior and inferior nerve fibers are formed into arcuate bundles that course around the papillomacular bundle to enter the optic nerve superiorly and inferiorly, respectively. Peripherally in the retina, they join at a structure called the horizontal raphe. Fibers do not cross this raphe. The nasal most extent of a superior or inferior arcuate defect is the horizontal meridian (Fig. 2-1).

- Papillomacular bundle: Retinal nerve fibers from the macula enter the optic disc temporally. Involvement of the papillomacular bundle produces a central (Fig. 2-2A) or a cecocentral (Fig. 2-2B) scotoma.

- Nasal nerve fiber bundles: These enter the nasal aspect of the optic disc and travel in a straight (nonarcuate) course. The resulting defect is a wedge-shaped temporal scotoma arising from the blind spot and does not necessarily respect the temporal horizontal meridian.

Lesions of the optic disc can produce visual field defects identical to those of the retina. Because the retinal fibers extend posteriorly through the optic nerve toward the chiasm, they rotate 90 degrees, and the macular fibers come to occupy the central core of the optic nerve. Therefore, lesions in the retrobulbar prechiasmal optic nerve tend to produce more central scotomas, whereas lesions of the intracranial prechiasmal optic nerve may even present a visual field defect that begins to respect the vertical meridian (see Chapter 5).

Testing Strategies

A variety of testing strategies are available to explore the extent of the visual field. The specific technology used is less important than the goal that the method employed arrives at the correct answer as to the form and extent of any scotoma.

Discussion of the types of visual field examinations performed routinely in neuro-ophthalmologic practice follows.

Confrontation Visual Fields

Confrontation visual field tests should be performed on all patients, even those without afferent complaints. Confrontation visual field tests provide a rapid and practical method of visual field assessment that can be performed with minimal equipment and may be the only method of testing readily available. The test is quickly performed and easily understood by most patients. It will identify gross scotomas and has only moderate sensitivity and specificity for identifying small or subtle scotomas. A normal confrontation visual field test does not preclude the need for more automated visual field testing.

Several techniques have been described for performing confrontation visual fields. We describe a few options below. For all tests of confrontation visual fields, it is important for the examiner and patient to be seated face to face at a distance of approximately 2 to 3 feet from each other and the patient asked to occlude one eye using the palm of his or her hand, a patch, or other occluding device. The patient is asked to fixate on the examiner's opposite eye (if the patient's right eye is being examined, the patient fixates on the examiner's left eye) or nose.

The patient needs to be told that confrontation visual field test is a test of side vision and that they need to maintain central fixation at all times (i.e., to look at the examiner's eye).

• Kinetic red target: A 5-mm red-topped pin is moved inward from beyond the boundary of each quadrant along a line bisecting the horizontal and vertical meridians. The patient is asked to report when the pin is first perceived to be red.

• Finger counting: The patient is asked to count 1, 2, or 5 static fingers presented sequentially in each of the four quadrants approximately 20 degrees eccentric to fixation and equidistant from the quadrant borders. Simultaneous presentation of fingers in two quadrants can be used to speed up testing (Fig. 2-3). A modified version of the game "Simon Says" can be used for young children who cannot yet count fingers. The child is asked to mimic the examiner by holding up the same number of fingers as she observes (Fig. 2-4).

• Red comparison: Two identical red mydriatic bottle tops, approximately 20 mm in diameter, are presented in a fashion analogous to the finger comparison test in all four quadrants and the patient asked if the bottle tops appeared equally red. Simultaneous comparison of color between hemifields and asking specifically about desaturation is useful in distinguishing subtle anomalies. Any quadrant in which the bottle top appeared less red is considered abnormal.

• Static finger wiggle: Two index fingers are presented simultaneously on either side of the vertical meridian approximately 20 degrees eccentric to fixation and equidistant from the quadrant borders in the superior and then inferior quadrants. The patient is asked to report which finger wiggled.

The probability of detecting a visual field defect is dependent on the size and density of the field defect, with the probability increasing with worsening visual field defect. Confrontation tests that utilize a red target (either red comparison or kinetic red testing) tend to have the highest sensitivities.

Kinetic testing with a red target has been shown to provide the highest sensitivity and specificity (of any individual test), and the sensitivity and specificity improve slightly if combined with static finger wiggle.

Static Automated Perimetry

Automated perimetry has several advantages as a testing procedure. It is a readily available means of visual field testing in most ophthalmology offices. It is not excessively technician dependent, although some technician interaction during the testing procedure will ensure a more reliable result. It is a standardized method of testing and is an excellent way to follow visual fields to test for progression.

Computerized threshold static perimetry involves determining the dimmest stimulus that can be seen at a number of predetermined test point locations. At each test point, retinal sensitivity is determined and expressed in decibels (dB). The dB value refers to retinal sensitivity, not stimulus intensity, and varies between 0 dB (the brightest stimulus [10,000 apostilbs] not seen) and 51 dB (the dimmest stimulus [0.08 apostilbs] seen). Mean deviation indicates the extent to which the whole visual field departs from age-matched normal controls and is expressed in dB.

The most frequent testing strategies used are the threshold strategies using a Humphrey field analyzer (Carl Zeiss Meditec Inc., Dublin, CA) using the SITA (Swedish Interactive Threshold Algorithm)-Standard 24-2 (or 30-2) program with a white Goldmann size III stimulus. SITA uses a database of expected threshold values for patients with a more sophisticated knowledge of the relationship between different points and how they influence the outcome at other points. Hence, determination of the threshold is achieved by a few testing points.

Several programs on static threshold perimeters are available. We routinely employ three of them:

• The full threshold 30-2, which consists of 76 testing points and examines the full 30 degrees of visual field. The test points are spaced approximately 6 degrees apart.

• The full threshold 24-2, which is similar to the 30-2 except that it eliminates the edge points, except for the two most nasal points along the horizontal meridian. Thus, 54 test points in the central 24 degrees are tested. The test points are likewise 6 degrees apart.

• In order to magnify small, centrally located defects that might be missed on the 24-2 and the 30-2 that allow 4-degree test spacing between points, the 10-2 program is used. This strategy tests all points within the 10 degrees of fixation in 2-degree intervals.

• It is also critical to measure the foveal threshold (normal, 30–37 dB) because it is an estimate of central visual function.

Several factors influence automated perimetry:

• Refractive error

• Pupil size

• Ptosis (may produce a superior visual field defect)

• Media opacities

• Patient factors: concentration, anxiety, learning effects, fixation instability

- Poor testing setup: lens rim obstruction, misalignment
- Testing conditions: background luminance, stimulus size

Kinetic Manual Perimetry (Goldmann Manual Perimetry)

The perimeter designed by Goldmann is a bowl perimeter on which it is possible to perform both static and kinetic perimetry. The test can also explore the full extent of the visual field and is useful for testing for defects that occur outside the central 30-degree zone. The disadvantages of this technology are that it is becoming less available and is highly dependent on the skill of the perimetrist.

In this test, a super threshold object is moved from a peripheral area where the patient cannot perceive it toward the center of the visual field. The patient is instructed to signal as soon as the moving light is perceived. The speed at which the target moves is controlled by the examiner and must be constant.

Tangent Screen

Many of the perimetric principles used today derive from testing with the tangent screen. This is a black felt covered board that measures the central 30 degrees of the visual field. The patient is seated in front of this large board while white or colored objects of specific sizes are brought in from the periphery to the center until the patient signals perception of the object. There are several disadvantages to this technique. The patient can tell from where the examiner is standing and where the examiner's arm is, and the direction from whence the target is coming. In addition, the illumination is not standard. Finally, with loss of popularity of this method of testing visual fields, tangent screens are becoming less available.

With the tangent screen, the distance that the patient sits from the testing surface can be changed. This is an important element in trying to detect nonphysiologic patterns of visual loss, such as tunnel vision.

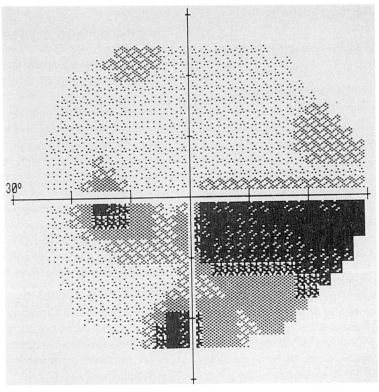

FIGURE 2-1. **Arcuate defect.** A left inferior arcuate defect denser nasally and respects the horizontal raphe.

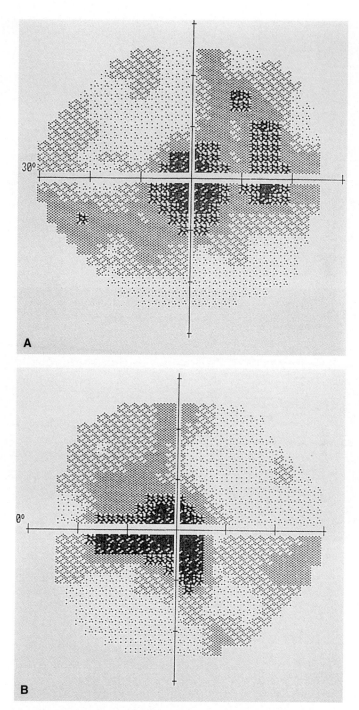

FIGURE 2-2. Central scotomas. A. Central scotoma right eye. The physiologic blind spot is separate from the scotoma. **B.** Cecocentral scotoma left eye involves the area of fixation and the physiologic blind spot.

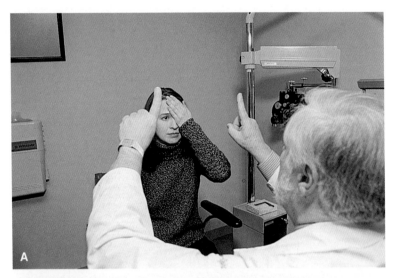

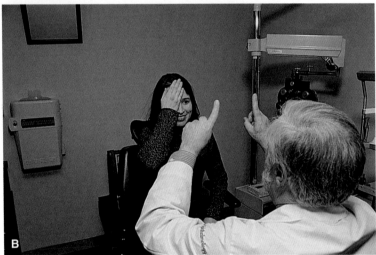

FIGURE 2-3. **Finger counting confrontation visual fields A to D.**

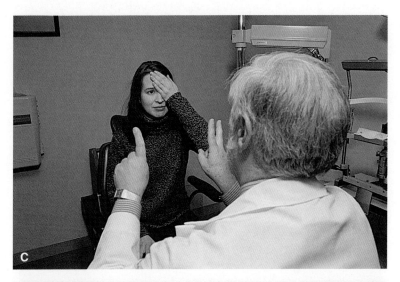

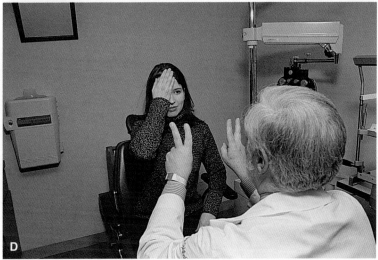

FIGURE 2-3. (*continued*)

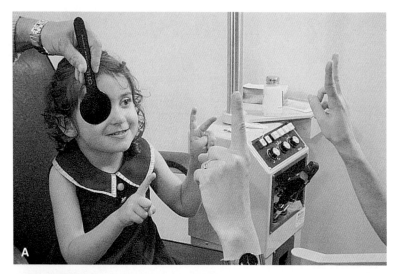

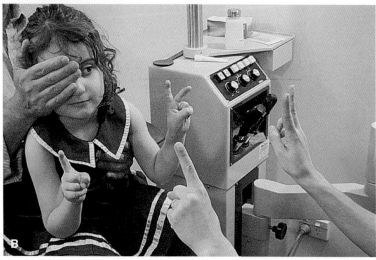

FIGURE 2-4. "Simon Says" **confrontation visual fields.** **A.** The parent covers one eye as the child is asked to "do this" as fingers (usually 1, 2, or 5) are presented in the appropriate areas of visual field. **B.** If the child has difficulty fixing on the examiner's face, her head is turned so that the eye is maximally abducted and she cannot move the eye laterally. This gives an accurate estimation of the temporal visual field.

CONCLUSION

N euro-ophthalmologists tend to disagree about the types of visual fields that are best able to detect scotomas. Our bias is to perform 24-2 or 30-2 threshold tests because both are adequate for detecting most visual field defects as nearly 80% of the visual cortex correlates to the central visual field. In some patients, the only information that can be obtained about the visual field is by confrontation techniques.

Magnetic Resonance Imaging for the Ophthalmologist

Rahul M. Nikam, Kiran Shankar Talekar, and Adam E. Flanders

INTRODUCTION

The superior contrast resolution and multi-planar capabilities of magnetic resonance imaging (MRI) make it uniquely qualified for the assessment of visual pathways. The predecessor to MRI, computed tomography (CT), also produces high-resolution digital images of the brain and orbital structures. However, because CT is based on the same physical principles as the X-ray, it accentuates bony anatomy at the expense of the soft-tissue detail. For example, at locations where soft-tissue components of the orbital contents are in close approximation to bony elements (e.g., the orbital apex, optic foramen), the details of the soft-tissue structures are lost.

Mobile hydrogen protons generate images in MRI, and these hydrogen protons are far more abundant in the soft-tissue structures than in bone. Therefore, the soft tissues are accentuated in MRI at the expense of the bony anatomy.

Thus, MRI is well suited for the detection of subtle abnormalities affecting the optic pathways. Disease processes that produce subtle pathologic changes in the optic pathways, such as optic neuritis, are easily identified with an MRI.

MRI uses a strong static magnetic field and radio waves to generate images; it has no known potential harmful effects in biologic tissues. Compared to CT, MRI does not use ionizing radiation; therefore, there is no potential risk of presenile cataracts due to radiation exposure for imaging the orbit. MRI does impose several safety limitations, which preclude imaging of patients with certain implanted ferrous instrumentation, such as cardiac pacemakers, neurostimulators, and older model cerebral aneurysm clips. In addition, approximately 10% of patients will experience an episode of claustrophobia during an MRI that may prevent completion of the entire examination. Sedation may be necessary to complete the examination.

High-field MRI units (1.5 Tesla or greater) using a standard head (brain) coil can produce images of the optic pathways with exceptional detail. No special equipment is required. Although low-field-strength open MRI units have an advantage in imaging claustrophobic patients, their capabilities in resolving small structures (e.g., optic nerves and cranial nerves) are limited because of their low inherent magnetic field strength, longer imaging times, and lower spatial and contrast resolution. Therefore, use of these devices for ophthalmologic imaging should be reserved only as a last resort in preference to a high-field-strength unit.

FUNDAMENTALS OF MAGNETIC RESONANCE IMAGING

MRI is based on the principles of nuclear magnetic resonance. In brief, the images generated with MRI are created by exploiting the principle that the mobile protons in biologic tissues (primarily water and fat) align themselves and resonate along the direction of a strong static magnetic field at a known frequency (Larmor frequency). In a clinical MRI unit, the static magnetic field may vary between 0.3 and 3.0 Tesla (3,000–30,000 gauss—or up to 100,000 times the earth's own magnetic field). During the MR examination, the resonating protons are exposed to a burst of radiofrequency energy that briefly excites them to a higher energy state. After excitation, the protons spontaneously undergo a process of relaxation and release weak radiofrequency energy, which is detected by an antenna (coil) inside the bore of the MRI unit. Through a series of sophisticated mathematical computations, the radiofrequency map emitted by the excited tissue is converted into a spatial signal map that appears as an image.

TERMINOLOGY AND MAGNETIC RESONANCE IMAGING PULSE SEQUENCES

In the MRI unit, different tissues and disease processes exhibit *tissue-specific relaxation properties* that allow one tissue to be distinguished from another. These fundamental relaxation properties are expressed as a rate or units of time and are known as *T1* and *T2* (Fig. 3-1). Tissues can be described by their T1 and T2 relaxation rates, proton density, and rate of movement (diffusion or blood flow). MRI pulse sequences have evolved from the most basic saturation recovery sequences to the ultrafast echo planar imaging sequences. A variety of pulse sequences exist, which are designed to make use of tissue-specific characteristics that improve the conspicuity of a particular tissue relative to the background tissues. Similar pulse sequences may have different acronyms depending on the vendor and are therefore confusing. Although a detailed discussion of these pulse sequences is beyond the scope of this chapter, a list of the commonly used sequences is tabulated below. The basic pulse sequences take advantage of differences in the T1 or T2 relaxation properties, otherwise known as T1-weighted (T1W) or T2-weighted (T2W) pulse sequences. The term "weighted" is used because although the T1 or T2 relaxation characteristics provide the majority of the tissue information, there are other tissue-specific parameters that provide minor but observable contributions to the "look" of the images. It is useful to learn how to recognize these basic image types. It is also important to realize that because MRI signal and enhancement characteristics are not entirely disease specific, MRI interpretation is largely dependent on the location and morphology of the abnormality in conjunction with the clinical history.

T1-Weighted Imaging

It is based on T1 relaxation time of the tissues. In the orbit it gives a good general anatomic outline with the normal retrobulbar fat imparting excellent contrast. It also serves as a baseline to study contrast enhancement characteristics. The T1 signal ranges from very hyperintense for fat to very hypointense for cerebrospinal fluid (CSF). Certain lesions containing fat (dermoid and lipoma), subacute blood (Figs. 3-2A and 3-3B, D), and melanin are characteristically hyperintense on T1. Fat suppression techniques help distinguish fat and fat-containing lesions from other T1 hyperintense lesions. White matter is more hyperintense than gray matter due to abundance of myelin. Therefore, disease processes severely affecting myelin, like progressive multifocal leukoencephalopathy (PML), which targets oligodendrocytes (Fig. 3-4C), are characterized by a very hypointense T1 signal.

Gadolinium-Enhanced T1

This is vital in characterizing lesions. With the possible exception of imaging for optic atrophy, use of contrast material is mandatory when imaging the optic pathways. This sequence is acquired with fat suppression technique while imaging the orbit, because normal fat may obscure pathologic enhancement due to its inherent T1 hyperintensity. The MR contrast agent contains heavy metal gadolinium. Intravenous contrast material is used to improve the visibility of an abnormality (e.g., optic nerve sheath meningioma; Fig. 3-5B and D), to characterize the activity of a pathologic process (e.g., multiple sclerosis [MS]; Fig. 3-6B), or to make pathology visible (e.g., optic neuritis; Fig. 3-7D and E, and other cranial neuropathies; Fig. 3-8B). Meningeal pathologies may only be seen on postcontrast sequences (Figs. 3-9B–D and 3-10). The mechanism for contrast enhancement in MRI is similar to the process on CT; it augments areas of increased vascularity or vascular permeability (e.g., damaged blood–brain barrier), which are nonspecific markers for a disease process. Beware of normally enhancing structures, including the pituitary gland (Figs. 3-1K, 3-11B, and 3-12C), pituitary stalk (Fig. 3-7E), veins (like superior ophthalmic veins), and adjacent nasal mucosa (Fig. 3-13B). Symmetric enhancement is to be expected in the extraocular muscles (Fig. 3-1I and J) and lacrimal glands. Additionally, susceptibility artifacts from air in the nasal cavity and paranasal sinuses and from dental works may mimic enhancement, especially on 3-Tesla MRI.

T2

It is based on T2 weighting of the tissues (Fig. 3-1B and H). This sequence is very sensitive for detecting pathology but is not entirely specific. CSF and most pathologies (due to higher water content compared to normal tissues) are hyperintense, for example, demyelination (Figs. 3-4B and 3-6D), tumors (Fig. 3-5C), infection (Fig. 3-14B), and strokes (Fig. 3-15C). Cavernous hemangiomas are characteristically extremely bright on T2 (Fig. 3-16A), whereas tumors like lymphoma (Fig. 3-17A) and meningioma may be less hyperintense secondary to high cellularity. Heavily T2W high-resolution sequences can be obtained in patients with cranial neuropathies to study the cisternal segments of the nerves (Fig. 3-1L–N).

Short T1 Inversion Recovery and T2 Fat-Saturated Sequence

In these techniques, hyperintense signal from normal fat is suppressed on an essentially T2W image (Fig. 3-1D–G), making lesions and edema evident, which is vital in detecting subtle T2 hyperintensity in the optic nerve (Fig. 3-7A–C and 3-18B). In general, the ability to perceive an abnormality is markedly improved with the use of a fat suppression technique. Additionally, it is vital in detecting calvarial marrow abnormalities including osteomyelitis and tumors.

Fluid-Attenuated Inversion Recovery

The fluid-attenuated inversion recovery (FLAIR) is also essentially T2W image but with active suppression of signal arising from bulk water (CSF) more than from bound water (interstitial edema or demyelination). This is the most sensitive technique to demonstrate periventricular white matter disease (e.g., demyelinating lesions; Fig. 3-6A and C) and subarachnoid disease processes (e.g., subarachnoid hemorrhage and leptomeningeal inflammation or carcinomatosis). Other examples included are infarct (Fig. 3-15A), tumor (Figs. 3-13A), and inflammatory neuritis (Fig. 3-8A).

T2-Weighted Gradient Echo

This is obtained with the specific purpose of detecting susceptibility artifact primarily from blood products (Fig. 3-19B). However, other materials including calcification, gas, and metallic structures like surgical clips and aneurysm coils cause susceptibility artifact.

Proton Density Weighted

Proton density–weighted image contrast is purely based on differences in the number of protons between tissues. It is no longer a common sequence. Some argue that it is helpful in detecting demyelinating lesions. Figure 3-20A shows an unusual application of this sequence demonstrating abnormal signal in an aneurysm.

Magnetic Resonance Angiography and Venography

Protons in motion exhibit a specific type of signature that can be exploited with MRI. These MR techniques are used to image flowing blood. The signal from fast-moving particles, such as in blood, is augmented, whereas signal from the stationary tissues is suppressed. The images are acquired without intravenous contrast agent and are postprocessed to produce an angiographic-like image. This method has evolved to a level where it is now used to replace conventional catheter angiography in specific applications. Magnetic resonance angiography is a useful noninvasive procedure in diagnosing intracranial aneurysms (Fig. 3-20B and C), arterial stenosis (Fig. 3-21C), dissection (Fig. 3-22A), occlusion, carotid cavernous fistula (Fig. 3-23B and C), and all but very small arteriovenous malformations. Magnetic resonance venography is useful in diagnosing venous thrombosis (Fig. 3-19C) and bilateral transverse sinus stenosis in some cases of pseudotumor cerebri (Fig. 3-18E).

Diffusion-Weighted Imaging

Diffusion-weighted imaging (DWI) is one of the most clinically useful pulse sequences based on the physiologic process of molecular diffusion. Diffusion simply means the translation that particles and molecules experience because of random collision. (It should not be mistaken with flow where particles are displaced in bulk.) Pathologies that obstruct free diffusion, most importantly infarcts (due to intracellular water accumulation and shrinkage of extracellular space), lead to what is widely referred to as "restricted diffusion," which is seen as hyperintense signal on the B-1000 diffusion sequence (Figs. 3-15B and 3-21A) and more importantly a dark signal on the apparent diffusion coefficient (ADC) maps (Fig. 3-21B). A hyperintense signal on DWI has two components: a true restricted diffusion component and a T2 component. In the simplest terms, an ADC map is obtained by taking out the T2 signal from a DWI and thereby represents the true restricted diffusion. This technique is the most sensitive method for identification of acute cerebral cortical infarction (Figs. 3-15 and 3-21). In infarcts, DWI can be abnormal within few minutes of the ictus without a corresponding abnormality on the conventional MR images. The intensity of the signal decreases over several days and can persist for up to 4 to 6 weeks. Although DWI is most useful in diagnosing strokes, it can be helpful in defining abscess (Fig. 3-14C and D) and certain cellular tumors like lymphoma and retinoblastoma.

Functional Magnetic Resonance Imaging

Functional neuroradiology expands upon the high-resolution anatomic imaging of the brain. Its two most promising techniques are blood-oxygen-level–dependent functional MRI (BOLD-fMRI) for mapping the eloquent cortex (e.g., visual cortex) (Fig. 3-24A) and diffusion tensor imaging (DTI) (Fig. 3-24B–F) for mapping the white matter connections (e.g., optic radiations). Accurate lesion-localizing abilities of fMRI and DTI are specifically important in neuro-ophthalmology where lesions at different locations within the visual system can produce field defects and/or selective functional losses, depending on the pathways and visual areas affected.

BOLD-fMRI is based on the difference in the magnetic properties of deoxyhemoglobin and oxyhemoglobin. Fundamentally, in fMRI a specifically designed visual task results in alteration of neuronal activity of the visual cortex, which in turn alters the regional cerebral hemodynamics, namely, cerebral blood flow and volume, thereby altering the ratio of deoxyhemoglobin to oxyhemoglobin. This results in a signal that although miniscule can be effectively measured and overlaid on an anatomic image to generate clinically useful fMRI maps. The resulting brain map can be color-coded to identify each quadrant of the visual field and to distinguish central (foveal) from peripheral vision. This is especially important in surgical planning.

Diffusion Tensor Imaging

DTI on the other hand is an advancement of diffusion MRI technique, which is based on the estimation of "diffusion anisotropy." The free random motion of water molecules in CSF is called "isotropic diffusion." However, diffusion in brain parenchyma is not isotropic, especially in white matter, where the presence of natural barriers to diffusion like cell membrane, myelin sheath, and parallel arrangement of axons restricts diffusion across them and facilitates diffusion preferentially along main direction of the axons and the fiber tracts. Such preferentially oriented diffusion is called "anisotropic diffusion." Using DTI, it is possible to deduce the preferred diffusion directions and use these to reconstitute the nerve fiber trajectory, a method referred to as fiber tractography (Fig. 3-24B–F). Various DTI parameters that can be deduced include fractional anisotropy (FA), which is a measure of directionality of diffusion, and radial diffusivity (RD) and mean diffusivity (MD), which measure the rate of diffusion. It has been suggested that DTI values offer objective measure of axon and myelin integrity. Typically, FA decreases and RD and MD increase with myelin or axonal pathologies. This allows for detection of physiologic damage to white matter even when no structural lesions are visible, for example, in MS. These parameters have been shown to correlate well with visual outcomes in optic neuritis from several causes including remote optic neuritis and have been found to be useful to detect early degeneration of pathways in glaucoma before it is clinically manifest. Naturally, it is very useful for planning tumor resection and temporal lobe surgery for intractable seizures to avoid injury to optic radiations. Table 3-1 enlists various orbital pathologies illustrated in the text, whereas Table 3-2 enumerates the commonly encountered orbital emergencies.

TABLE 3-1. Orbital Pathologies

Anatomy		Figure 3-1
Demyelinating diseases	Optic neuritis	Figure 3-7
	Multiple sclerosis	Figure 3-6
	Demyelinating plaque presenting as INO	Figure 3-25
	Neuromyelitis optica	Figure 3-26
	Progressive multifocal leukoencephalopathy	Figure 3-4
Inflammation	Idiopathic orbital inflammation	Figure 3-27
	Thyroid orbitopathy	Figure 3-28
	Sarcoidosis	Figures 3-8 and 3-29
Infection	Orbital cellulitis	Figure 3-30
	Brain parenchymal abscess	Figure 3-14
Neoplasms	Optic nerve sheath meningioma	Figure 3-5
	Pediatric optochiasmatic glioma	Figure 3-31
	Optic nerve glioma	Figure 3-13
	Orbital lymphoma	Figure 3-17
	Cavernous hemangioma	Figure 3-16
	Pituitary macroadenoma	Figure 3-3
	Craniopharyngioma	Figure 3-32
	Tuberculum sellae meningioma	Figure 3-11
	Cavernous sinus meningioma	Figure 3-10
	Glioblastoma multiforme	Figure 3-9
	Left superior colliculus glioma	Figure 3-33
Vascular pathologies	Left posterior cerebral artery territory infarction	Figure 3-15
	Lacunar infarct in midbrain presenting with left trochlear nerve palsy	Figure 3-21
	Posterior communicating artery aneurysm	Figure 3-20
	Carotid cavernous fistula	Figure 3-23
	Cavernous sinus thrombosis	Figure 3-12
	Acute superior sagittal sinus thrombosis	Figure 3-19
	Subacute superior sagittal sinus thrombosis	Figure 3-2
	Right ICA dissection presenting as Horner syndrome	Figure 3-22
	Idiopathic intracranial hypertension	Figure 3-18
Miscellaneous	Wernicke encephalopathy	Figure 3-34
	Functional magnetic resonance imaging	Figure 3-24
	Diffusion Tensor Imaging	Figure 3-35

INO, internuclear ophthalmoplegia; ICA, internal carotid artery

TABLE 3-2. Common Orbital Emergencies Encountered in Our Clinical Practice Are

Inflammation	Optic neuritis	Figure 3-7
	Multiple sclerosis	Figure 3-6
	Neuromyelitis optica	Figure 3-26
	Idiopathic orbital inflammation	Figure 3-27
	Sarcoidosis	Figures 3-8 and 3-29
Infection	Orbital cellulitis	Figure 3-30
Vascular pathologies	Infarction	Figures 3-15 and 3-21
	Intracranial aneurysms	Figure 3-20
	Carotid cavernous fistula	Figure 3-23
	Cavernous sinus thrombosis	Figure 3-12
	Dural sinus thrombosis	Figures 3-2 and 3-19
	Horner syndrome	Figure 3-22

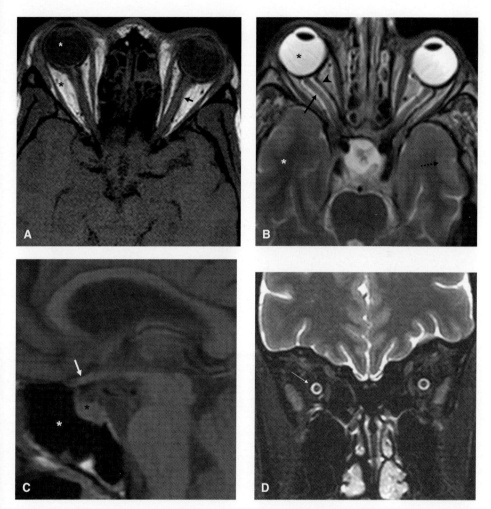

FIGURE 3-1. Normal anatomy. A. Axial T1-weighted image (T1WI). The vitreous body is low in signal (white asterisk). The orbital fat is hyperintense (black asterisk). The optic nerve is seen throughout its entire course (*black arrow*). **B.** Axial T2-weighted image (T2WI) shows the hyperintense (bright) vitreous body (black asterisk). Optic nerve (*long black arrow*) surrounded by the nerve sheath seen as linear dark signal (*arrow head*) which contains the cerebrospinal fluid (CSF). Normal gray matter (*dotted black arrow*) is mildly hyperintense relative to normal white matter (white asterisk). **C.** Midline sagittal T1WI shows the optic tract (*white arrow*) coursing through the suprasellar cistern. Normal pituitary (black asterisk) and aerated sphenoid sinus (white asterisk). **D.** Coronal short T1 inversion recovery (STIR) image from the midorbit shows the hyperintense CSF contained by the optic sheath (*arrow*) surrounding the lower signal intensity optic nerve. Note how fat is suppressed on this sequence.

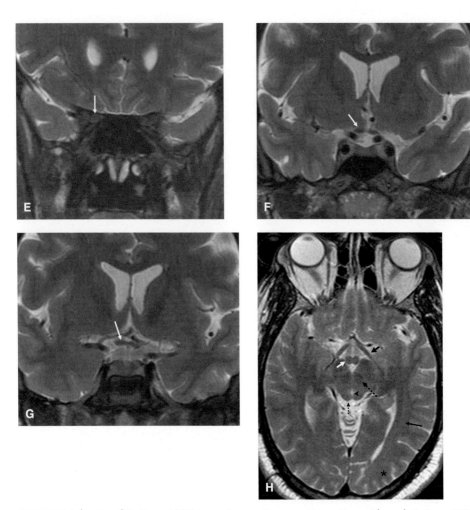

FIGURE 3-1. (*continued*) **E.** Coronal STIR image shows optic nerve within optic canal (*arrow*). **F.** Coronal STIR shows the prechiasmatic optic nerves (*arrow*). **G.** Coronal STIR through optic chiasm (*arrow*). **H.** Axial T2W at the level of midbrain shows optic tracts as they enter the brain (*small black arrow*), the expected location of the optic radiation (*long black arrow*), and the occipital lobe (*asterisk*). Also seen are red nucleus (*long black dotted arrow*), cerebral aqueduct (*arrow head*), superior colliculus (*short black dotted arrow*), and mammillary bodies (*white arrow*).

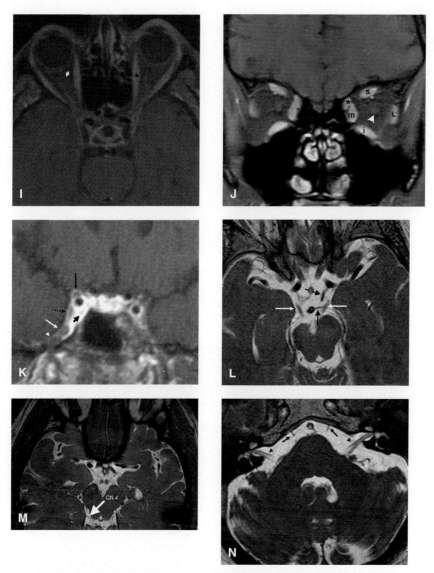

FIGURE 3-1. (*continued*) **I.** Postcontrast axial T1WI with fat suppression. Note normal intense enhancement of the extraocular muscles (asterisk) and no enhancement of the optic nerve (*white arrow*). **J.** Postcontrast coronal T1WI with fat suppression. Optic nerve (*white arrow head*), extraocular muscles—medial (m), lateral (L), superior (s), and inferior (i) recti and the superior oblique (asterisk). **K.** Postcontrast coronal T1WI with fat suppression shows the cranial nerves within the right cavernous sinus: oculomotor nerve (*long black arrow*), trochlear nerve (*dotted arrow*), abducens nerve (*short bold black arrow*), V-1 (ophthalmic) division of the trigeminal nerve (*long white arrow*), and V-2 (maxillary) division (*white arrow head*). **L.** Axial high resolution heavily T2WI at the level of upper midbrain shows oculomotor nerves within the cistern (*white arrows*). Note the proximity of oculomotor nerves to superior cerebellar artery flow voids (seen on the left—*black solid arrow*) and left posterior communicating artery (*dotted black arrow*). **M.** Axial high resolution heavily T2WI image at the level of lower midbrain shows trochlear nerves as they wind around the midbrain (*long arrow*). **N.** Axial high resolution heavily T2WI at the level of pons shows the abducens nerves entering Dorello's canal (*black arrows*) and the seventh to eighth nerve complexes (*arrow heads*).

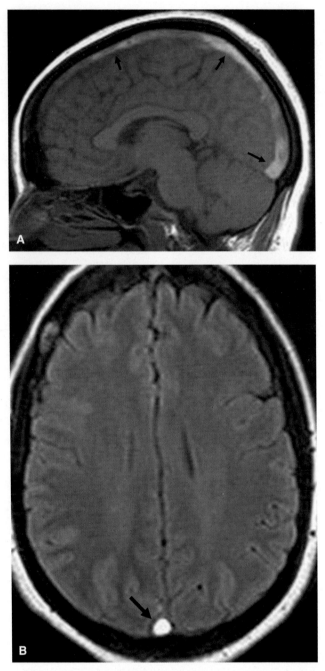

FIGURE 3-2. **Subacute superior sagittal sinus (SSS) thrombosis. A.** Sagittal T1-weighted imaging shows abnormal hyperintense signal (*arrows*) in the SSS representing a subacute clot. **B.** Axial fluid-attenuated inversion recovery image shows abnormal hyperintense signal in place of a normal flow void (*arrow*) suggesting thrombosis.

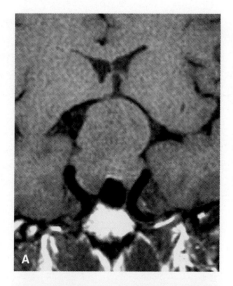

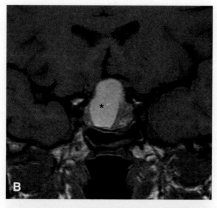

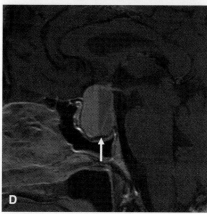

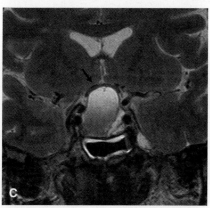

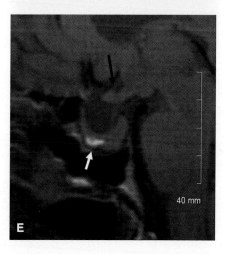

40 mm

FIGURE 3-3. Pituitary tumor causing optic chiasm compression and visual deficit. A. Coronal T1-weighted imaging (T1WI) shows a bilobed sellar and suprasellar mass. This is a macroadenoma which by definition is more than 1 cm in size. The optic apparatus which is not separately identified is presumably compressed by the mass. **B.** Different patient with pituitary apoplexy presenting with sudden-onset visual deficit. Coronal T1WI showing a mass with hyperintense T1 signal compatible with hemorrhage (asterisk). Notice the snowman-shaped bilobed appearance, which is the typical shape of a pituitary mass extending in the suprasellar cistern. **C.** Coronal T2-weighted imaging shows compression of the optic chiasm (*black arrow*). **D.** Sagittal T1WI shows a widened sella and a fluid–fluid level (*white arrow*) within the mass compatible with layering blood in this case of apoplexy. **E.** Follow-up sagittal T1WI shows contraction of the hemorrhagic cavity (*white arrow*) with reduced pituitary height in a widened sella which will likely evolve into an empty sella. Notice the slight sagging of the optic chiasm (*black arrow*); in severe cases the optic chiasm may herniate into the sella, which is known to cause visual deficit.

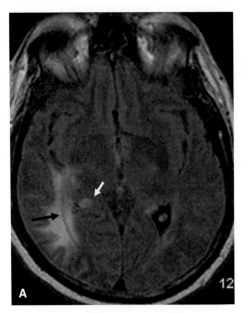

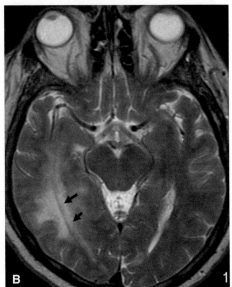

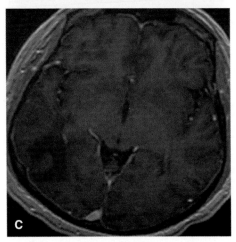

FIGURE 3-4. **Progressive multifocal leukoencepha-lopathy (PML)** presenting with visual field deficit. Axial fluid-attenuated inversion recovery (FLAIR) image (**A**) and Axial T2-weighted imaging (**B**) show right tempo-ro-occipital white matter signal abnormality sparing the cortex (making an infarct unlikely). Hippocampus is also involved (*white arrow* on FLAIR). The right optic radiation is involved and can be seen as a relatively lower intensity curvilinear band (*black arrows* in **A** and **B**), which explains the visual deficit, compared to normal appearance on image 1H. **C.** Postcontrast axial T1-weighted imaging shows characteristic very low T1 signal, lack of mass effect, and lack of enhancement in the lesion, which are characteristic features of PML. This was a case of bone marrow transplant for chronic lymphocytic leukemia.

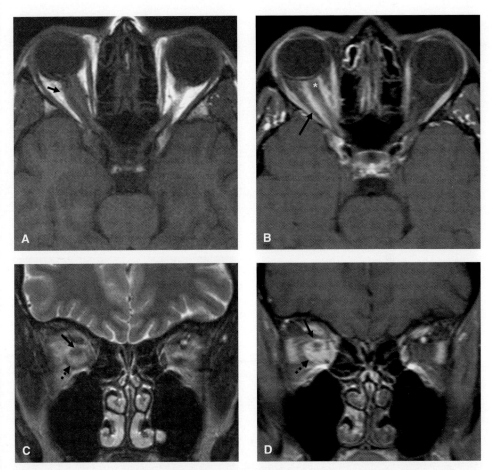

FIGURE 3-5. Optic nerve sheath meningioma. A. Axial T1-weighted imaging (T1WI) shows enlarged right optic nerve sheath complex (*arrow*). **B.** Corresponding axial postcontrast T1WI with fat suppression shows tram-track–like appearance due to intense enhancement of the meningioma (*black arrow*) which surrounds a nonenhancing nerve (white asterisk); compare with the case of optic nerve glioma (3–13) in which the nerve itself is abnormal. **C.** Coronal T2-weighted imaging shows normal intensity of the nerve (*solid arrow*) versus a mildly heterogeneously hyperintense tumor (*dotted arrow*). **D.** Coronal postcontrast T1WI shows a nonenhancing nerve (*solid arrow*) with surrounding eccentric avidly enhancing meningioma (*dotted arrow*). Meningiomas typically enhance very intensely.

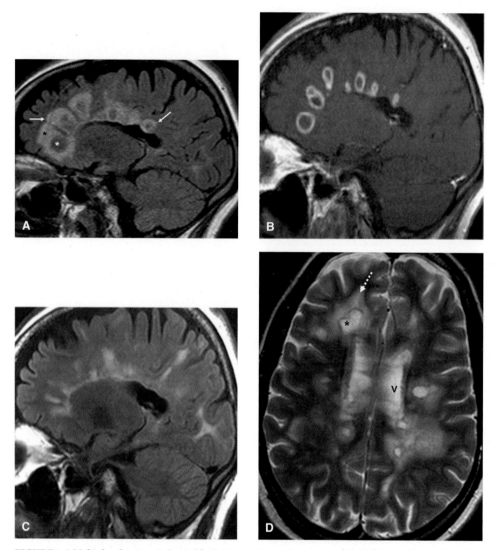

FIGURE 3-6. Multiple sclerosis. A. Sagittal fluid-attenuated inversion recovery (FLAIR) shows the periventricular lesions (*arrows*) which are arranged perpendicular to the ventricular margin, Dawson fingers. Note that the center (white asterisk) is darker than the periphery (black asterisk), which represents rim of edema consistent with an actively demyelinating plaque. **B.** Sagittal postcontrast T1-weighted imaging; contrast is administered to study the activity of the lesions, because in this case the plaques show ring enhancement representing active demyelination. **C.** Follow-up sagittal FLAIR shows the lesions to be smaller representing a more quiescent stage. **D.** Different patient. Axial T2-weighted imaging at the level of top of lateral ventricles (v) demonstrates multiple, periventricular white matter high-signal-intensity lesions consistent with demyelinating plaques. Notice how the lesion on right reveals a more hyperintense center (asterisk) representing the plaque with rim of slightly less hyperintense signal (*dotted arrow*) representing edema with active demyelination.

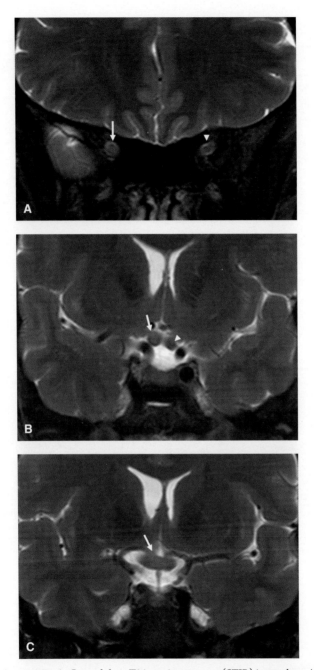

FIGURE 3-7. Optic neuritis. A. Coronal short T1 inversion recovery (STIR) image shows increased signal and swelling of the right orbital optic nerve (*arrow*) compared with normal left nerve (*arrow head*). **B.** Coronal STIR shows increased signal in the prechiasmatic right optic nerve (*arrow*) compared to the left (*arrow head*). **C.** Coronal STIR shows increased signal in the chiasm (*arrow*).

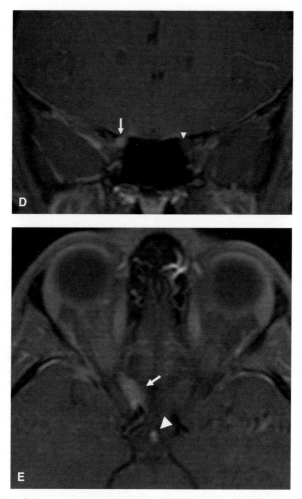

FIGURE 3-7. (*continued*) **D.** Coronal postcontrast T1-weighted imaging (T1WI) with fat suppression shows abnormal enhancement of the canalicular right optic nerve (*arrow*) compared to left (*arrow head*). **E.** Axial postcontrast T1WI with fat suppression shows abnormal enhancement of the canalicular and prechiasmatic right optic nerve (*arrow*). Note normal enhancement of the pituitary stalk (*white arrow head*).

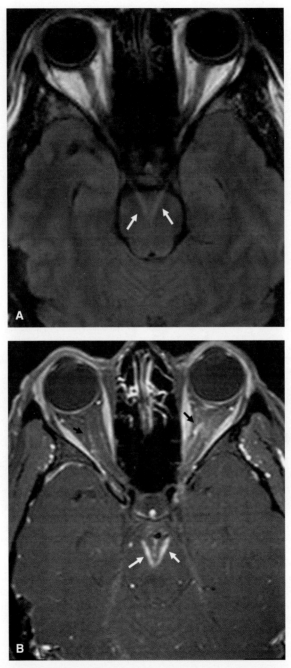

FIGURE 3-8. Neurosarcoidosis presenting with sudden-onset left eye vision loss. **A.** Axial fluid-attenuated inversion recovery at the level of midbrain shows linear abnormal hyperintense signal in the region of the root entry zones of oculomotor nerves (*arrows*). **B.** Postcontrast axial T1-weighted imaging with fat suppression shows abnormal enhancement along the oculomotor nerves (*white arrows*); also, note abnormal enhancement in optic nerve sheaths (*black arrows*), especially on the left explaining the visual loss.

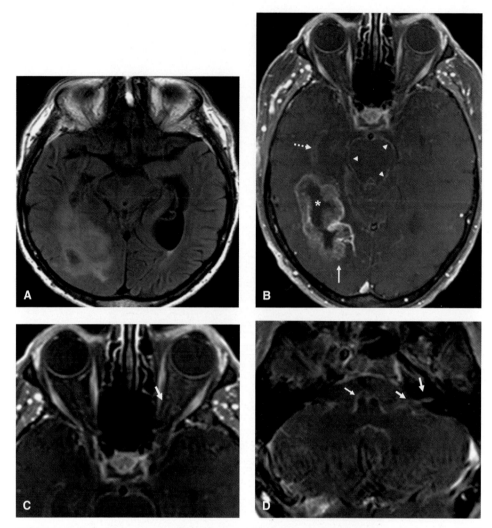

FIGURE 3-9. Right temporo-occipital glioblastoma with carcinomatous meningitis producing a visual field cut. **A.** Axial fluid-attenuated inversion recovery image of the brain reveals an infiltrative mass in the right temporo-occipital region. **B.** Postcontrast axial T1-weighted image with fat suppression demonstrates a heterogeneously enhancing mass (*solid white arrow*) with necrosis (asterisk) consistent with a glioblastoma (GBM). Note cerebrospinal fluid seeding of the tumor leading to carcinomatous meningitis with ependymal enhancement in the right temporal horn (*dotted arrow*) and abnormal enhancement coating the brainstem (*arrow heads*) implying a grave prognosis. **C.** Abnormal enhancement within the optic sheath especially on left (*arrow*). **D.** Abnormal enhancement coating the medulla and the 7 to 8 nerve complexes on left including within the internal auditory canal (*arrows*).

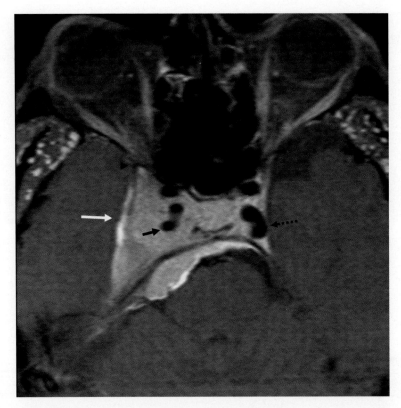

FIGURE 3-10. Right cavernous sinus meningioma presenting with diplopia. Postcontrast axial T1-weighted image shows an intensely enhancing extra-axial mass (*white arrow*) at the petrous apex and in the cavernous sinus with anterior extension up to the superior orbital fissure (*black arrow head*). Note that the mass encases and narrows the right ICA flow void (*solid black arrow*) when compared to the left (*dotted black arrow*), a feature differentiating meningioma from pituitary adenoma, which is a common tumor that encases the ICA without narrowing.

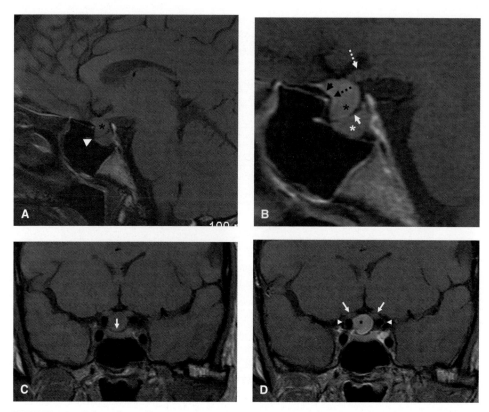

FIGURE 3-11. Tuberculum sellae meningioma impinging on the optic apparatus. A. Sagittal T1-weighted image (T1WI) shows an isointense lesion (black asterisk) extending in the sella but separated from the pituitary by a normal hypointense diaphragma sellae (*arrow head*). **B.** Postcontrast sagittal T1WI shows the meningioma (black asterisk) enhancing even more intensely than the normal pituitary (white asterisk). Note the exquisite depiction of anatomic relationship of the tumor to tuberculum sellae which is seen as a somewhat triangular bony protuberance with its bony cortex being characteristically very hypointense (*dotted black arrow*) and is seen separating sulcus chiasmatis (*short solid arrow*) from the sella turcica. Diaphragma sellae (*white arrow*). Optic chiasm (*dotted white arrow*). **C.** Coronal T1WI—diaphragma sellae (*white arrow*). **D.** Coronal postcontrast T1WI shows relationship of the meningioma (black asterisk) to prechiasmatic optic nerves (*solid white arrows*) and internal carotid artery flow voids (*white arrow head*). Visualization of an intact diaphragma sellae between the mass and pituitary excludes a pituitary adenoma.

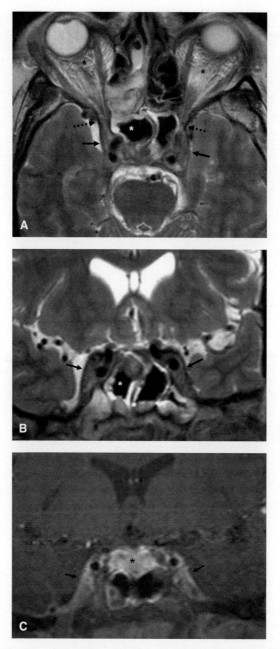

FIGURE 3-12. Bilateral cavernous sinus thrombosis. A. Axial T2-weighted image (T2WI) shows abnormal signal and enlargement of the cavernous sinuses (*solid black arrows*) which extend up to the superior orbital fissure (*dotted black arrows*). Note abnormal hyperintense signal in the orbital fat (black asterisk) compatible with either inflammation or congestion. There is marked proptosis. Also, note the inflammatory mucosal thickening within the paranasal sinuses (white asterisk). **B.** Coronal T2WI shows abnormal signal and enlargement of the cavernous sinuses (*solid black arrows*). Sphenoid sinus mucosal thickening (white asterisk). **C.** Postcontrast coronal T1-weighted image—cavernous sinuses are enlarged and enhance heterogeneously and less intensely than expected (*arrows*); compare with pituitary enhancement (black asterisk) which normally should be less intense than the cavernous sinus enhancement.

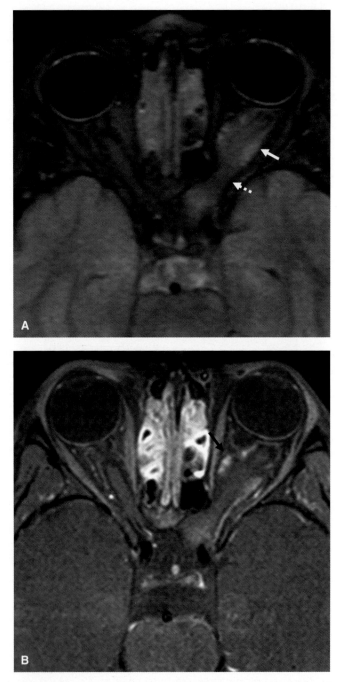

FIGURE 3-13. Optic nerve glioma. A. Axial fluid-attenuated inversion recovery shows diffuse bilobed enlargement of the left optic nerve (*solid arrow*) with a waist at the optic canal (*dotted arrow*). **B.** Axial postcontrast T1-weighted image with fat suppression shows mild linear enhancement along the medial aspect of the neural mass (*arrow*). Compare this appearance with case of optic nerve sheath meningioma. Note nonspecific ethmoid mucosal enhancement.

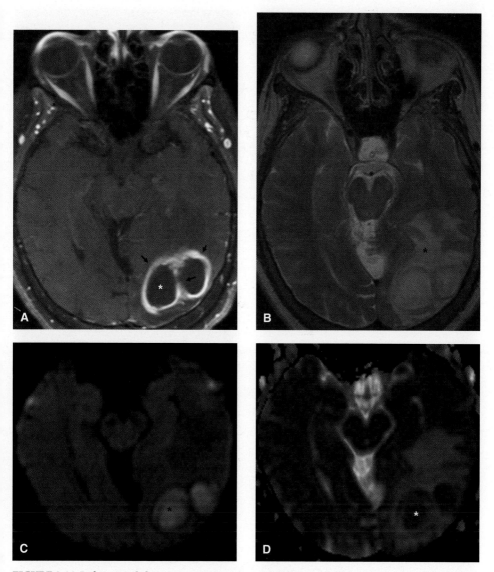

FIGURE 3-14. Left occipital abscess presenting with visual deficit. A. Axial postcontrast T1-weighted image shows bilobed peripherally enhancing lesion with a fairly uniform thickness wall and a septation (*arrows*) with central necrosis (asterisk). **B.** Axial T2-weighted image shows that the lesion is primarily hyperintense with a wall that is hypointense, which is commonly seen with abscesses. Note the extensive associated vasogenic edema (asterisk). **C.** Axial B-1000 diffusion image shows hyperintense signal in the area of necrosis (asterisk). **D.** Apparent diffusion coefficient map shows corresponding dark signal compatible with true restricted diffusion (asterisk). Restricted diffusion associated with necrosis is almost diagnostic for an abscess with purulent material.

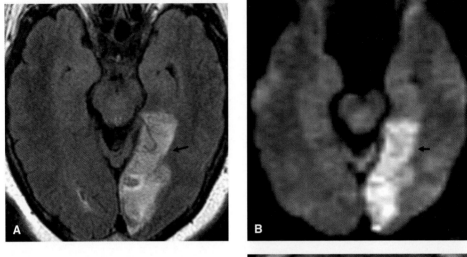

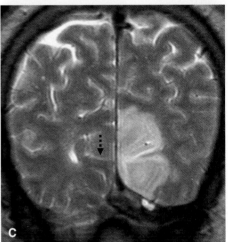

FIGURE 3-15. **Left occipital infarct. A.** Axial fluid-attenuated inversion recovery image shows hyperintense signal in left occipital lobe (*arrow*) confined to the posterior cerebral artery territory involving gray and white matter with only mild mass effect. **B.** Restricted diffusion as seen on the B-1000 diffusion image (*arrow*). **C.** Coronal T2-weighted image shows hyperintensity confined to the left posterior cerebral artery (PCA) territory. Note location of the calcarine fissure on the right (*dotted arrow*); it is effaced on the left.

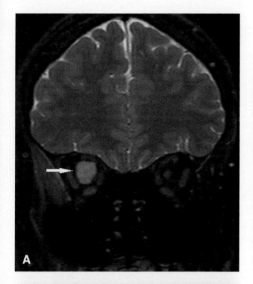

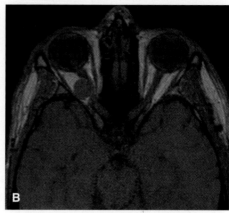

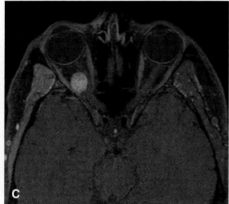

FIGURE 3-16. Cavernous hemangioma. A. Coronal short T1 inversion recovery image through the orbits demonstrates a well-defined hyperintense lesion in the intraconal right orbit (*arrow*). The optic nerve seems to be displaced medially by this mass. **B.** On precontrast T1-weighted axial image through the orbit, the intraconal mass appears slightly hyperintense with displacement of optic nerve medially. **C.** On postcontrast T1-weighted fat-saturated axial image through the orbit, the right orbital mass demonstrates intense homogeneous enhancement. On dynamic postcontrast imaging (not shown), this mass showed early patchy enhancement with progressive pooling of contrast, compatible with cavernous hemangioma.

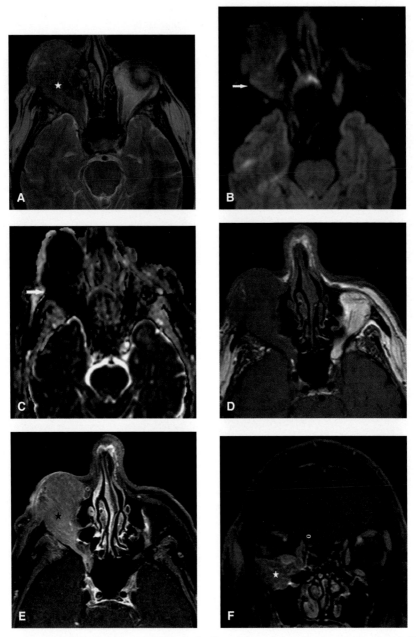

FIGURE 3-17. **Orbital lymphoma. A.** Axial T2-weighted image through the orbits demonstrate a large infiltrating mass involving the right orbit extending up to the orbital apex (asterisk). **B, C.** On axial diffusion–weighted image (**B**) through the orbit, the mass appears slightly hyperintense with corresponding hypointense signal on apparent diffusion coefficient map (**C**) (*arrows*), suggestive of restricted diffusion. Diffusion restriction is characteristically seen with highly cellular tumor. **D, E, F.** Axial pre- and axial and coronal postcontrast T1-weighted images with fat suppression through the orbits demonstrate homogeneous enhancement of right orbital mass (asterisk). This constellation of findings is suggestive of highly cellular tumor such as lymphoma. Biopsy of the right orbital mass confirmed diffuse large B-cell lymphoma.

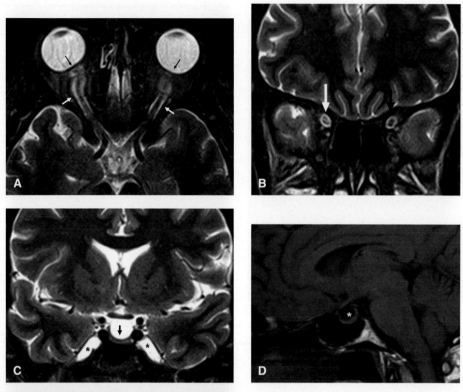

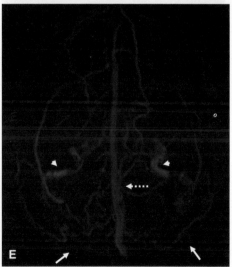

FIGURE 3-18. Pseudotumor cerebri. A. Axial fat-suppressed T2-weighted image (T2WI) shows papilledema—flattening of the posteromedial aspects of the globe at the point of optic nerve attachment (*black arrows*) and ectasia of optic nerve sheaths both vertically and side to side (*white arrows*), resulting in dilated cerebrospinal fluid spaces surrounding the optic nerves. **B.** Coronal short T1 inversion recovery (STIR) image through the orbits shows increased signal in the right optic nerve (*white arrow*) representing optic neuropathy; compared with normal signal of left optic nerve (*black arrow*). **C.** Coronal STIR image through chiasm shows an empty sella (*arrow*) and dilated Meckel caves (asterisk). **D.** Sagittal T1-weighted image shows empty sella (asterisk). Note position of optic chiasm (*arrow*). **E.** Magnetic resonance venogram—maximum intensity projection image—view from top. Note the loss of flow signal in the transverse sinuses bilaterally (their expected positions are marked by *solid white arrows*); normal flow in superior sagittal sinus (*dotted arrow*) and flow signal in sigmoid sinuses (*short arrows*).

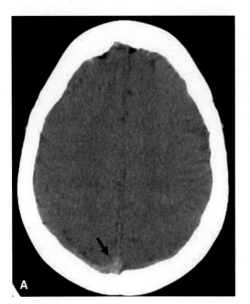

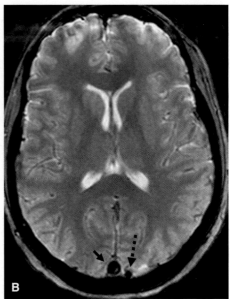

FIGURE 3-19. **Acute superior sagittal sinus (SSS) thrombosis. A.** Axial CT image shows a hyperdense clot in the SSS (*arrow*). **B.** Axial T2 gradient echo sequence shows signal blooming in the SSS (*small solid arrow*) and in a draining cortical vein (*long dotted arrow*) suggesting thrombosis—in this very early case this was the only sign of sinus thrombosis on routine MRI sequences. **C.** Sagittal maximum intensity projection image derived from 3D phase contrast venography shows no flow signal in SSS (expected position marked by *solid arrows*). Note that the inferior sagittal sinus (*bold arrow head*) which is not usually seen on magnetic resonance venogram has opened up. Note a patent straight sinus (*dotted arrow*) and sigmoid sinus (asterisk).

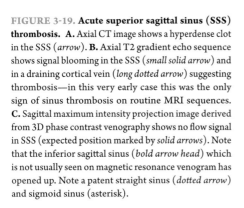

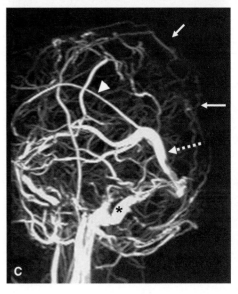

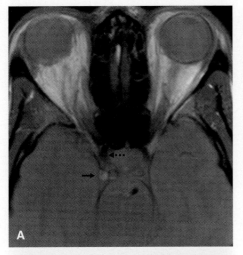

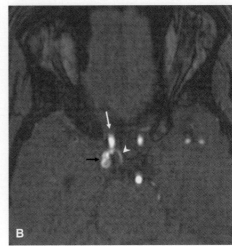

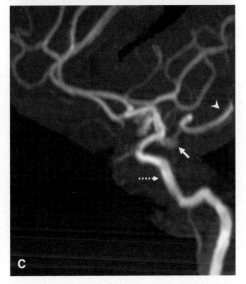

FIGURE 3-20. **Right posterior communicating artery aneurysm (PCoA)** presenting with oculomotor nerve palsy. **A.** Axial proton density–weighted image shows an abnormal rounded hyperintense signal (*solid arrow*) posterior to ICA flow void (*dotted arrow*). **B.** Axial magnetic resonance angiography source image shows a saccular aneurysm projecting posteriorly (*solid black arrow*) from the posterior wall of ICA (*solid white arrow*) along the lateral margin of origin of the PCoA (*arrow head*). **C.** Maximum intensity projection image shows the aneurysm (*solid arrow*) arising from the ICA (*dotted arrow*) at the origin of PCoA (*arrow head*).

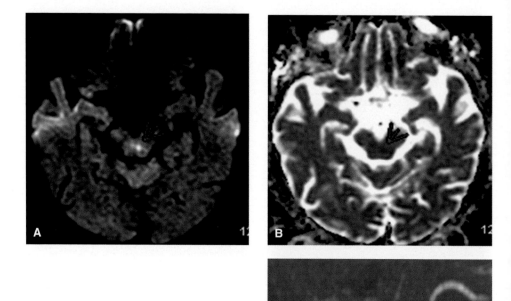

FIGURE 3-21. **Lacunar infarct in the midbrain** in a diabetic presenting with left trochlear nerve palsy. **A.** Punctate bright signal on B-1000 diffusion image (*black arrow*) in the left periaqueductal region. **B.** Corresponding dark signal on apparent diffusion coefficient map (*black arrow*) confirming that it is true restricted diffusion. There was no corresponding T2 hyperintensity suggesting that it was a hyperacute infarct. **C.** Maximum intensity projection magnetic resonance angiography image shows moderate focal midbasilar stenosis (*arrow*).

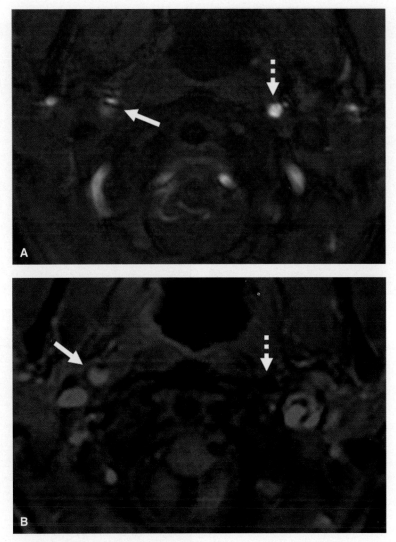

FIGURE 3-22. Right ICA dissection presenting with Horner syndrome. A. Axial 2D time of flight source image shows a dissection flap with pseudoaneurysm along posterolateral aspect of the right ICA (*solid arrow*) just below the skull base which is the commonest location for ICA dissection compared to left (*dotted arrow*). **B.** Axial fat-suppressed T1-weighted image shows increased T1 signal within the false lumen/pseudoaneurysm (*solid arrow*) representing a subacute subintimal hematoma. Note small intact flow void of the true lumen along anterior margin of the pseudoaneurysm. Normal flow void of left ICA (*dotted arrow*).

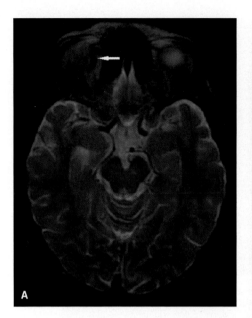

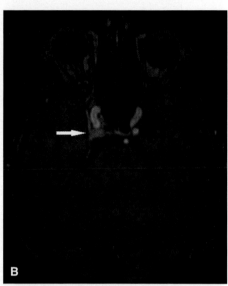

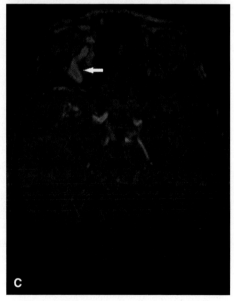

FIGURE 3-23. **Carotid cavernous fistula. A.** Axial T2-weighted fat suppression image through the superior aspect of the orbits demonstrates asymmetrically dilated right superior ophthalmic vein with a prominent flow void (*arrow*). **B.** Noncontrast, time of flight magnetic resonance angiography source image through the cavernous sinuses shows abnormal flow-related enhancement (hyperintense signal) in the region of right cavernous sinus (*arrow*) concerning for carotid cavernous fistula. **C.** Time of flight magnetic resonance angiography source image through the orbits depicts flow-related enhancement in dilated right superior ophthalmic vein (*arrow*).

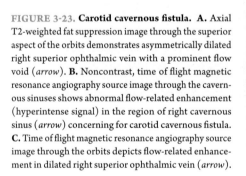

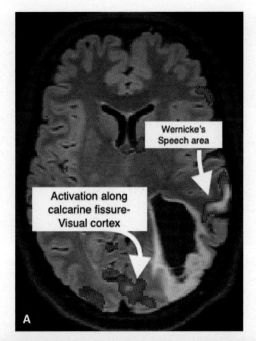

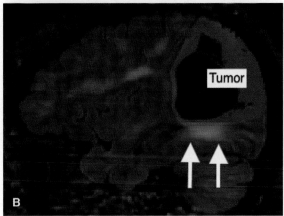

FIGURE 3-24. Diffusion tensor imaging (DTI) and functional magnetic resonance imaging (fMRI) in pre-surgical planning. Left parieto-occipital mass in a 33-year-old female presenting with seizure during pregnancy. **A.** Blood-oxygen-level–dependent fMRI activation superimposed on fluid-attenuated inversion recovery (FLAIR) image showing the Wernicke speech area located at the anterior tumor margin. Activation along calcarine fissure presumably representing visual cortex activation. **B.** Sagittal fused FLAIR and colored fractional anisotropy image showing complex mass in left parieto-occipital lobes with the anteroposteriorly oriented green colored fibers (*arrows*) at the inferior tumor margin likely representing a combination of optic radiation, inferior longitudinal fasciculus, and inferior fronto-occipital fasciculus.

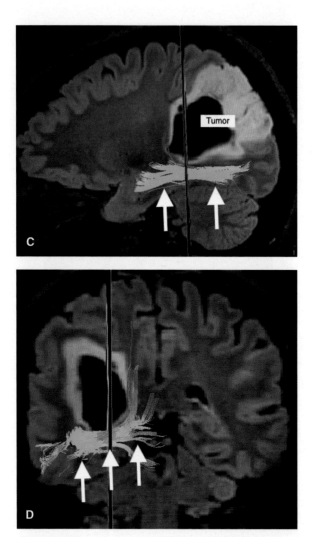

FIGURE 3-24. (*continued*) **C, D,** and **E.** Sagittal, coronal, and axial DTI images, respectively, superimposed on FLAIR image, derived by drawing regions of interest (seeds) better delineate the presumed tracts (*arrows*). The coronal images better delineate the probable course of optic radiation extending to the calcarine fissure.

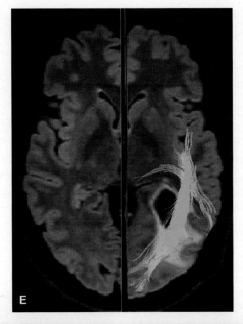

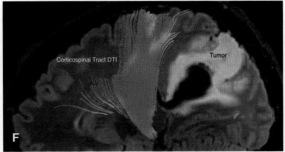

FIGURE 3-24. (*continued*) **F.** DTI of presumed corticospinal tract located anterior to the tumor.

RECOMMENDED IMAGING PROTOCOL

A suggested imaging protocol for use in imaging the optic pathways should include the following:

- Sagittal T1 of entire brain by 5-mm slice thickness

- Axial T1W images of the orbits parallel to the optic nerves by 3-mm slice thickness

- Coronal short T1 inversion recovery or T2 fat suppressed the orbits by 3-mm slice thickness

- Axial FLAIR of the entire brain by 5-mm slice thickness

- Axial DWI of the entire brain by 5-mm slice thickness

- Intravenous gadolinium (0.1 mmol/kg)

- Postcontrast fat-suppressed axial and coronal T1W images through the optic nerves up to the optic tracts by 3-mm slice thickness

- Postcontrast axial of the entire brain by 5-mm slice thickness

- Optional sequences include coronal T1W imaging, axial T2W imaging (preferably with fat suppression), and oblique sagittal T1W imaging postcontrast oriented along the optic nerves.

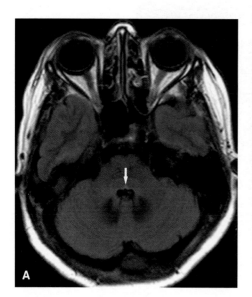 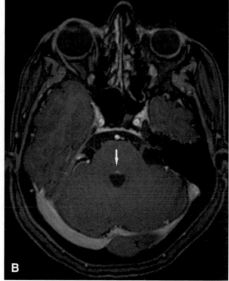

FIGURE 3-25. **Demyelinating plaque presenting with internuclear ophthalmoplegia. A.** Axial fluid-attenuated inversion recovery weighted image at the level of pons shows a subtle hyperintense lesion in the dorsal pons, at the site of medial longitudinal fasciculi (*arrow*). **B.** Postcontrast, axial volumetric T1-weighted image at the same level through the pons demonstrates enhancement of the dorsal pontine lesion, compatible with active demyelinating plaque (*arrow*). The most common causes of internuclear ophthalmoplegia are demyelinating disease and infarction involving the medial longitudinal fasciculus in dorsomedial pons and midline midbrain tegmentum.

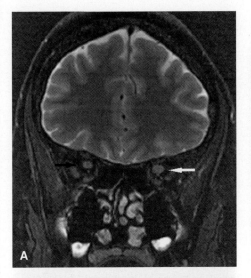

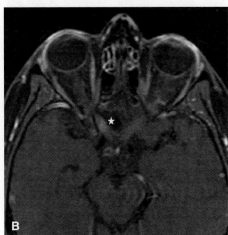

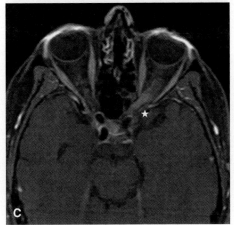

FIGURE 3-26. **Neuromyelitis optica. A.** Coronal short T1 inversion recovery weighted through the orbits demonstrates enlargement of left optic nerve with abnormal hyperintense signal (*white arrow*). Also, note involvement of right optic nerve (*black arrow*), but to a lesser extent. **B, C.** Postcontrast T1-weighted images with fat suppression at the level of optic nerves demonstrate enhancement of intracanalicular and prechiasmatic segments of right optic nerve (fig. B, asterisk) and enhancement of orbital, intracanalicular, and prechiasmatic segments of left optic nerve (fig. C, asterisk).

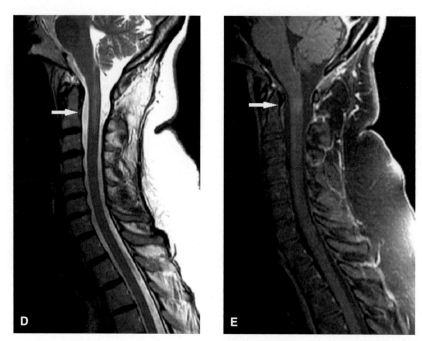

FIGURE 3-26. (*continued*) **D.** Sagittal T2-weighted image of the cervical spine shows hyperintense signal abnormality within the spinal cord extending from cervicomedullary junction through C1–C2 intervertebral disc level. **E.** Postcontrast sagittal T1-weighted image with fat suppression of the cervical spine demonstrates mild patchy enhancement within the spinal cord at C1 level. This constellation of findings is consistent with neuromyelitis optica. Neuromyelitis optica or Devic disease is a severe, progressive demyelinating disease with predominant affection of optic nerves and spinal cord. Recurrent optic neuritis and/or long segment transverse myelitis is considered a hallmark of neuromyelitis optica, and should be considered in differential in patients with first attack of bilateral optic neuritis.

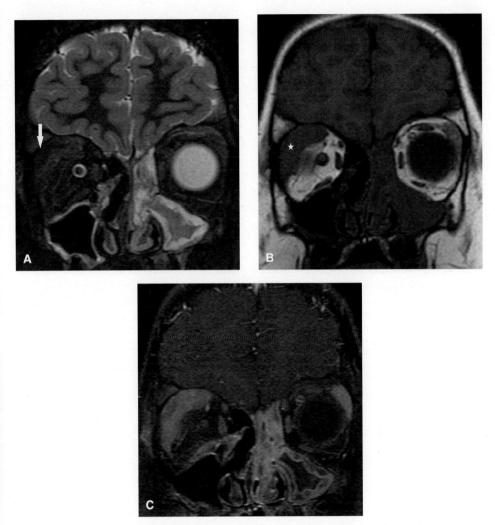

FIGURE 3-27. Idiopathic orbital inflammation (orbital pseudotumor). A. Coronal short T1 inversion recovery weighted image through the orbits shows a hypointense mass (*arrow*) centered in the superolateral aspect of the right orbit, in the region of lacrimal gland with involvement of superior and lateral recti muscles. Incidentally seen is opacification of left maxillary sinus and ethmoid air cells. **B.** The entire extent of the right orbital mass (asterisk) is better visualized on coronal T1-weighted image, and demonstrates isointense signal to extraocular muscles. Also, there is minimal infiltration of adjacent intraconal fat. **C.** This mass demonstrates homogeneous postcontrast enhancement, as seen on coronal T1-weighted image with fat suppression through the orbits. This constellation of findings is consistent with idiopathic orbital inflammation. A substantial proportion of idiopathic orbital inflammations are associated with immunoglobulin G4-related disease. These orbital lesions may be unilateral or bilateral and can involve either the entire orbit or selected components, including the extraocular muscles, lacrimal system, and optic nerves.

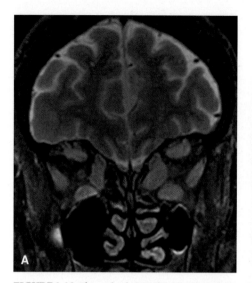
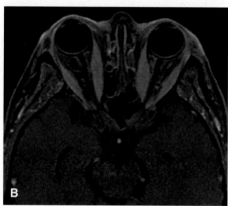

FIGURE 3-28. **Thyroid orbitopathy. A.** Coronal short T1 inversion recovery weighted image through the orbits demonstrates enlargement of bellies of extraocular muscles, with more pronounced involvement of inferior and medial recti muscles. **B.** Coronal, contrast-enhanced T1-weighted image with fat suppression depicts enlarged and enhancing extraocular muscles. Note the relative sparing of anterior tendinous insertions, considered specific for thyroid orbitopathy (in contrast to orbital pseudotumor in which the anterior tendinous insertions are affected). The involvement of extraocular muscles in decreasing order of frequency in thyroid orbitopathy is as follows: inferior rectus, medial rectus, superior rectus, lateral rectus, and oblique muscles (can be remembered by the mnemonic I M SLOw).

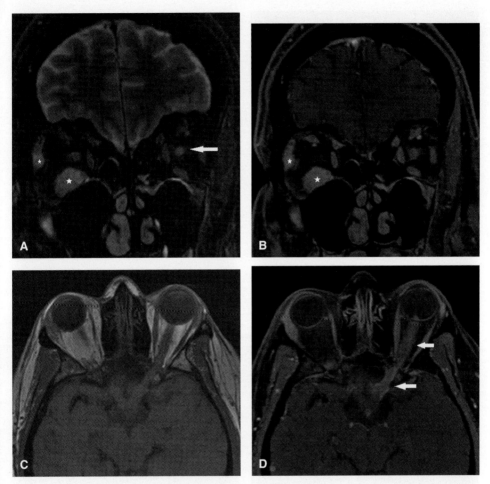

FIGURE 3-29. Sarcoidosis. A. Coronal short T1 inversion recovery weighted image through the orbits demonstrates enlargement with hyperintense signal abnormality involving right inferior rectus muscles (asterisk). The right lateral rectus muscle also demonstrates abnormal contour and signal (asterisk). Also note hyperintense signal abnormality within the left optic nerve (*arrow*). **B.** Postcontrast coronal T1-weighted image with fat suppression shows enhancement of right inferior rectus and lateral rectus muscles (asterisk). **C, D.** Precontrast axial T1-weighted and postcontrast axial T1-weighted fat suppression images through the orbits demonstrate abnormal enhancement of entire course of left optic nerve (fig. D, *arrows*). Biopsy of the right inferior rectus muscle revealed noncaseating granulomas consistent with sarcoidosis.

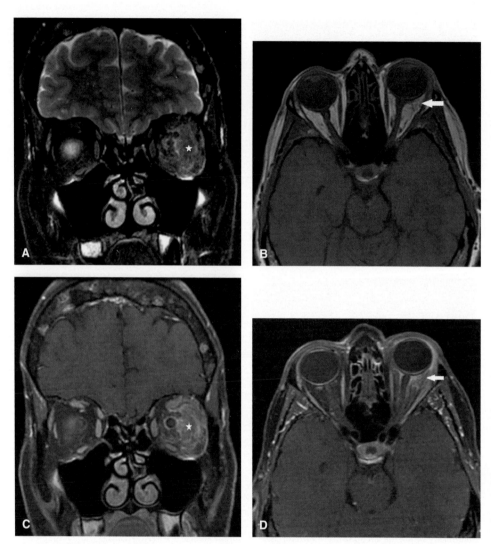

FIGURE 3-30. **Orbital cellulitis. A.** Coronal short T1 inversion recovery weighted image through the orbits shows heterogeneous signal abnormality and infiltration of left orbital fat (asterisk). **B.** Axial T1-weighted image without fat suppression demonstrates infiltration of retrobulbar fat (*arrow*). T1-weighted images are superior for evaluation of fat infiltration as uninvolved fat demonstrates homogeneously hyperintense signal on T1-weighted images. **C, D.** Coronal and axial T1-weighted images with fat suppression show heterogeneous enhancement of the left orbital fat (asterisk and *arrow*).

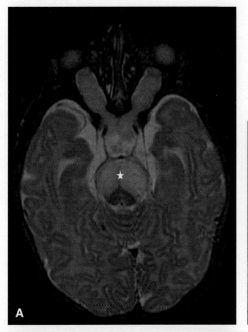

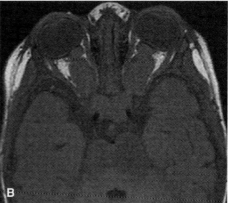

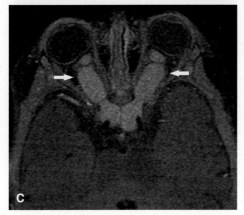

FIGURE 3-31. **Optochiasmatic glioma. A.** Axial T2-weighted image with fat suppression through the optic nerves demonstrates diffuse enlargement of bilateral optic nerves. Also, note the infiltration signal abnormality in the midbrain (asterisk). **B, C.** Axial pre- and postcontrast T1-weighted images through the optic nerves demonstrate enhancement of diffusely enlarged optic nerves (*arrows*). Majority of the optochiasmatic gliomas are pathologically juvenile pilocytic astrocytoma, and are associated with neurofibromatosis Type I.

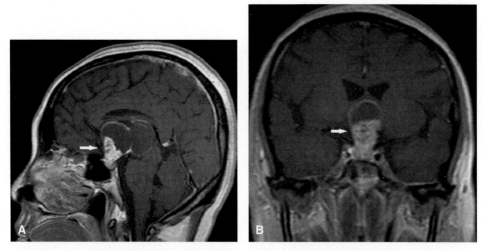

FIGURE 3-32. **Craniopharyngioma.** Postcontrast sagittal (**A**) and coronal (**B**) T1-weighted images through the sella demonstrate a solid and cystic mass in the suprasellar region (*arrows*), typical of craniopharyngioma.

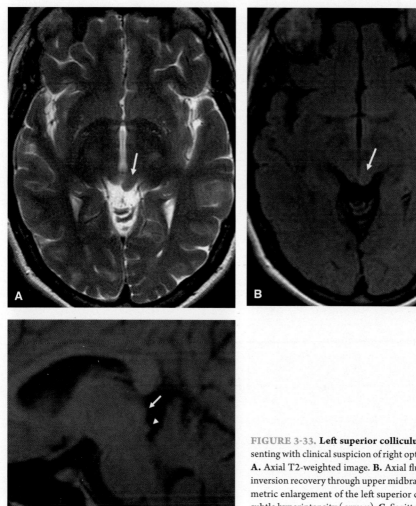

FIGURE 3-33. **Left superior colliculus glioma** presenting with clinical suspicion of right optic neuropathy. **A.** Axial T2-weighted image. **B.** Axial fluid-attenuated inversion recovery through upper midbrain show asymmetric enlargement of the left superior colliculus with subtle hyperintensity (*arrows*). **C.** Sagittal T1-weighted image shows an enlarged left superior colliculus (*arrow*) compared with the left inferior colliculus (*arrow head*).

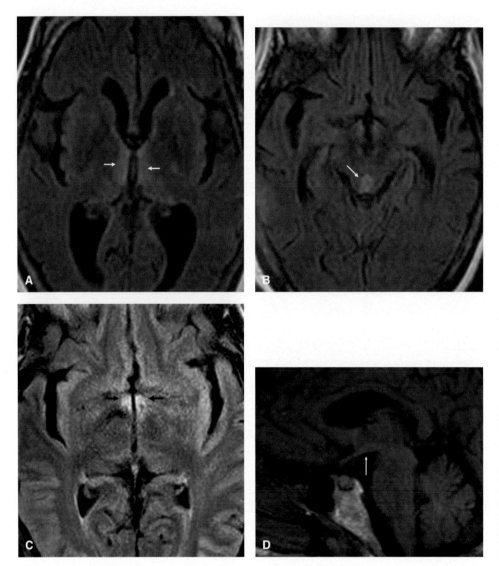

FIGURE 3-34. **Wernicke encephalopathy** in a chronic alcoholic presenting with confusion and ophthalmoplegia. **A.** Axial fluid-attenuated inversion recovery (FLAIR) at the level of third ventricle shows increased signal in the medial thalami (*arrows*), which form the lateral walls of the third ventricle. **B.** Axial FLAIR at the level of upper midbrain shows increased signal in the periaqueductal region (*arrow*), which is the expected location of oculomotor nerve nucleus. **C.** Axial FLAIR in the region of floor of third ventricle (different patient) shows increased signal in the region of the mammillary bodies (*arrows*). **D.** Sagittal T1-weighted image shows atrophy of mammillary bodies (*arrow*) which is typical.

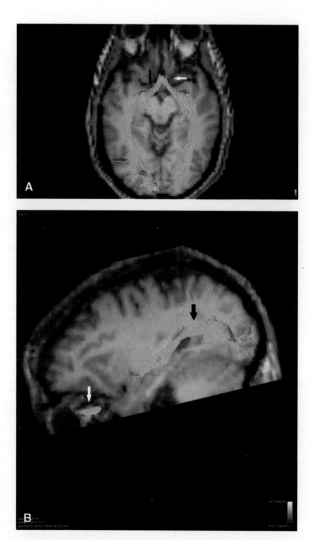

FIGURE 3-35. **Tractography** in a normal subject using higher order diffusion tensor technique (NODDI: neurite orientation dispersion and density imaging). **A.** Optic chiasm (*white arrow*), optic tract (*black arrow*), and optic radiation (*red arrow*). **B.** Optic nerve (*white arrow*) and optic radiation (*black arrow*). (Courtesy: Dr. Mahdi Alizadeh PhD and Dr. Firoze Mohamed PhD.)

Transient Visual Loss/Retinal Artery Occlusion

TRANSIENT VISUAL LOSS

INTRODUCTION

Transient visual loss (TVL) refers to the abrupt and temporary loss of vision that may be monocular or binocular. In general, the most important cause of transient monocular visual loss is retinal or ocular ischemia due to vascular occlusion or embolization. The most common cause of transient binocular visual disturbance is migraine. We will use the terms TVL and transient visual obscuration (TVO) interchangeably.

The investigation of the patient with a history of TVL is challenging because at the time the patient is evaluated the examination is often normal. Therefore, the *history* is of critical importance. Certain characteristics are of particular relevance in determining the cause of TVL.

Unilateral versus bilateral: Determining if the cause of visual loss was in one or both eyes can be challenging because the history may be misleading. Patients with a transient homonymous hemianopia may describe monocular visual loss in the eye with the temporal defect not appreciating the nasal component of the homonymous hemianopia.

Age of patient: In patients less than 50 years, the most likely cause of TVL is migraine, retinal embolization, or, less commonly, vasospasm. In older patients, one needs to consider giant cell arteritis (GCA).

Duration of symptoms: TVL that lasts seconds (and often associated with postural changes) most likely is related to papilledema or optic disc drusen. Other ocular causes such as recurrent microhyphaema should be considered as well. Retinal ischemia is more consistent with visual loss that lasts 5 to 15 minutes, whereas ocular hypoperfusion from vascular insufficiency may last from seconds up to 30 minutes.

Precipitated by any activity: Visual loss precipitated by exercise may be caused by vasospasm, pigment dispersion syndrome, or demyelinating disease. *Uhthoff phenomenon* (transient visual blurring with physical activity or elevation in body temperature) frequently occurs in patients with a current or previous episode of optic neuritis (see Chapter 5).

Other associated signs and symptoms: It is important to identify associated features that may provide clues to the underlying cause of the TVL. Features that suggest the abnormality is related to posterior circulation ischemia include bilateral or homonymous visual loss and associated brainstem or cerebellar symptoms.

Macular disorders should be considered if the TVL is in the form of persistent after images or prolonged recovery of vision following exposure to intense lights.

ETIOLOGY

MONOCULAR TVL

In the investigation of patients with transient monocular visual loss, a key step is to exclude nonvascular causes.

Anterior Segment Causes

Dry eye syndrome can produce transient blurring or TVO. The patient will often experience relief by blinking, rubbing the eye, or using lubricating drops.

Transient *hyphemas* cause TVOs. Typically, this is associated with the UGH (uveitis, glaucoma, hemorrhage) syndrome. Often the examination will be unremarkable except that gonioscopy shows blood in the inferior angle (Fig. 4-1). The UGH syndrome usually follows cataract surgery especially with sulcus-fixated implants or glaucoma surgery. Other abnormalities of the media in either the anterior chamber or vitreous, such as floaters, may also cause transient visual disturbances.

Intermittent elevation of intraocular pressure may cause transient corneal edema and TVO. This is usually associated with halos and pain. This may be seen with plateau iris syndrome (Fig. 4-2) or intermittent angle closure.

Orbital Causes

Orbital masses may produce a specific type of TVO or TVL termed *directional amaurosis*. When the patient gazes in a particular direction, the symptom occurs and disappears when the eye is removed from that position. The cause is decreased ocular blood flow due to optic nerve compression by the mass (Fig. 4-3).

Vascular Causes

Retinal ischemia is the most frequent cause of monocular TVL. The typical event lasts from 10 to 20 minutes and then clears. The most frequent cause is thromboembolism in patients over 50 years of age, with the carotid artery being the most frequent origin of the embolus. The investigation of these patients is outlined below.

A form of TVL due to retinal and choroidal ischemia occurs after exposure to light (*light-induced amaurosis*). This is usually due to carotid stenosis causing the retina to display prolonged recovery from light exposure (Fig. 4-4).

● Recent guidelines proposed by the American Stroke Association for investigation of TVL recommend that an immediate workup be initiated for a source of emboli as TVL is considered a significant risk factor for cerebral stroke. It has been recommended that patients be referred to stroke units for the workup. Noninvasive vascular imaging of the carotid arteries (for unilateral visual loss), vertebral arteries (for bilateral visual loss), and the aortic arch should be performed. Tests that reliably image these structures include duplex carotid ultrasonography, magnetic resonance angiography (MRA), or computed tomographic arteriography (CTA). MRA and CTA allow the visualization and characterization of the plaque and are also useful for detecting carotid artery dissection. Brain imaging to identify associated cerebral ischemia is also recommended because up to 25% of patients with acute retinal ischemia may have acute brain infarctions identified on diffusion-weighted imaging (DWI). The risk is higher with embolic retinal ischemia. Patients who have acute cerebral ischemia must be managed according to stroke guidelines.

● Venous stasis can also produce TVL. This is often associated with an elevated optic disc, venous congestion, and dot hemorrhages in the retinal periphery (Fig. 4-5).

Optic Nerve Causes

Congenital optic disc anomalies may cause TVO. Optic disc *drusen* may produce TVOs similar to those of papilledema (see the following paragraph). Some optic disc *colobomas* (e.g., a contractile morning glory malformation) may also produce TVOs.

Papilledema may cause TVOs. They typically last for seconds, may be in one or both eyes, and most often occur when going from a sitting to a standing position (see also Chapter 5; Fig. 4-6).

GCA may produce TVL due to optic nerve, retinal, or choroidal ischemia. Any anterior ischemic optic neuropathy (AION) preceded by TVO should prompt an investigation for GCA (see also Chapter 5).

Demyelinating *optic neuritis* may be associated with TVO after exercise or a hot bath. The TVO lasts for minutes or rarely hours. This is called Uhtoff phenomenon and is seen in patients who have had optic neuritis. The exact cause of the phenomenon is not known, and treatment is controversial.

Retinal migraine is a disorder now thought to be *retinal vasospasm*. The visual loss lasts for minutes and retinal arterial narrowing and venous congestion can be observed during the episode.

Systemic Diseases

Any condition that produces decreased blood flow to the retina, choroid, or optic nerve can result in TVL. Some causes are intermittent systemic hypotension from any cause, hyperviscosity syndromes, vasculitidies, and vasospasm.

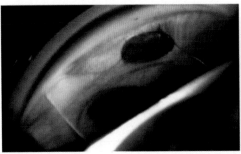
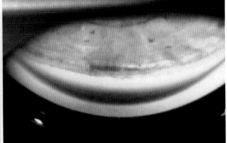

FIGURE 4-1. **Hyphema.** Transient monocular TVO following cataract surgery with an anterior chamber implant. Gonioscopy shows blood in the inferior angle. (Courtesy of L Jay Katz, MD.)

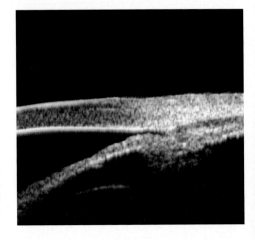

FIGURE 4-2. **Plateua iris syndrome.** A 42-year-old woman experienced monocular TVO associated with a large pupil and ocular pain. Anterior segment imaging documented plateau iris. Following iridotomy, the episodes disappeared.

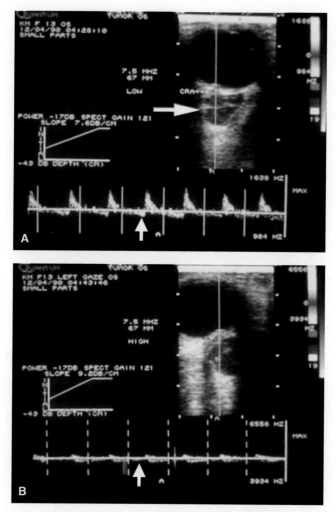

FIGURE 4-3. Orbital mass. Thirteen-year-old girl loses vision OS when looking to the left. In primary position her examination is normal, but on left gaze the vision OS slowly decreases to no light perception (NLP) with an amaurotic pupil. Orbital Doppler shows (**A**) a retrobulbar mass (*horizontal arrow*) with a normal arterial pulse (*vertical arrow*) in primary gaze and (**B**) complete loss of the pulse in left gaze.

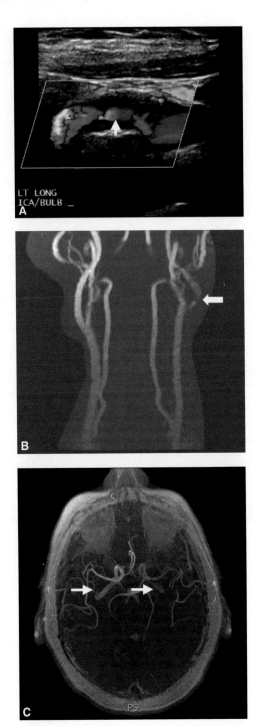

FIGURE 4-4. **Carotid stenosis.** A 62-year-old man loses vision OS for 45 seconds after prolonged exposure to light. **A.** Carotid Doppler shows marked stenosis (*arrow*). **B.** MRA shows stenosis and irregularity of the left carotid artery (*arrow*). **C.** Decrease flow in the intracranial artery on the left compared with the right (*arrows*). Following endarterectomy, the symptoms resolved.

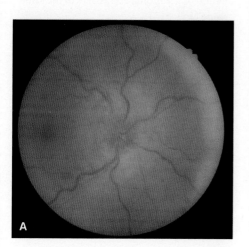
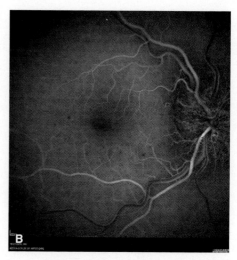

FIGURE 4-5. **Venous stasis.** A 53-year-old woman experience TVOs OD lasting less than a minute. Examination revealed (**A**) an elevated right optic disc (OS was normal) with small hemorrhages in the posterior pole more numerous in the retinal periphery and venous congestion. **B.** Fluorescein angiography shows delayed venous filling and accentuates the posterior pole hemorrhages.

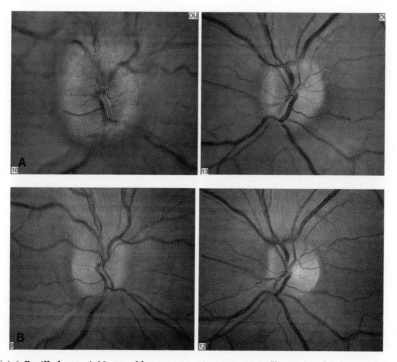

FIGURE 4-6. **Papilledema.** A 30-year-old woman experiences transient "brown outs" in her vision lasting seconds. They were initially posturally related but became unrelated to activity. **A.** Bilateral asymmetric papilledema diagnosed as PTC. **B.** Following treatment with acetazolamide and weight loss, the papilledema resolved and the TVOs disappeared.

BINOCULAR TVL

The most frequent cause of binocular TVL is *migraine*. This is a disorder of the young and causes binocular TVL almost exclusively. The visual loss may be in the form of a homonymous hemianopia or scintillating scotomas. Both last for approximately 20 minutes and then clear without a lasting defect. When a permanent scotoma results, this is *complicated* migraine.

The scintillating scotoma often starts small and in the periphery. It then expands and migrates across the entire visual field. It then slowly dissipates (see Fig. 7-9).

Scintillating scotomas may occur without headache (*acephalgic* migraine) or may be followed by headache of variable intensity (*migraine with aura*). The scotoma often alternates sides.

Diagnosis

Migraine is a clinical diagnosis. Not all patients with suspected migraine require neuroimaging. There are several signs that should prompt imaging to look for migraine mimickers:

Scintillating scotoma exclusively to the same side (Fig. 4-7)

Headache preceding the scotoma

Persistent neurologic defect following the migraine

Any other atypical finding

Occipital Lobe Abnormalities

Abnormalities of the occipital lobe, such as mass lesions, ischemia, or seizure, may all cause transient binocular visual loss. A structural abnormality such as a tumor or arteriovenous malformation should be excluded if the visual loss is always on the same side. Such patients require magnetic resonance imaging (MRI/MRA). Posterior cerebral ischemia may produce binocular visual loss and may be associated with transient diplopia, dysphagia, or drop attacks, suggesting associated brainstem ischemia. Occipital lobe seizures usually manifest as unformed positive visual phenomena, although blacking out of vision has also been reported.

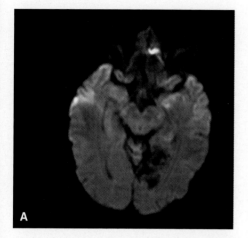 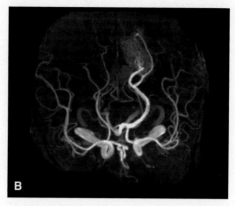

FIGURE 4-7. Arteriovenous malformation (AVM). A 25-year-old woman experienced a fortification scotoma to the right but always in the same location. **A.** MRI shows mass resembling an arteriovenous malformation (AVM) that was confirmed by (**B**) cerebral angiography.

RETINAL ARTERY OCCLUSION

INTRODUCTION

Occlusion of retinal arterioles in the form of a branch retinal artery occlusion (BRAO) or central retinal artery occlusion (CRAO) may be a precursor to further visual loss, stroke, or death.

EPIDEMIOLOGY AND ETIOLOGY

The causes of retinal artery occlusion may be embolic or thrombotic. Different etiologies are more prevalent in different age groups. For example, in the vasculopathic age group (over 50 years), carotid atheroma is a more likely cause than it would be in a younger population. In the younger age group, hyperviscosity syndromes, vasculitis, or cardiac abnormalities tend to be more frequent causes.

There are several types of retinal emboli:

• Platelet–fibrin emboli: These appear as nonrefractile white or gray emboli usually seen in the distal arterioles. The source of the emboli is thrombotic (carotid or aortic arch atheroma), cardiac, or cardiac prosthesis.

• Cholesterol: These are often multiple yellow, refractile emboli often located at the arterial bifurcation (Fig. 4-8). They suggest an atheroma in the ipsilateral carotid artery or aortic arch. The bifurcation of the common carotid into the internal and external carotid and the carotid siphon are the most common sites for atheroma formation. It is important to remember that emboli may occur on ulcerated atheromatous plaques with any degree of stenosis. However, in order for distal flow to be affected the carotid lumen must be reduced by 50% to 90%. Emboli may also originate from aortic arch atheromas. Risk factors for atheroma include diabetes mellitus, hypertension, hypercholesterolemia, and smoking.

• Calcium: These are usually isolated, large white emboli located in the proximal segment of the central retinal artery or its branches. They suggest calcified atheromatous plaque or cardiac valve (Fig. 4-9).

• Other

  ▪ Fat: It appears as multiple whitish spots associated with hemorrhages and/or cotton wool infarcts. They occur most frequently with damage/injury to long bones.

  ▪ Talc: These multiple yellow refractile emboli are associated with intravenous drug use.

  ▪ Infectious: Multiple white spots (Roth spots) suggest underlying infectious endocarditis.

  ▪ Neoplasm: Cardiac myxoma may produce multiple white gray emboli.

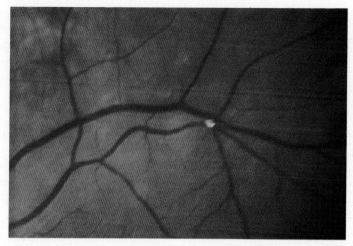

FIGURE 4-8. Cholesterol embolus. A bright plaque that appears larger than the artery in which it resides is seen at a retinal arteriole bifurcation. This glistening appearance suggests a cholesterol embolus of carotid artery origin.

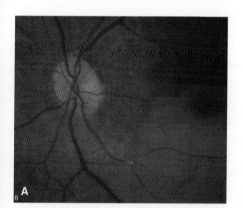
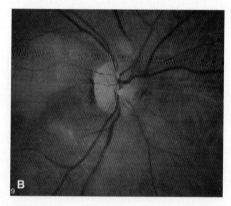

FIGURE 4-9. Calcium embolus. A. Hour-glass–shaped embolus lodged in the inferior temporal artery OS with adjacent retinal whitening. **B.** The following day, the patient presented with decreased vision OD with multiple large white emboli (not present the previous day) at the optic disc with retinal whitening.

CLINICAL CHARACTERISTICS

Symptoms

• The primary symptom is acute, usually unilateral painless visual loss, which is sudden, but may be stepwise and stuttering in onset. The visual loss may be partial, with a scotoma that may involve or spare fixation, or may be nearly total, with the preservation of a small island of peripheral vision. Some conditions, such as GCA or retinal emboli, are more likely to be associated with episodes of TVL before the visual loss becomes permanent. However, many conditions can be associated with prodrome of TVL. Exploration of the time course through detailed history taking may be helpful. For example, retinal ischemia from emboli is more likely to cause visual loss that last several minutes and typically not longer than 15 minutes. Ocular hypoperfusion or venous insufficiency may last longer—up to 30 minutes. Retinal artery vasospasm may last seconds to hours.

• The pattern of visual loss may also be helpful in determining if the underlying cause is retinal ischemia. Retinal emboli classically produce a monocular curtain-like visual loss, but may also cause tunnel-like contraction or sudden complete loss of vision.

• The presence of a cilioretinal artery will often determine the configuration of the scotoma and, at times, the level of visual acuity.

• Associated symptoms are also important to identify. Patients with visual loss over the age of 55 years should be directly questioned for symptoms of GCA. Neurologic symptoms may also be present. Cerebral ischemia in the posterior circulation may be associated with diplopia, dizziness, or drop attacks (loss of consciousness). If the patient has ipsilateral Horner syndrome or periorbital headache, the possibility of internal carotid artery dissection should be considered. Some symptoms suggest hypoperfusion such as postprandial or exercise induced visual loss.

Signs

• Decreased acuity if the macula area is involved.

• Visual field defects that correspond to the area of retinal infarction (Fig. 4-10).

• Relative afferent pupillary defect (RAPD) is usually detected.

• Areas of retinal whitening that correspond to the scotoma develop within hours but fades over days or weeks. The fundus may appear almost normal initially (Fig. 4-11).

• Intravascular embolic or thrombotic material, at times characteristic of the site of origin, is sometimes identified on ophthalmoscopy.

• Diabetic patients with carotid occlusions will have less diabetic retinopathy on the side of the occluded carotid artery (Fig. 4-12).

• Occlusion at different locations of the retinal vasculature may produce different clinical features:

   ▪ Asymptomatic cholesterol retinal emboli: These are found in 1% to 2% of the population over the age of 50. Their presence warrants an investigation for underlying vascular risk factors.

   ▪ Branch retinal artery occlusion: This is characterized by acute unilateral partial visual loss, a mild-moderate RAPD, attenuation of the involved branch retinal artery, often the presence of emboli, and localized retinal edema in the acute stage. There is usually a corresponding arcuate visual field defect. The underlying etiology of BRAO is less likely to be GCA.

- An important cause of recurrent BRAO is Susac syndrome, which is a vasculopathy of unknown etiology occurring predominantly in young woman that leads to occlusion of small retinal, cochlear, and cerebral arteries. Hence, it is characterized by BRAO, hearing loss, and encephalopathy with focal neurologic signs and psychiatric manifestations (see below).

- CRAO results in profound unilateral loss of visual acuity, generalized retinal edema (acutely), and the presence of a cherry-red spot, a profound RAPD, and attenuated retinal arterioles. Emboli may or may not be visible. If the patient has a patent cilioretinal artery, which originates in the posterior ciliary circulation and is present in approximately 30% of patients, then some vision may be preserved. If the artery supplies the fovea, central visual acuity may be preserved.

- Ophthalmic artery occlusion results in severe visual loss often to the level of no light perception. The fundus shows retinal edema, attenuated retinal vessels, but no cherry-red spot as the underlying choroid is also ischemic. GCA should be considered in all cases of ophthalmic artery occlusion.

- Ocular ischemic syndrome: Chronic hypoperfusion due to severe stenosis or occlusion of the ipsilateral internal carotid artery with poor collateral circulation may result in ocular ischemia. In some cases of internal carotid artery stenosis, the blood supply to the orbit may originate completely from the external carotid artery and its branches. Furthermore, there may be a reversal of flow through the ophthalmic artery, so that the blood flow also supports the ipsilateral cerebral hemisphere. Clinical features of ocular ischemic syndrome are as follows:

  - Venous stasis retinopathy: This is characterized by tortuosity and dilation of retinal veins and blot hemorrhages in the midperiphery. Patients are asymptomatic, although they may experience hemodynamic transient unilateral visual loss such as with exposure to bright lights or change in posture.

  - Dull periocular pain: This is often worse when patient is standing up but resolves when patient is lying down.

  - Low intraocular pressure

  - Intraocular inflammation

  - Dilated episcleral arteries

The prognosis of ocular ischemic syndrome is poor.

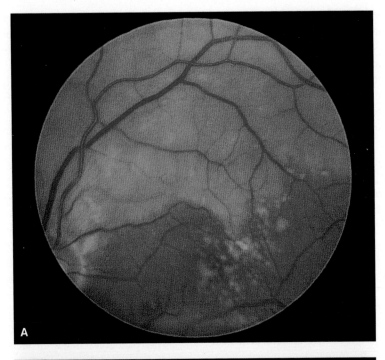

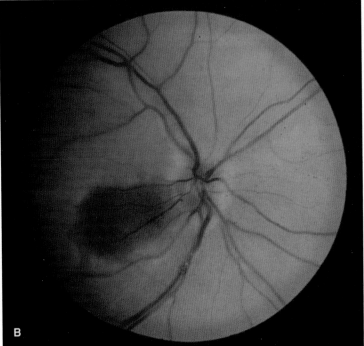

FIGURE 4-10. **Retinal artery occlusion. A.** BRAO with retinal whitening of the superior arcuate nerve fiber bundle. The patient had an inferior arcuate visual field defect. **B.** Patent cilioretinal artery prevents macula ischemia and preserves central vision.

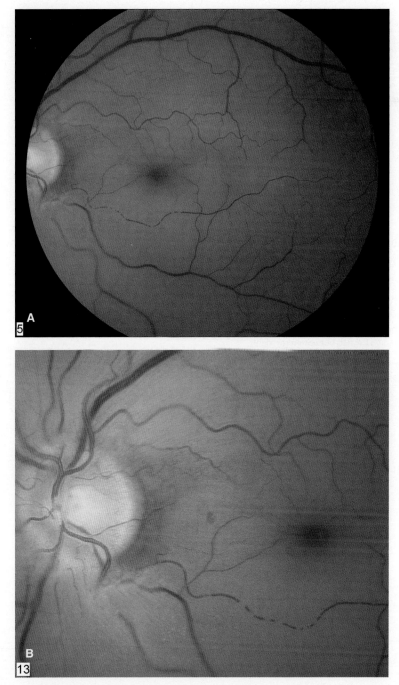

FIGURE 4-11. Retinal artery occlusion. A. CRAO with a cherry-red spot. **B.** Note "box car" appearance in inferior vessel from interruption of the blood flow.

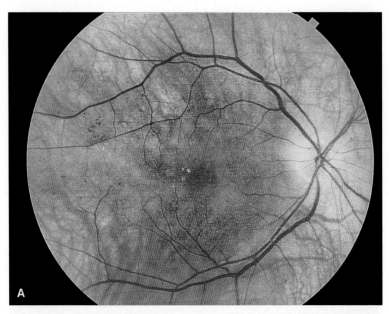

FIGURE 4-12. **Carotid artery occlusion.** A patient with diabetes has obvious diabetic retinopathy in the right eye (**A**), but none in the left (**B**). Because of this, carotid ultrasound was performed and carotid occlusion was documented on the left, but not on the right.

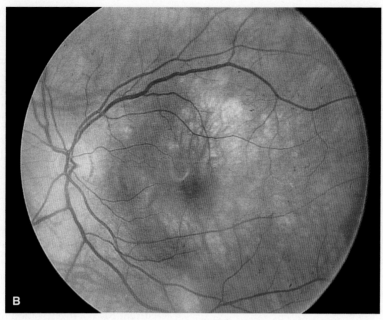

FIGURE 4-12. Carotid artery occlusion. A patient with diabetes has obvious diabetic retinopathy in the right eye (**A**), but none in the left (**B**). Because of this, carotid ultrasound was performed and carotid occlusion was documented on the left, but not on the right.

DIAGNOSTIC EVALUATION

Investigation depends on the age of the patient and the presence or absence of visible embolic material in the retinal circulation (Table 4-1). The presence of visible emboli dictates that the primary investigations should be aimed at finding the source of the emboli. The studies that should be performed are detailed below.

• Determination of carotid patency (MRA/CTA or carotid Doppler). The presence of a refractile embolus in the retinal circulation (Hollenhorst plaque) is highly suggestive of a cholesterol embolus originating in a carotid atheroma (Fig. 4-8).

• In younger patients, carotid atheromas are less likely to be the cause of retinal artery occlusion, and the investigation should focus primarily on the following:

• Cardiac evaluation including trans-esophageal echocardiography and rhythm monitoring

• Investigation for hyperviscosity states, collagen vascular diseases, especially including testing for the presence of anticardiolipin and antiphospholipid antibodies

• Testing for underlying vasculitis

• In older patients without embolic material present in the retinal arterioles, GCA must always be considered, and the appropriate questions to detect this disorder should be asked. The association of a BRAO or CRAO with anterior ischemic optic neuropathy in the same or contralateral eye is highly suggestive of GCA. Any suspicion that GCA is the cause of the retinal artery occlusion should prompt urgent treatment with systemic corticosteroids. The gold standard for the diagnosis of GCA is a positive temporal artery biopsy.

• Retinal artery occlusion, which occurs with ophthalmoplegia or orbital signs. These patients should be investigated for paranasal sinus fungal infection, for example, mucormycosis. Often the initial MRI or computed tomography (CT) scan is normal or minimally abnormal.

• Recurrent BRAO. Investigation for Susac syndrome, which is a systemic microangiopathy that typically shows the triad of encephalopathy, BRAO (which are typically bilateral and typically of more peripheral arterioles) (Fig. 4-13 and 4-14), and hearing loss. MRI with gadolinium shows characteristic lesions in the corpus callosum and occasionally multiple small lesions in the white and gray matter of the brain (Fig. 4-7).

TABLE 4-1. Investigation of Retinal Artery Occlusion (All Patients Should Have Brain MRI to Exclude Concurrent Stroke)

	Embolus Present	No Embolus Present
Under age 50	Cardiac echography	Cardiac echography
	Carotid Doppler/MRA/CTA	Cardiac rhythm monitor
		Hyperviscosity panel
Over age 50	Carotid Doppler/MRA/CTA	Cardiac echography
	Cardiac echography	Cardiac rhythm monitor
		Hyperviscosity panel
		ESR, temporal artery biopsy (GCA)

CTA, computed tomographic arteriography; ESR, erythrocyte sedimentation rate; GCA, giant cell arteritis; MRA, magnetic resonance angiography.

TREATMENT

There is no unanimity of opinion on the usefulness of treatment of acute retinal artery occlusion. Traditional treatments include lowering the intraocular pressure to promote better intraocular perfusion. This is done by anterior chamber paracentesis or by administering pharmacologic agents that block aqueous secretion. Ocular massage is recommended on the assumption that it may dislodge an embolus and allow reperfusion of the ischemic retina. Although no prospective studies prove that any of these maneuvers is helpful in restoring retinal blood flow, we believe that these maneuvers should be tried acutely, possibly up to 12 hours from the time of onset of the retinal artery occlusion. Some investigators recommend thrombolytics for CRAO in selected patients who present within a few hours of visual loss. To date, there is no study that proves the efficacy or safety of this intervention. In cases of suspected GCA, patients should be treated with high-dose intravenous methylprednisolone (1 g daily) while temporal artery biopsy is performed and interpreted.

Treatment will also vary depending on the underlying condition. There is controversy with regard to the management of carotid stenosis. Prospective multicenter studies indicate that patients with carotid stenosis greater than 70% benefit more from surgical endarterectomy than from medical treatment. This presumes, however, a low rate of intra- and perioperative morbidity and mortality (under 2%). Surgical candidates should be in reasonably good health and have the anticipation of multiyear survival. Patients with visual transient ischemic attacks (TIAs) may be at a lower risk for stroke than those with cerebral TIA. A more conservative therapeutic approach to patients with only visual symptoms may be indicated.

The treatment of ocular ischemic syndrome is carotid endarterectomy. Panphotolasercoagulation or intravascular anti-VEGF agents to ischemic retinal may be necessary to decrease neovascularization.

An important aspect of managing these patients is preventing the risk of cerebral stroke and cardiovascular patients. Studies have shown that there is approximately 10% risk of stroke within 3 months, most occurring within 48 hours. Patients also have a longer term risks with approximately 40% combined 10-year stroke, myocardial infarction, or vascular death (4% per year). Risk factors that stratify these patients into a high-risk category include male sex, age 75 years or older, previous history of cerebral stroke, intermittent leg claudication, stenosis of 80% to 94%, and absence of collateral vessels on cerebral angiography. Medical treatment for underlying carotid artery stenosis includes antiplatelet agents such as aspirin, aspirin-dipyridamole, or clopidogrel.

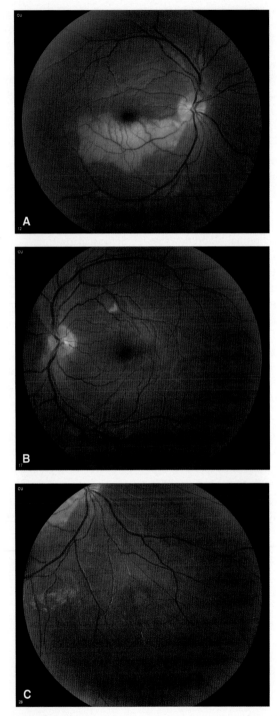

FIGURE 4-13. **Susac syndrome. A.** BRAO in right eye of patient with Susac syndrome. **B.** Infarct in left eye. **C.** Yellow deposits along arteriole in midperiphery (Gass plaque).

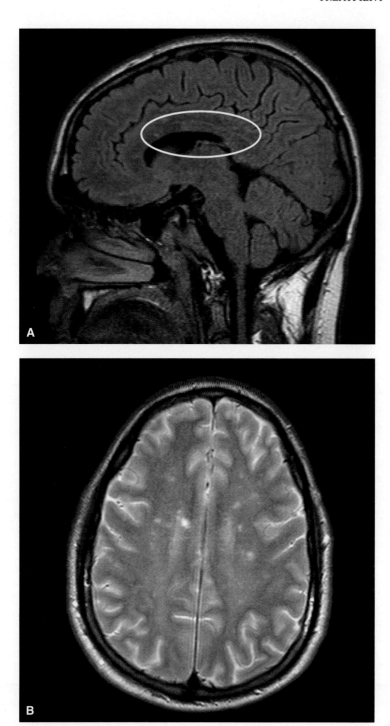

FIGURE 4-14. Susac syndrome. A. Sagittal MRI showing lesions in the corpus callosum (oval). **B.** Periventricular white matter lesions.

Optic Nerve Disorders

INTRODUCTION

Optic neuropathies are generally classified as acutely anterior, those in which the optic nerve head is swollen, and posterior, those in which there is decreased optic nerve function but a normal appearing optic nerve head.

OPTIC NEURITIS

Optic neuritis refers to inflammation of the optic nerve. The term "optic neuritis" most often refers to the optic neuropathy associated with demyelinating disease. This is the most common acute optic neuropathy in individuals under the age of 45 years. It is also a frequent presenting sign of multiple sclerosis (MS). Demyelinating optic neuritis can be considered in three categories: acute, chronic progressive, and asymptomatic (subclinical). Acute optic neuritis is the most common form of optic neuritis.

Epidemiology and Etiology

- MS: Optic neuritis may be the initial presentation of this disorder

- Age of onset: 20 to 50 years, mean age of 30 to 35 years
- Gender: More common in women (female:male ratio is 3:1)
- Incidence: Between 1 and 5 per 100,000
- Prevalence: Approximately 115 per 100,000

Clinical Characteristics

Symptoms

- Unilateral pain or discomfort around the orbit or with eye movement is present in approximately 90% of the patients. It may precede or occur concurrently with visual loss.

- Decreased visual acuity: The degree of visual loss varies widely and is usually monocular, although a small subgroup, particularly children, often have both eyes affected simultaneously.

- Decreased color vision

- Other: Positive visual phenomena (photopsias), such as flashes of lights, showers of sparks, or flashing black squares, may occur spontaneously or in response to loud noises.

- Uhthoff phenomenon: Worsening of visual function with heat or exercise

Signs

- Relative afferent pupillary defect (RAPD) if the process is unilateral or asymmetric

- Decreased visual acuity is the rule but need not be present.

- Acquired dyschromatopsia with the color deficit often greater than the degree of visual acuity loss.

- Virtually any type of optic nerve visual field defect can occur in optic neuritis (Fig. 5-1). Visual field defects are often found in the contralateral eye.

- Contrast sensitivity impairment is found in virtually all patients with optic neuritis.

- The optic disc appears normal (retrobulbar neuritis) in about two-thirds of the patients. Optic disc swelling (Fig. 5-2) will be present in 20% to 40% of the cases. The degree of swelling does not correlate with the severity of optic nerve dysfunction. Optic disc or peripapillary hemorrhages are uncommon.

- Vitreous cells, particularly overlying the optic disc, may be seen but are usually minimal.

- Peripheral venous sheathing occurs in some patients with demyelinating optic neuritis. Pars planitis is also associated with demyelinating optic neuritis.

Diagnostic Evaluation

- Neuroimaging: MRI with gadolinium is the modality of choice for investigating optic neuritis. The indication for neuroimaging in optic neuritis is to exclude a compressive lesion or to confirm the diagnosis (which is made on clinical grounds). An MRI is performed to:

  ▪ detect subclinical demyelinating plaques (Fig. 5-3),

  ▪ assist in determining the prognosis for developing MS, and

  ▪ evaluate patient's potential benefit from intravenous methylprednisolone and disease-modifying therapy.

- Cerebrospinal fluid (CSF) examination may be performed; however, this testing is not necessary and is being performed less frequently. However, it may be particularly helpful in atypical cases. The following abnormalities have been identified in patients with optic neuritis, although none is diagnostic of MS:

  ▪ Pleocytosis and elevated protein

  ▪ Oligoclonal bands

  ▪ Myelin basic protein

  ▪ Increased IgG index

- Visual-evoked responses are almost always abnormal, showing a prolonged latency on the side of the affected optic nerve.

- No serologic tests or CSF studies need to be performed unless the patient's course does not follow that of typical optic neuritis or the patient's history or examination suggests an underlying systemic illness (Table 5-1).

TABLE 5-1. Results of Investigations of Patients in Optic Neuritis Treatment Trial

Etiologic studies
  Antinuclear antibodies (ANA) positive in titer <1:320 in 13%; one patient developed a connective tissue disorder within 2y
  Chest radiograph: No case of sarcoidosis or tuberculosis was identified
  Cerebrospinal fluid analysis: No lumbar puncture offered any unsuspected information
  Fluorescent treponemal antibody absorption: No case of active syphilis was identified

Treatment

- Fortunately, visual recovery without treatment is the rule following an episode, with approximately 90% of the patients recovering to 20/40 or better vision within weeks. The Optic Neuritis Treatment Trial (ONTT) evaluated the benefits of treatment with corticosteroids. The study identified the following:

  - Oral prednisone

    - showed no benefit to recovery of vision,

    - resulted in doubling the risk of further attack of optic neuritis in the same or fellow eye.

  - Intravenous methylprednisolone (250 mg every 6 hours for 3 days) followed by oral prednisone (1 mg/kg/day) for 11 days, then a 3-day taper

    - hastened visual recovery by 2 weeks,

    - did not change the final extent of visual recovery,

    - is helpful for the management of periocular pain,

    - delayed neurologic symptoms and signs of MS for 2 years. The beneficial effect wore off after 2 years.

Natural History

- Initially, the visual loss may worsen over several days to 2 weeks.

- Improvement initially is rapid and starts approximately 3 weeks after onset.

- Recovery of vision is nearly complete by 5 weeks after onset.

- Improvement may continue up to 1 year.

- Despite the excellent prognosis of optic neuritis, patients usually remain aware of visual deficits in the affected eye after recovery.

- The ONTT showed that optic neuritis recurred in the affected or fellow eye in 35% of cases within 10 years. Most eyes with a recurrence regained normal or almost-normal vision.

The present recommendations for the investigation and treatment of patients with optic neuritis are based on the results of two early multicentered studies: the ONTT and Controlled High-Risk Avonex Multiple Sclerosis Prevention Study (CHAMPS). Both studies investigated the risk of developing clinically definite multiple sclerosis (CDMS) in patients with optic neuritis alone (ONTT) or with their first demyelinating episode that could be optic neuritis (CHAMPS). The details of the ONTT are listed in **Table 5-2**.

TABLE 5-2. Optic Neuritis Treatment Trial

Multicentered control clinical trial
> 389 patients with isolated acute unilateral optic neuritis between 18 and 46 y

Inclusion criteria:
> Clinical syndrome consistent with unilateral optic neuritis (including RAPD, visual field defect in affected eye)
> Visual symptoms of 8 d or less
> No previous episode of optic neuritis in the affected eye
> No previous corticosteroid treatment for optic neuritis or multiple sclerosis (MS)
> No evidence of systemic disease other than MS as a cause of optic neuritis

Randomized to three treatment groups
> Oral prednisone 1 mg/kg/day for 14 d, plus 3 d oral taper
> Intravenous methylprednisolone 250 mg QID for 3 d followed by 1 mg/kg/day for 11 d orally, plus a short taper
> Oral placebo for 14 d

TABLE 5-3. Optic Neuritis Treatment Trial Baseline Data

Gender: 77% female

Race: 85% Caucasian

Age: Mean 32 ± 7 y

Symptoms
  Photopsias, 30%
  Orbital pain, 92%
  Pain worsened with eye movement, 87%

Signs
  Baseline visual acuity
    20/20, 11%
    20/50–20/40, 25%
    20/50–20/190, 29%
    20/200–20/800, 20%
    Finger counting, 4%
    Hand motion, 6%
    Light perception, 3%
    No light perception, 3%

Color vision
  Ishihara color plates abnormal, 88%
  Farnsworth–Munsell 100 Hue abnormal, 94%

Visual field
  Focal defects (altitudinal, arcuate, nasal step, central, or paracentral defects), 52%
  Diffuse defects, 48%

Contrast sensitivity: Abnormal, 98%

Ophthalmoscopic appearance
  Optic disc swelling, 35%
  Optic disc or peripapillary hemorrhages, 6%

Abnormal fellow eye
  Visual activity, 13.8%
  Contrast sensitivity, 15.4%
  Color vision, 21.7%
  Visual field, 48%

TABLE 5-4. Visual Recovery

No significant difference between three arms of treatment groups at 1 y in mean visual acuity (VA), color vision, contrast sensitivity, or visual field
Patients treated with IV methylprednisolone recovered VA significantly faster than other two treatment arms; this effect was greatest in the first 15 d
Most of visual recovery occurs within first 6 wk although continues up to 1 y

Patients treated with oral prednisolone had an increased rate of recurrent attacks of optic neuritis in the previously affected eye and in the fellow eye

Median VA in all three treatment groups was 20/16

Less than 10% have VA 20/50 or worse

Of patients with baseline VA of worse than 20/200, 6% had this level of vision at 6 mo

Of patient with initial VA of light perception or no light perception, 64% had a final VA of 20/40 or better
After 15 y, 72% have visual acuity of 20/20 in affected eye
At 15 y, visual function is more likely to be abnormal if patient has multiple sclerosis

The visual defects and their response to the treatment protocols are given in **Tables 5-3** and **5-4**, respectively. The ONTT also calculated the risk of developing CDMS in patients with optic neuritis. The risk and the effect of treatment on these risks are shown in **Table 5-5** and **Figure 5-4**, respectively. **Table 5-6** shows the risk at the yearly follow-up periods.

The only accurate predictor of increased risk to develop CDMS was the presence of lesions on the initial MRI scan (**Fig. 5-5**). The CHAMPS (**Table 5-7**) extended the ONTT by including other neurologic events (50% of the patients had optic neuritis) and investigated the efficacy of interferon beta-1a versus placebo both on the development of CDMS and on the development or evolution of MRI lesions (**Fig. 5-6**). The results and conclusions of CHAMPS are also presented in Table 5-7. Subsequent studies have shown that other disease-modifying agents may be used in place of interferon beta-1a.

Progression to MS

The cumulative probability of developing MS by 15 years after optic neuritis was 50% and

TABLE 5-5. Cumulative Risk of Development of Multiple Sclerosis

Based on initial MRI results (at 15 y)

The overall risk of multiple sclerosis (MS) at 15 y is approximately 50%

If the MRI is normal with no T2 white matter lesions, the risk of MS after 15 y is 25%

If the MRI shows one (or more) T2-weighted white matter lesions larger than 3 mm in diameter, the risk is 56% at 5 y and 72% at 15 y

Patients in the group treated with IV methylprednisolone had a reduced rate of development of MS during the first 2 y *only* in patients who had abnormal brain imaging at time of diagnosis

strongly related to the presence of lesions on a baseline brain MRI. If a patient has a normal MRI at presentation, the risk of developing MS was 25% compared to 72% of risk in patients with one or more lesions. However, patients with normal MRI results and no conversion to MS by year 10 had only a 2% risk of conversion by year 15 (Fig. 5-5B).

After 10 years, the risk of developing MS was very low for patients without baseline lesions but remained substantial for those with lesions. Among patients without lesions on MRI, baseline factors associated with a substantially lower risk for MS included male sex, optic disc swelling, and certain atypical features of optic neuritis.

Atypical Optic Neuritis

Atypical features of optic neuritis include lack of pain, persistent pain or failure of visual recovery by 1 month, significant swelling of the optic disc with peripapillary hemorrhages or exudates, inflammatory ocular features (e.g., uveitis, phlebitis, choroiditis, pars), bilateral vision loss, involvement of other cranial nerves (CNs), and steroid-responsive optic neuropathy. Such patients require more extensive investigations based on the findings of the clinical history examination.

TABLE 5-6. Cumulative Probability of Clinically Definite Multiple Sclerosis by Treatment Group

	Treatment Group		
Time Period	Intravenous N = 133 (%)	Placebo N = 126 (%)	Oral Prednisone N = 129 (%)
6 mo	3.1	6.7	7.1
1 y	6.4	12.6	10.4
2 y	8.0	17.6	17.0
3 y	18.5	21.0	24.5
4 y	24.6	26.3	27.8
5 y	26.4	31.1	32.1

TABLE 5-7. The Controlled High-Risk Subjects AVONEX Multiple Sclerosis Prevention Study (CHAMPS)

Design

Multicentered randomized double-blind controlled clinical trial

Eligibility criteria
 18–50 y
 First isolated, well-defined neurologic event consistent with demyelination involving the optic nerve (optic neuritis), spinal cord (incomplete transverse myelitis), or brain stem or cerebellum
 MRI abnormality: Two or more silent lesions of the brain at least 3 mm in diameter characteristic of MS
 Onset of symptoms 14 d or less before intravenous corticosteroid therapy and no more than 27 d before randomization

Treatment groups
 Interferon beta-1a 30 μg weekly by intramuscular injection following intravenous methylprednisolone 1 g/day for 3 d with an 11-d subsequent oral prednisone 1 mg/kg
 Placebo intramuscular injection weekly following intravenous methylprednisolone 1 g/day for 3 d with an 11-d subsequent oral prednisone 1 mg/kg

Results

Cumulative probability of development of CDMS during the 3-y follow-up period was significantly lower in the interferon beta-1a group (adjusted rate ratio, 0.49; 95% CI, 0.33–0.73)

MRI changes at 18 mo: The median increase in lesion volume was 1% in the interferon beta-1a group compared to 16% in the placebo group

Side effects of treatment
 Influenza-like syndrome: 54% of interferon beta-1a group vs. 26% of placebo group
 Depression: 20% of interferon beta-1a group vs. 13% of placebo group

Conclusions

Weekly intramuscular interferon beta-1a initiated at the time of a first clinical demyelinating event may be beneficial in patients who have MRI evidence of prior subclinical demyelination, reducing the risk of CDMS by approximately half

Interferon beta-1a is well tolerated, with no serious treatment-related adverse effects

CDMS, clinically definite multiple sclerosis.

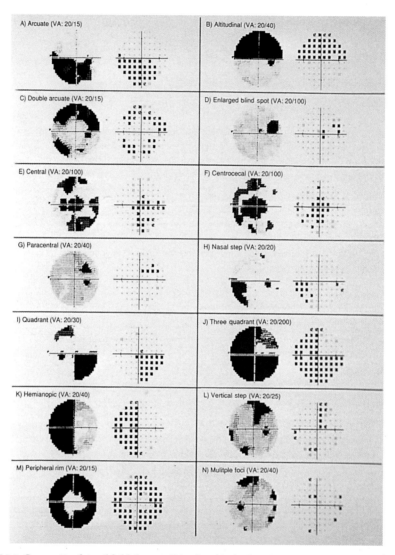

FIGURE 5-1. Composite of visual field abnormalities found in the Optic Neuritis Treatment Trial. (Keltner JL, Johnson CA, Spurr JO, Beck RW. Baseline visual field profile of optic neuritis: the experience of the Optic Neuritis Treatment Trial. *Arch Ophthalmol.* 1993;111:233, with permission).

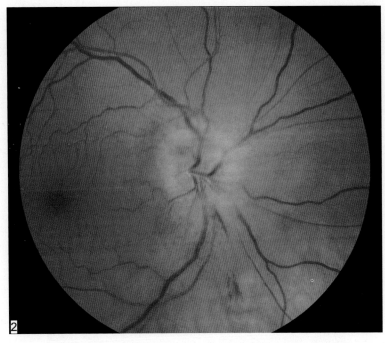

FIGURE 5-2. Optic disc swelling. The right optic disc is elevated and hyperemic with opacification of the retinal nerve fiber layer.

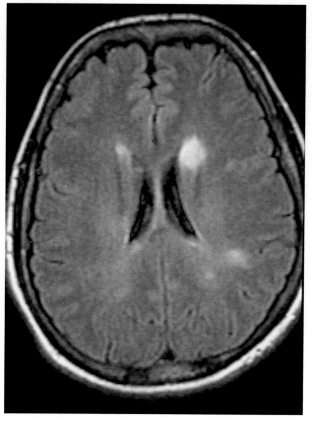

FIGURE 5-3. **A–D. Multiple sclerosis.** Axial MRI shows enhancing periventricular plaques characteristic of multiple sclerosis.

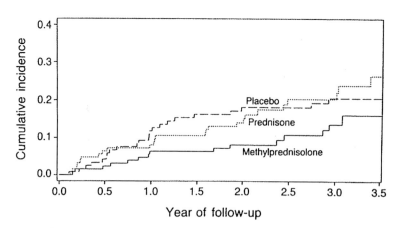

FIGURE 5-4. **Incidence of development of clinically definite multiple sclerosis** per treatment group in the initial phase of the Optic Neuritis Treatment Trial. (Beck RW, Cleary PA, Anderson MM Jr, et al; for the Optic Neuritis Study Group. A randomized controlled trial of corticosteroids in the treatment of acute optic neuritis. *N Engl J Med.* 1992;326:581–588, with permission).

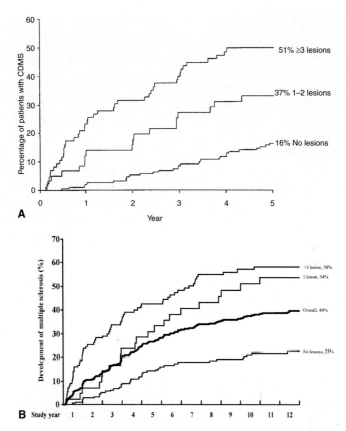

FIGURE 5-5. **A. Percentage of patients developing clinically definite multiple sclerosis** is directly related to the number of lesions on MRI. (Optic Neuritis Study Group. The 5-year risk of MS after optic neuritis: experience of the Optic Neuritis Treatment Trial. Optic Neuritis Study Group. *Neurology.* 1997;49:1404–1413, with permission). **B.** At 13 years.

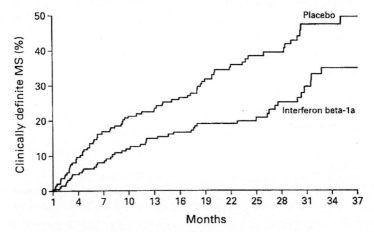

FIGURE 5-6. **Percentage of patients developing clinically definite multiple sclerosis** over 37 months was less in the treated group. (Jacobs LD, Beck RW, Simon JH, et al, and the CHAMPS Study Group. Intramuscular interferon beta-1a therapy initiated during a first demyelinating event in multiple sclerosis. *N Engl J Med.* 2000;343:898–904, with permission).

NEUROMYELITIS OPTICA

Some patients who present with acute optic neuritis may have neuromyelitis optica (NMO) or Devic disease. This is a rare, idiopathic, autoimmune, severe inflammatory disorder that results in astrocyte loss and demyelination in the optic nerves and spinal cord. NMO may assume a relapsing course, which may lead to a mistaken diagnosis of MS.

Epidemiology and Etiology

● It is thought that specific autoantibodies (NMO-IgGs) target aquaporin-4 (AQP4), a water channel on astrocytes within the central nervous system (CNS).

● Although the exact series of pathologic events is not known, the autoantibody undermines the integrity of the myelin surrounding the optic nerves and the spinal cord, leading in most cases to significant visual impairment and neurologic compromise.

● NMO has a predilection for women and Asian individuals.

Clinical Characteristics

● The clinical course of NMO is variable.

● Core clinical features of NMO include unilateral or bilateral optic neuritis, transverse myelitis, or both. The myelopathy may precede the neuropathy or follow the visual loss.

● The visual impairment from optic neuritis in NMO is more often bilateral, although at times sequential, than MS on presentation.

● Neuro-ophthalmic features include
  ▪ pain on eye movement
  ▪ central loss of vision
  ▪ profound visual field defects
  ▪ dyschromatopsia
  ▪ retinal nerve fiber layer thinning on optical coherence tomography

● Other neurologic features include
  ▪ decreased coordination
  ▪ paraplegia or quadriplegia
  ▪ sensory impairment
  ▪ bladder and bowel impairment
  ▪ fatal respiratory failure

Natural History

● The prognosis of NMO is generally poor. The cycle of remission and relapse in NMO tends generally to be more frequent and severe. Visual loss is profound and often permanent with associated paraplegia.

● Treatment consists of high-dose intravenous steroids with a slow taper. Recent evidence suggests long-term immunosuppressive therapy or monoclonal antibody treatment is beneficial. Plasmapheresis may be used acutely in severe cases or with paraplegia.

Diagnostic Evaluation

● If acute optic neuritis is associated with any of the following, testing for AQP4-IgG should be considered (**Table 5-8**):
  ▪ Bilateral visual loss
  ▪ Profound visual loss
  ▪ Painless visual loss
  ▪ Irreversible visual loss (lack of vision improvement by 1 month)
  ▪ Recurrent optic neuritis
  ▪ Extensive enhancement of the optic nerve on MRI
  ▪ History of systemic autoimmune disease
  ▪ Asian descent
  ▪ Presence of hiccoughs

● Neuroimaging: The diagnosis of NMO is usually made with an abnormal cervical spine MRI (long T2-weighted hypersignal over more than three segments) and a brain

MRI that is typically normal. The brain MRI may show T2-weighted hypersignals that are atypical for MS, for example, not involving the periventricular white matter (Fig. 5-7).

● Serologic tests: Patients usually have a positive NMO immunoglobulin (AQP4 antibody) on serologic testing. The AQP4-IgG test alone has 76% sensitivity and 94% specificity.

Variability in the clinical profile of NMO has led to the concept of **NMO spectrum disease (NMOSD)**. An international classification for the diagnosis of NMOSD is:

● With AQP4-IgG

  ▪ At least one core clinical characteristic

  ▪ Positive test for AQP4-IgG

  ▪ Exclusion of alternative diagnoses

● Without AQP4-IgG or with unknown AQP4 IgG status

  ▪ At least two core clinical characteristics meeting all of the following:

    ▶ One clinical characteristic must be optic neuritis or acute myelitis

    ▶ Dissemination in space (two or more different core clinical characteristics)

    ▶ Fulfillment of additional MRI requirements

    ▶ Exclusion of alternative diagnoses

● CSF: CSF usually demonstrates a neutrophil-predominant white blood cell (WBC) count that exceeds 50 cells/month and elevated protein. Furthermore, the CSF is free of oligoclonal bands in approximately 75% of the patients.

● Serologic tests: Seropositivity for NMO-immunoglobulin G (IgG) autoantibodies is highly specific for NMO.

Treatment

● Acute attack: Treatment is with high-dose intravenous methylprednisolone (i.e., 1 g/day for 3–5 days). Some patients require additional plasmapheresis or intravenous immunoglobulin treatment if there is no response to intravenous methylprednisolone. Other immunosuppressive agents (azathioprine or rituximab) are introduced following the acute treatment. Refractory or aggressive disease can be treated with plasmapheresis.

● Relapse prevention: Immunomodulation with long-term prednisone, azathioprine, or rituximab has been shown to be helpful.

TABLE 5-8. Diagnostic Criteria for Neuromyelitis Optica Spectrum Disorder

Criteria	Finding
Clinical	Acute optic neuritis, myelitis, Area postrema syndrome (episode of otherwise unexplained hiccups or nausea and vomiting), acute brain stem syndrome, symptomatic narcolepsy or acute diencephalic clinical syndrome with NMOSD-typical diencephalic MRI lesions
Imaging	Normal appearing brain MRI
	Optic nerve MRI with T2-hyperintense lesion or T1-weighted gadolinium-enhancing lesion extending over 1/2 optic nerve length or involving optic chiasm
	Area postrema syndrome: requires associated dorsal medulla/Area postrema lesions
	Acute brain stem syndrome: requires associated periependymal brain stem lesions
	Spinal MRI demonstrates cord enlargement and cavitation involving at least three contiguous vertebral segments
CSF	Decreased serum/CSF albumin ratio with normal IgG synthesis rate and general absence of oligoclonal bands
Serologic	Seropositivity for AQP4-IgG autoantibodies

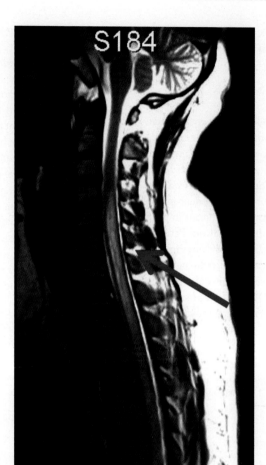

FIGURE 5-7. Neuromyelitis optica. Sagittal T2-weighted MRI demonstrating involvement of more than three contiguous vertebral segments of the spinal cord (*arrow*) in a patient with neuromyelitis optica.

ANTI–MYELIN OLIGODENDROCYTE GLYCOPROTEIN (ANTI-MOG) SYNDROME

Anti–myelin oligodendrocyte glycoprotein (anti-MOG), a protein exclusively expressed on the surface of oligodendrocytes and myelin in the central nervous system, antibody (anti-MOG antibody) positive optic neuritis has been established as a new subset of optic neuropathy. Anti-MOG antibodies are important in both pediatric and adult demyelination. Patients with MOG antibody–associated demyelination appear to have a unique clinical, radiologic, and therapeutic profile. Recent studies indicate a high prevalence of anti-MOG antibody positivity in patients with chronic relapsing inflammatory optic neuropathy.

Epidemiology and Etiology

There is an equal preponderance of males and females, whereas NMO has a significantly higher female preponderance. The recent finding of MOG antibodies in patients with the clinical syndrome of NMO or NMO spectrum disease (NMOSD) has led to some controversy regarding the nomenclature and classifications of these patients. Using the revised diagnostic criteria for NMO, it is possible for a patient to be diagnosed with "definite NMO" without being AQP4 antibody positive. As a consequence, both MOG and AQP4 antibody–positive patients who present with optic neuritis and/or transverse myelitis are classified under the umbrella terminology of "NMO/NMOSD" as a syndrome. However, AQP4 antibody–associated disease is an astrocytopathy with a distinct histologic and immunopathologic profile, whereas MOG antibody–associated disease targets oligodendrocytes.

Anti-MOG antibodies have also been associated with pediatric inflammatory demyelinating diseases, including acute disseminated encephalomyelitis.

Clinical Characteristics

Clinical Features	Anti-MOG Antibody Positive	Aquaporin-4 Antibody Positive
Optic neuritis	More commonly bilateral	Unilateral
Optic nerve head	More common anterior optic neuritis with optic nerve swelling	Retrobulbar or anterior
Eye pain	50%	Less common
Response to pulse steroid treatment	Excellent	Poor—often resistant to steroid
Optic nerve MRI	Intraorbital T2 hyperintensity with long segments but not involving chiasm. Perineural enhancement	Intracanalicular, chiasm and optic tract more likely involved. Long T2 hyperintense lesions
Brain MRI	Normal fluffy brain lesions like ADEM	
Relapse rate of optic neuritis	High—especially if rapid taper of steroids	Observed but not as frequent as anti-MOG positive, although variable
CNS symptoms	Less common	Transverse myelitis more common
Relapse rate of CNS symptoms	Low	Higher

ADEM, acute disseminated encephalomyelitis.

The most frequently observed manifestation is optic neuritis, in particular bilateral optic neuritis. Some studies have reported higher rates of eye pain compared to idiopathic optic neuritis or NMO. Anti-MOG positive patients have lower rates of myelitis and CNS recurrence compared to NMO patients.

Natural History

Patients with anti-MOG antibody positive optic neuritis tend to respond rapidly and dramatically to intravenous steroid treatment but often have residual visual field defects. They have a high risk of recurrence, especially if steroid treatment is tapered rapidly. Often these patients are diagnosed as demyelinating optic neuritis and the diagnosis of anti-MOG antibody syndrome is considered only when the steroids are tapered as per the ONTT protocol and a rapid relapse occurs. Although it is known that in anti-MOG antibody positive patients there are frequent relapses of optic neuritis, there is so far no report indicating that myelitis itself has a tendency to relapse.

Diagnostic Evaluation

- Live cell-based assays using full-length human MOG as the antigen have been shown to be the gold standard for the detection of biologically relevant MOG antibodies in human demyelination.

- Orbital MRI: extensive T2 hyperintensity and T1 gadolinium enhancement that predominates in the anterior parts of the nerve

- Brain MRI is generally normal or will show nonspecific T2 hyperintensities

- OCT: The average RNFL thickness was greater in the anti-MOG positive ocular neuritis eyes compared with the anti-AQP4-positive ocular neuritis eyes

Treatment

Treatment guidelines for anti-MOG antibody positive optic neuritis have not yet been established. MOG antibody–positive patients have a rapid response to steroids and plasma exchange. Following treatment and clinical resolution, there is a tendency to relapse rapidly on steroid withdrawal or cessation. This necessitates the consideration of a longer course of oral steroid therapy as well as maintenance immunosuppression with mycophenolate or azathioprine for some patients.

Some therapeutic agents used for the management of MS including interferon, natalizumab, and fingolimod have been shown to have a detrimental effect when used in AQP4 antibody–associated disease; their effect in MOG antibody–associated demyelination is as yet unknown.

LEBER STELLATE NEURORETINITIS

Leber stellate neuroretinitis is characterized by loss of vision associated with concomitant swelling of the optic nerve and hard exudates arranged in a star configuration at the macula (Fig. 5-8). The macular star can appear at initial presentation or several days later. Although this is primarily a retinal disorder, it is included in this section because it is frequently confused with optic neuritis.

Epidemiology and Etiology

- Neuroretinitis is considered an infectious or immune-mediated process. Up to 50% of patients have an antecedent viral illness, usually affecting the respiratory tract, a few weeks before the onset of visual symptoms.

- Neuroretinitis usually affects children and young adults, although it may occur in persons of all ages.

- The vast majority of patients with neuroretinitis have no cause identified or it is associated with cat scratch disease (*Bartonella henselae*). Other various infections have been implicated and include syphilis, Lyme disease, and toxoplasmosis.

- Many causes of optic disc swelling, for example, papilledema and hypertensive optic neuropathy, may have retinal exudates in a stellate formation; however, the star formation is usually incomplete (Fig. 5-9; see Fig. 5-23). Therefore, the presence of disc edema and a macula star is not pathognomonic for neuroretinitis.

Clinical Characteristics

Symptoms

- Painless loss of vision

Signs

- Visual acuity: Ranges from 20/20 to light perception
- RAPD if unilateral or asymmetric
- Decreased color vision
- Typical fundus picture:
  - Optic disc swelling: Mild to severe
  - Macular star and exudates deposited within Henle layer, giving a typical star or hemistar appearance to the macula. This usually appears after the appearance of optic disc swelling.

- Fluorescein angiography shows leakage of dye from vessels on the disc, whereas macular vasculature is usually entirely normal. This investigation is not necessary for the diagnosis.

Natural History

- Neuroretinitis is usually a self-limiting condition, with the optic disc swelling resolving in 6 to 8 weeks. The macular star can take several months and even up to 1 year to resolve. The majority of patients regain good vision.

- If visual symptoms persist, the patient usually complains of metamorphopsia or blurred central vision.

Diagnostic Evaluation

- History of being scratched by a kitten, which maximally exposes the patient to cat scratch fever. In this circumstance, titers for *B. henselae* should be drawn.

- A swollen optic nerve and exudates, and a star or hemistar figure in the macula may be seen in other conditions, for example, hypertensive optic neuropathy or papilledema (see p. 108; Fig. 5-9). In these conditions, the macula star often is located only nasal to the macula, suggesting it spills over from optic nerve head swelling. Therefore, the patient's blood pressure should be obtained.

- It should be noted that this fundus picture is not recognized as the equivalent of optic neuritis. It does not increase the risk of developing MS.

Treatment

- Treatment depends on etiology.

- Antibiotic therapy may be administered for cat scratch fever.

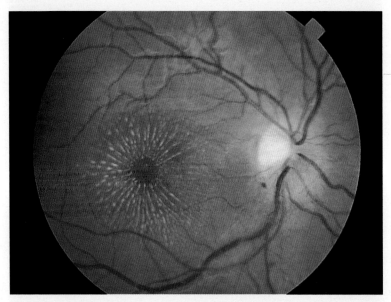

FIGURE 5-8. **Leber stellate neuroretinitis.** The optic disc is swollen with nerve fiber layer edema and a hemorrhage at the 7 o'clock position off the disc. The exudates in the macula form a star.

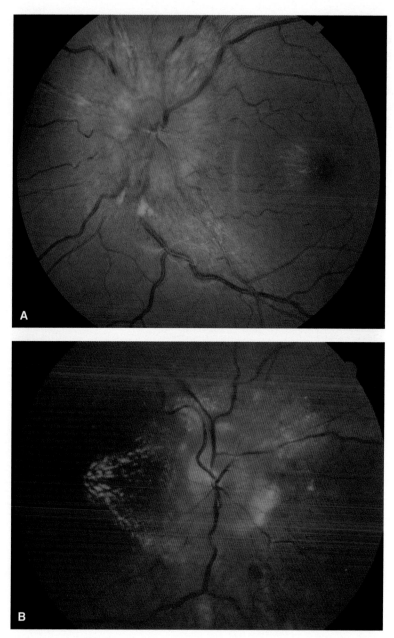

FIGURE 5-9. **Optic disc swelling. A.** Patient with pseudotumor cerebri because of minocycline ingestion with a swollen disc and a hemimacular star.

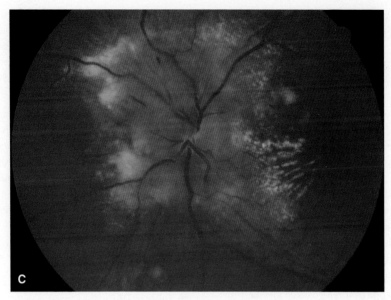

FIGURE 5-9. (*continued*) **B** and **C**. Patient with hypertensive optic neuropathy with hemimacular star.

SARCOID OPTIC NEUROPATHY

Sarcoidosis is a multisystem granulomatous inflammation with ocular, neurologic, and neuro-ophthalmic manifestations. Optic neuropathy may develop at any time during the course of systemic sarcoidosis or it can be the initial manifestation of the disease.

Etiology

● Sarcoidosis is a granulomatous inflammatory process that is identified pathologically by a noncaseating granuloma. Epithelioid and giant cells are characteristic findings on histopathologic studies.

● The optic neuropathy of sarcoidosis is produced by one of three possible mechanisms:

▪ Compression produced by a granuloma (Fig. 5-10) or by pachymeningitis (Fig. 5-11)

▪ Infiltration by inflammatory cells. Sarcoid granulomas may be seen in the optic disc (Fig. 5-12).

▪ Ischemia because of obliterating arteritis

Clinical Characteristics

Symptoms

● Unilateral or bilateral decreased vision that is usually slowly progressive but may progress rapidly

● Decreased color perception

Signs

● Decreased visual acuity

● An RAPD if unilateral or asymmetric

● Acquired dyschromatopsia

● Central scotoma or other variations of nerve fiber bundle defects are plotted on perimetric evaluation.

● Signs of anterior granulomatous uveitis with flare, cells, or mutton fat keratic precipitates present

● Optic disc may be normal if the process is retrobulbar, swollen and hyperemic if the optic disc is inflamed, or show the presence of a sarcoid granuloma. Optic atrophy is often the end result of these optic neuropathies.

● A vitreous inflammatory reaction can be seen at times. Lesions at the level of the retinal pigment epithelium (RPE) produce white areas in the fundus (Fig. 5-13). The retinal changes described in the past as venous sheathing (candle wax drippings) are actually retinal or choroidal lesions that at times coalesce (Fig. 5-14).

● Nonoptic nerve manifestations of sarcoidosis are listed in Table 5-9.

● Other ocular signs of sarcoidosis are listed in Table 5-10.

Diagnostic Evaluation

● MRI will show enhancement of the optic nerve or the portion of the anterior visual pathway that is involved (Fig. 5-15). The meninges may be thickened and show abnormal enhancement.

● Serum ACE levels may be abnormally high.

● Chest X-ray or imaging will often show hilar adenopathy or pulmonary nodules or infiltrates.

● Pulmonary function studies often are abnormal.

● Gallium scan documents involvement of the lung and lacrimal glands in many patients.

● Definitive diagnosis is established by biopsy. Tissue is usually obtained from the enlarged hilar lymph nodes via bronchoscopy or from the lacrimal glands if they appear involved by the process (Fig. 5-16). Blind conjunctival biopsy has a very low yield, whereas biopsy of a conjunctival lesion (granuloma) visible on the slit lamp examination has a much higher yield.

Treatment

- Corticosteroids are the mainstay of treatment in this disorder. They should be given systemically for the optic neuropathy.

- If uveitis coexists, it should be treated with a topical or periocular corticosteroid.

- If corticosteroids fail to halt or reverse the process, agents such as methotrexate should be tried.

- Recently, there is increasing evidence that rituximab, an anti-CD20 antibody, is beneficial.

TABLE 5-9. Other Neuro-ophthalmic Manifestations of Sarcoidosis

Afferent visual pathway

    Chiasmal involvement

    Bitemporal hemianopia, junctional scotoma, and bilateral optic nerve involvement

    Postchiasmal visual pathway: The pattern of the visual field defects depends on the area of the visual pathway that is involved; mechanism of damage can include compression, infiltration, or vascular occlusion related to angiitis

Efferent visual pathway

    Abducens nerve palsy most common; may be unilateral or bilateral

    Supranuclear gaze palsy and ocular flutter have been described

Pupils (uncommon)

    Tonic pupil

Orbital involvement

    Orbital mass (granuloma)

    Infiltration of extraocular muscles

    Diffuse infiltration of orbit

TABLE 5-10. Other Ocular Features of Sarcoidosis

Lids and anterior segment

    Lupus pernio: Eyelids involved with purple sarcoid indurating rash

    Lacrimal gland infiltration and enlargement

    Band keratopathy

    Conjunctival follicles

    Episcleritis and scleritis with nodules

Uvea

    Anterior uveitis: Usually granulomatous with mutton fat keratic precipitates (a frequent finding)

    Pars planitis

    Vitritis

Posterior segment

    Choroiditis with yellow or white nodules

    Retinal neovascularization

    Choroidal granulomas

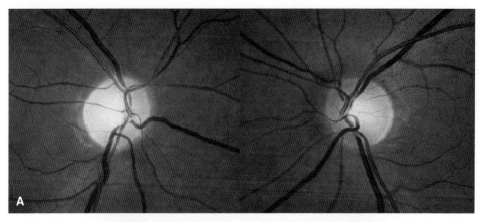

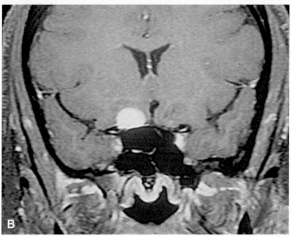

FIGURE 5-10. **Sarcoidosis. A.** Right optic nerve is pale with marked loss of the retinal nerve fiber layer. The left optic disc is normal. **B.** MRI shows enhancing mass (sarcoid granuloma) in the area of the planum sphenoidale compressing the right optic nerve.

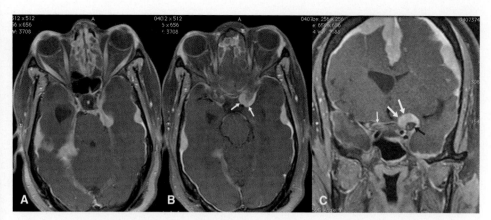

FIGURE 5-11. Neurosarcoidosis with pachymeningitis in a 42-year-old African American woman with previous right visual loss to no light perception (NLP) from neurosarcoidosis who presented with progressive left visual loss over 2 weeks. **A.** On T1-weighted MRI with gadolinium and fat suppression, an enhancing lesion (**B** and **C,** *wide white arrows*) is compressing and infiltrating the left optic nerve at the optic canal, consistent with a sarcoidal mass. The contralateral intracanalicular optic nerve was atrophic but not involved in the inflammatory process, although its meningeal sheath enhanced mildly (**C,** *thin white arrow*). The anterior clinoid process is identified by the *black arrow*. Diffuse, bulky pachymeningeal sarcoidal lesions were also present in all regions of the brain. The patient's vision improved on pulse intravenous corticosteroids and she was referred to a rheumatologist for maintenance antimetabolite therapy. (Courtesy of Jurij Bilyk, MD.)

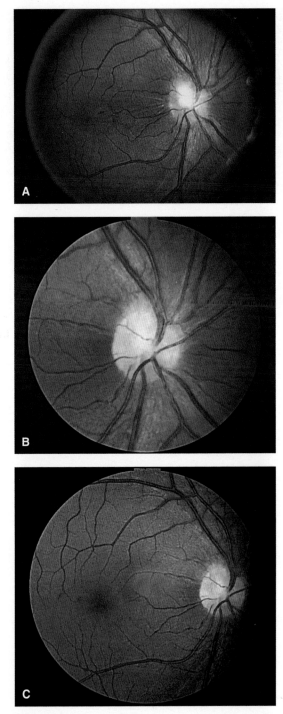

FIGURE 5-12. **Sarcoidosis.** Right optic disc of patient with biopsy-proven sarcoidosis showing a granuloma of the optic disc (**A**) that disappeared after 2 years of treatment with systemic corticosteroids (**B** and **C**).

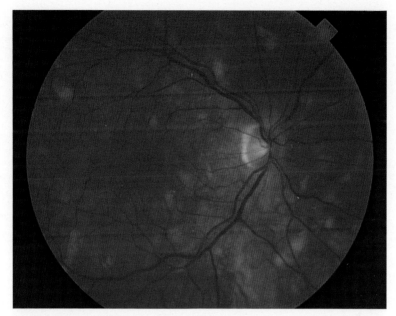

FIGURE 5-13. **Sarcoidosis.** White lesions in the posterior pole at the level of the retinal pigment epithelium (Courtesy of Tamara Vrabek, MD.)

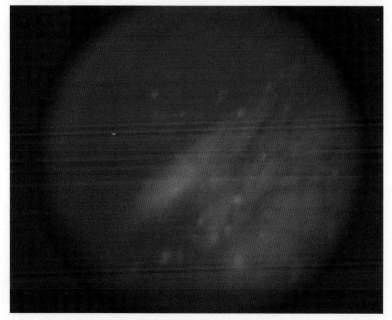

FIGURE 5-14. **Sarcoidosis.** Retinal pigment epithelium atrophy that may coalesce to form "candle wax spots" in the fundus of patients with sarcoidosis. (Courtesy of Tamara Vrabek, MD.)

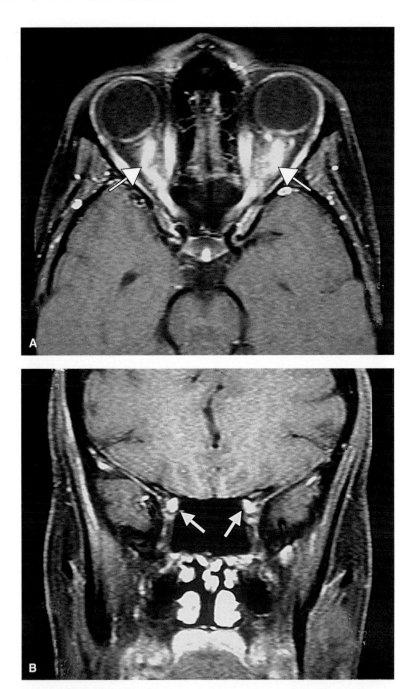

FIGURE 5-15. **Sarcoidosis.** MRI axial (**A**) and coronal (**B**) images of patient with sarcoidosis and decreased vision bilaterally showing enhancement of both optic nerves along (*arrows*) their entire course.

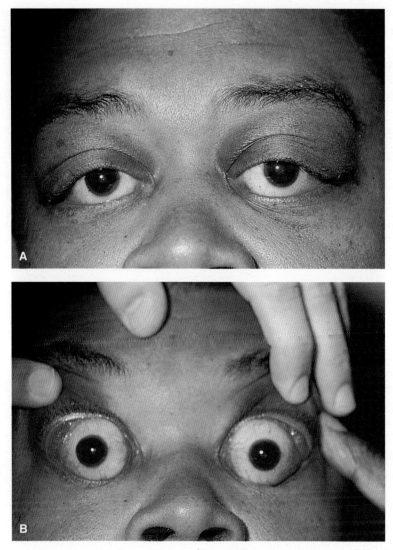

FIGURE 5-16. Sarcoidosis. A. Sarcoidosis producing fullness bilaterally in the area of the lacrimal glands. **B.** Elevation of the lids shows prolapse of the enlarged lacrimal glands.

SYPHILITIC OPTIC NEUROPATHY

Abnormalities of the optic nerve may be encountered in both secondary and tertiary syphilis. Optic neuropathy involvement in syphilis may be optic neuritis, neuroretinitis, or perineuritis. Syphilitic optic neuropathy may occur in isolation or associated with other features of intraocular inflammation.

Etiology

● Optic neuritis occurs during the secondary and tertiary stage of infection. We consider that syphilitic optic neuropathy implies neurosyphilis.

Clinical Characteristics

● The general ocular signs of syphilis are listed in **Table 5-11**.

Symptoms

● Decreased vision, which may be unilateral or bilateral

● Decreased color perception

Signs

● Central scotomas

● An RAPD if unilateral or asymmetric

● At times, a vitreous cellular reaction can exist, especially with papillitis and in HIV-positive patients.

● Neuroretinitis can occur in patients with secondary and tertiary syphilis. In secondary syphilis, it can occur as part of syphilitic meningitis and may be either a unilateral isolated phenomenon (with or without uveitis) or bilateral.

● Meningitis involves other CNs or signs of meningeal irritation.

● The syphilitic patient, in addition, may manifest the following optic nerve abnormalities:

■ Optic perineuritis (perioptic neuritis): The optic disc is swollen but visual acuity is normal and there are no other clinical signs of optic neuropathy. This is usually a manifestation of secondary syphilis.

■ Papillitis: This anterior optic neuritis may be indistinguishable from demyelinating optic neuritis (**Fig. 5-17**). It usually produces rapid visual loss. However, papillitis secondary to syphilis does not show spontaneous resolution. It may be seen in both secondary and tertiary syphilis.

■ Neuroretinitis: May be accompanied by vitritis and is encountered in both secondary and tertiary syphilis.

TABLE 5-11. Ocular Manifestations of Syphilis

Primary: Chancre on eyelid
Secondary
Uveitis
Panuveitis
Choroiditis
Choriretinitis
Optic neuritis
Retinitis and retinal vasculitis
Papilledema
Anterior segment
Episcleritis
Scleritis
Dacryoadenitis
Dacryocystitis
Interstitial keratitis
Iris papules and gumma
Tertiary
Optic neuropathy
Argyll Robertson pupil
Interstitial keratitis
Chronic uveitis
Ocular motor neuropathies, especially CN III

■ Retrobulbar optic neuritis: Appears as a typical optic neuropathy except that visual loss may be rapid and profound in secondary syphilis. In tertiary disease, it is a slowly progressive phenomenon.

■ Papilledema: May accompany the meningitis in secondary and tertiary disease. Its appearance may be confused with optic perineuritis until lumbar puncture documents increased intracranial pressure (ICP).

Diagnostic Evaluation

● The best method to prove a syphilitic infection is to demonstrate the spirochete in a tissue biopsy or CSF. This is not usually feasible, so indirect methods of testing for syphilis are routinely employed. Syphilitic optic neuropathy implies neurosyphilis and suspected cases should undergo CSF analysis.

● The serologic tests for syphilis are listed in **Table 5-12.** Specific testing recommendations appear in **Table 5-13.**

TABLE 5-12. Tests for Syphilis

Treponemal tests

Use

    High specificity and sensitivity in all stages of syphilis
    Once reactive, these tests do not revert to normal
    Used for confirming diagnosis of syphilis
    Used routinely for suspected late syphilis
    False positive can occur with other treponemal infections
    False negative can occur with HIV infection

Tests

    Immunofluorescence: FTA-ABS, fluorescent treponemal antibody absorption
    Hemagglutination
        MHA-TP: Microhemagglutination treponemal test for syphilis
        HATTS: Hemagglutination treponemal test
        TPHA: Widely used in Canada and Europe but not available in the United States

Nontreponemal (reagin) tests

Use

    Initial screening or to quantitate the serum reagin antibody titer, but there are significant false negatives in primary, latent, or late syphilis
    Reflects activity of disease: For example, a rise in titers seen between primary and secondary syphilis; persistent fall in titers following treatment provides evidence of an adequate response to therapy
    Nontreponemal tests usually become nonreactive after treatment. However, a significant number may continue to have low titers for long periods of time

Tests

    VDRL: Venereal Disease Research Laboratories test
        Advantages: Standard test used for cerebrospinal fluid; less expensive
        Disadvantage: Uses heated serum; reagent must be prepared fresh daily
    False positive with nontreponemal tests can occur with: autoimmune diseases, pregnancy, vaccination, IV drug abuse, tuberculosis and nonsyphilitic treponemal infections
    False negative can occur with HIV infection
    RPR: Rapid plasma reagin
        Advantages: Easy to perform; uses unheated serum; test of choice for rapid serologic diagnosis
        Disadvantage: More expensive than VDRL

TABLE 5-13. CSF Testing in Syphilitic Optic Neuropathy

Indications for lumbar puncture

    Seropositive patient with neurologic or neuro-ophthalmic signs and symptoms

    All patients with untreated syphilis of unknown duration

    HIV-positive patients who are also seropositive

Test to perform

    CSF VDRL

        Very specific if fluid is not contaminated with blood

        Low sensitivity: May be nonreactive in progressive symptomatic syphilis

CSF protein, cell count

Treatment

- It is strongly advised that staging and treatment of syphilis be conducted by, or in consultation with, an infectious disease specialist because there is no universally established criteria for the diagnosis of neurosyphilis. However, a general overview of the indications for and the methods of treatment are as follows.

Indications for Treatment

- Fluorescent treponemal antibody-absorption (FTA)-ABS positive and Venereal Disease Research Laboratory (VDRL) test negative
  - If active syphilitic signs and abnormal CSF
  - Concurrent HIV: These patients may have negative FTA-ABS and VDRL (diagnosis is then made on clinical grounds)
- FTA-ABS positive and VDRL positive
  - If previous VDRL titer (>1:8) did not decrease fourfold within 1 year of appropriate treatment
  - If previous titer is not available, present titer greater than 1:4, and treatment was more than several years ago

Treatment Regimen

- Neurosyphilis may be diagnosed in the presence of a positive serum FTA-ABS and either
  - CSF-VDRL positive,
  - greater than 5 WBC/mm^3 in CSF,
  - CSF protein greater than 45 mg/dL.
- Treatment consists of the following:
  - Intravenous aqueous crystalline penicillin G 2 to 4 million U, q4h, for 10 to 14 days, followed by intramuscular benzathine PCN, 2.4 million U weekly for 3 weeks.
  - If the CSF is normal, only the IM benzathine PCN, 2.4 million U weekly for 3 weeks is required.
  - There is an indication that the dosage of penicillin should be higher in HIV-positive patients.
- Follow-up: Patients with neurosyphilis need repeated lumbar punctures every 6 months until the white cell count returns to normal. If it does not decrease, retreatment may be indicated.

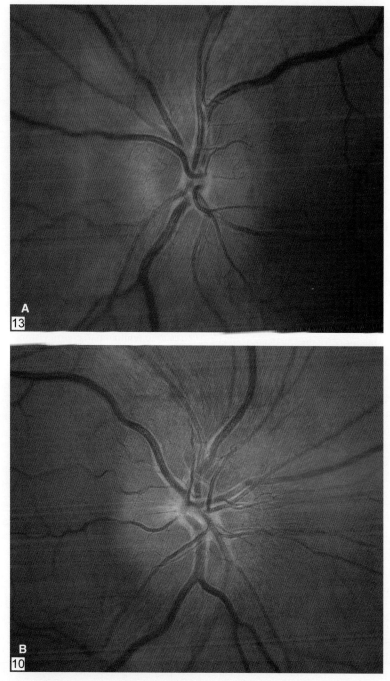

FIGURE 5-17. Syphilis. A. Patient with bilateral papillitis because of syphilis. **B.** The optic disc returned to normal after completion of intravenous penicillin therapy.

NONARTERITIC ANTERIOR ISCHEMIC OPTIC NEUROPATHY

Nonarteritic anterior ischemic optic neuropathy (NAION) is a frequently encountered disorder characterized by painless loss of vision associated with optic disc swelling. Its name indicates that it is not caused by giant cell arteritis (GCA).

Pathogenesis and Etiology

● NAION is thought to be the result of vascular insufficiency in the posterior ciliary circulation affecting the distal optic nerve, although this has not been proven.

● The incidence of NAION is between 2 and 10 per 100,000 persons over the age of 50 years. The average age of onset is between 55 and 65 (range 40 to 70) years, although it is becoming more frequently diagnosed in younger patients with known risk factors.

● Risk factors that are thought to be important include the following:

▪ Small cup-to-disc ratio and small optic discs (also referred to as congenitally anomalous discs or "discs at risk") (Fig. 5-18). This is probably the most important risk factor associated with NAION.

▪ Hypertension

▪ Diabetes mellitus

▪ Hypercholesterolemia

▪ Other vascular risk factors: Conditions associated with small vessel disease and co-agulopathies may be important, although the evidence is not conclusive.

▪ Profound blood loss (spontaneous, a result of surgery, or severe hypotension) may also produce posterior ischemic optic neuropathy (PION). Other than in these clinical situations or in GCA, the diagnosis of PION should be made with caution because the cause is often a compressive lesion (Fig. 5-19).

▪ Postcataract surgery

▪ Optic disc drusen (appears to predispose to NAION) (Fig. 5-20)

▪ The association of phosphodiesterase type 5 drugs [sildenafil (Viagra), tadalafil (Cialis)] with NAION is controversial. The World Health Organization has labeled the association "possible."

▪ Sleep apnea

Clinical Characteristics

Symptoms

● Patients present with painless loss of vision, although some may be asymptomatic. The level of visual loss can vary from 20/20 with a visual field defect to light perception.

● It would be very unusual for NAION to result in no light perception vision.

Signs

● Decreased visual acuity: In the Ischemic Optic Neuropathy Decompression Trial (IONDT), approximately one-half of the patients had initial visual acuity better than 20/64 and one-third had worse than 20/200.

● RAPD: An RAPD will be present unless there is optic nerve or significant retinal pathology in the contralateral eye.

● Dyschromatopsia: The degree of decreased color vision is usually proportional to the level of visual acuity loss, unlike optic neuritis in which the color vision is usually disproportionately affected.

● Anterior visual pathway visual field defect: The most common visual field defect is an inferior altitudinal loss, although any optic nerve defect may be seen.

● Disc edema (Fig. 5-17A): The swelling of the optic disc is either diffuse or sectoral. The swelling is usually hyperemic more than pale, with flame-shaped hemorrhages occurring commonly. The optic disc edema occurs before or concurrent with visual loss. The diagnosis of NAION may not be made in the presence of a normal optic disc.

- A congenitally anomalous optic disc ("disc at risk") in the contralateral eye

- Sequential NAION occurs, usually weeks or months apart. The clinical picture has been called the "pseudo Foster Kennedy Syndrome" because of the appearance of unilateral disc edema and contralateral optic atrophy (Fig. 5-21B).

Diagnostic Evaluation

- The diagnosis is a clinical one and may be made when patients have a swollen, hyperemic optic disc, usually with peripapillary hemorrhages and signs of optic neuropathy. Clinical features suggesting other causes of an anterior optic neuropathy (GCA, inflammatory optic neuropathies) should be excluded.

- GCA needs to be excluded as the cause of AION in all patients over the age of 55 years. This involves a thorough history and examination to identify other symptoms and signs of GCA, as well as performing appropriate investigations [erythrocyte sedimentation rate (ESR), C-reactive protein (CRP), temporal artery biopsy (TAB)].

- Other investigations that could be considered useful are aimed at identifying underlying vascular risk factors (blood pressure, fasting glucose, cholesterol level), although

there is no evidence that controlling these risk factors prevents contralateral eye involvement. Additional associations with NAION that have been made include sleep apnea and homocysteinemia.

- The edema of NAION resolves within 6 to 8 weeks. If the disc edema is present for greater than 2 months, further investigations to identify another cause for the optic neuropathy should be undertaken.

Natural History

- The visual dysfunction may be maximal at onset or it may worsen over days or even weeks in up to 35% of the patients. The IONDT investigators claim that approximately 40% of the patients will recover three or more lines of vision.

- The disc edema resolves over several weeks, with optic atrophy associated with attenuation of the arterioles at the disc margin.

- The estimated risk of developing NAION in the contralateral eye ranges from 12% to 40%. There is less than a 5% risk of having a second event in the same eye.

- Following an episode of NAION, there is no significant excavation of the optic cup, although there is thinning of the retinal nerve fiber layer (Fig. 5-22A–D).

Treatment

- No therapy has been proven to be effective in NAION. Some recommend the use of corticosteroids even though there is no strong scientific data to support this.

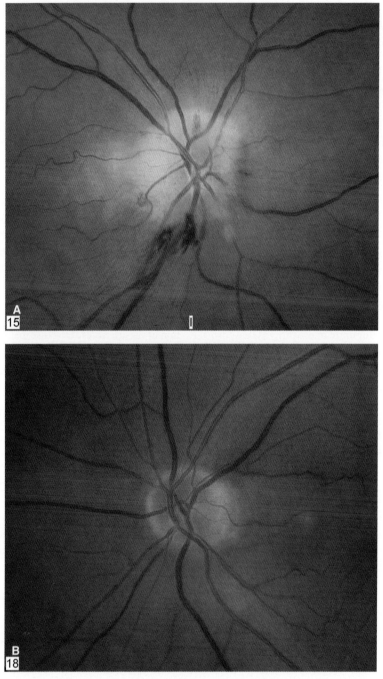

FIGURE 5-18. **Nonarteritic ischemic optic neuropathy. A.** The right optic disc is elevated with retinal nerve fiber layer edema and hemorrhage inferiorly. **B.** The left disc has a "disc at risk" appearance.

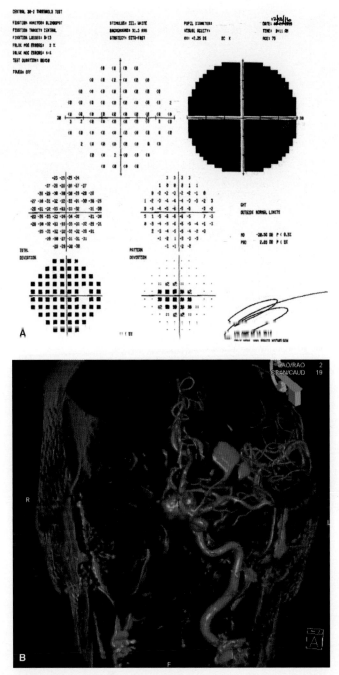

FIGURE 5-19. A 79-year-old woman had decreased vision OD following cataract surgery. The optic disc was initially normal and the diagnosis of posterior ischemic optic neuropathy was made. **A.** Perimetry shows profound central defect OD and a normal field OS. **B.** MR angiography and **C.** Arteriography demonstrates an aneurysm compressing the right optic nerve.

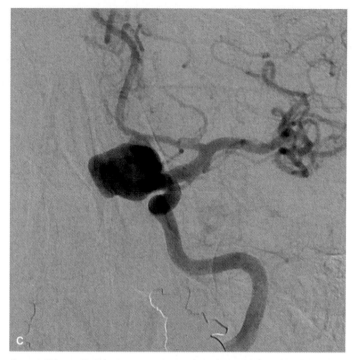

FIGURE 5-19. (*continued*)

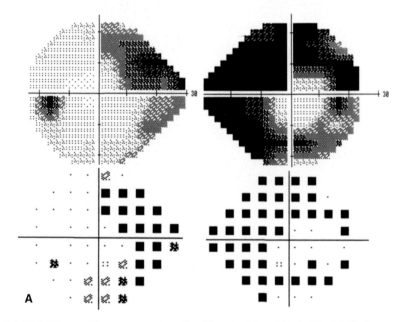

FIGURE 5-20. **A 35-year-old woman experienced sudden visual loss OD. A.** Visual fields show marked loss OD and nasal steps OS.

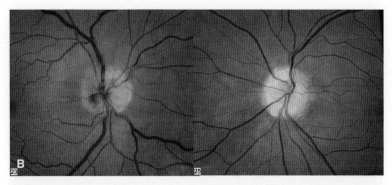

FIGURE 5-20. (*continued*) **B.** The right optic disc shows acute hemorrhagic infarction. Both discs have buried drusen.

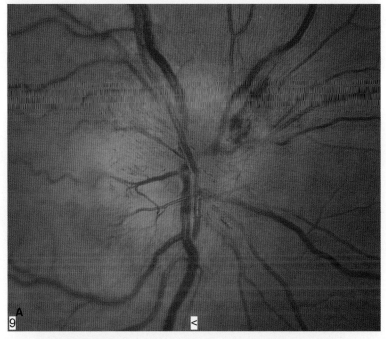

FIGURE 5-21. **Pseudo Foster Kennedy syndrome** with unilateral acute NAION and contralateral optic atrophy following a previous episode of nonarteritic anterior ischemic optic neuropathy.

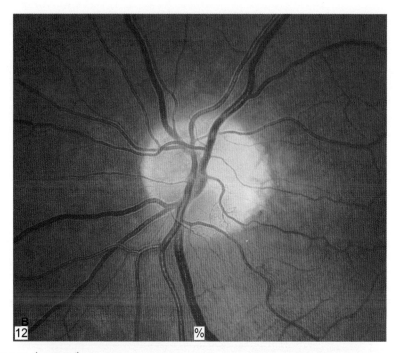

FIGURE 5-21. (*continued*)

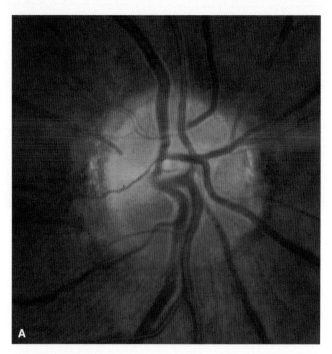

FIGURE 5-22. **Nonarteritic ischemic optic neuropathy. A.** Right optic nerve head 6 months following nonarteritic anterior ischemic optic neuropathy (NAION).

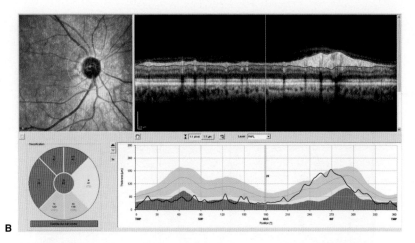

B

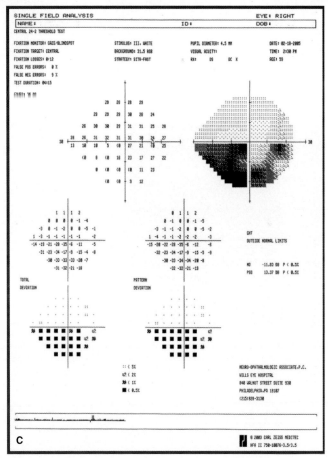

C

FIGURE 5-22. (*continued*) **B.** Spectral domain optical coherence tomography of optic nerve head and thinning of the retinal nerve fiber layer. **C.** Humphrey visual field test (SITA 24–2) of patient with NAION in right eye. (© 2003 Carl Zeiss Meditec.)

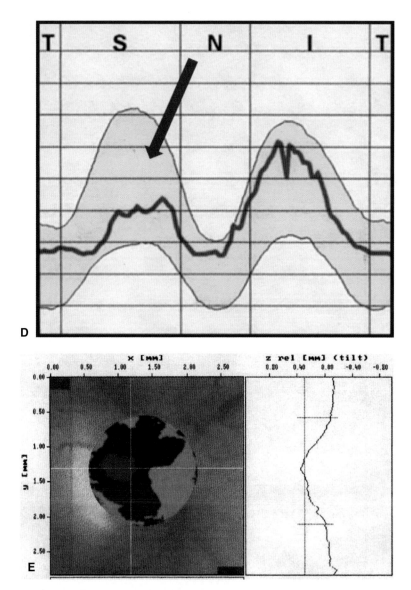

FIGURE 5-22. (*continued*) **D.** Corresponding scanning laser polarimetry demonstrating thinning of retinal nerve fiber layer superiorly (*arrow*). **E.** Heidelberg retinal tomograph of the left eye that experienced NAION 6 months earlier demonstrating there is no significant asymmetry between involved and uninvolved eye.

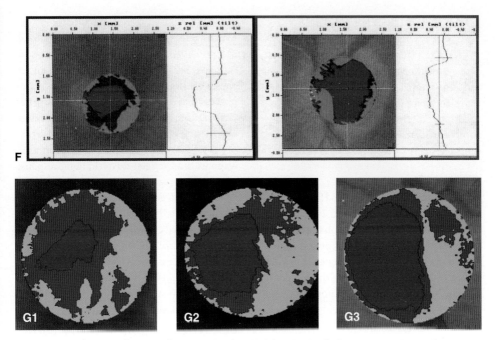

FIGURE 5-22. (*continued*) **F.** Right (uninvolved eye) and left (involved eye) after arteritic anterior ischemic optic neuropathy from giant cell arteritis demonstrating the excavation of the optic nerve head 3 months following an acute event. **G.** Series of three Heidelberg retinal tomographic images of a right optic nerve head following arteritic anterior ischemic optic neuropathy (1, 3, 4 months) demonstrating sequential enlargement of the optic cup.

GIANT CELL ARTERITIS

G iant cell (temporal, cranial) arteritis is a systemic necrotizing vasculitis of medium and large arteries that has several of the most important neuro-ophthalmologic manifestations encountered. The underlying cause remains poorly elucidated and the optimum treatment controversial.

Epidemiology

The incidence of GCA in the United States is stated to be 17.8/100,000 in men and 24.2/100,000 in woman over 50 years of age on the basis of a study performed in Olmsted County, Minnesota. However, because the incidence of GCA in non-Caucasians, including the Hispanic, African American, and Asian populations, is much less, its true national incidence may be less. Some reports also describe a seasonal variation in the occurrence of GCA, whereas other investigators have found no such fluctuation.

Age is an all-important factor. All the incidence statistics are calculated for patients over the age of 50 years. It is extraordinarily rare for GCA to occur in patients younger than 50 years, and most patients afflicted with this disorder actually are in their 60s or older.

Pathogenesis and Etiology

The exact cause of GCA is not known. There is some evidence to suggest that GCA has a genetic predisposition as there is an increased incidence in Northern Europeans and their descendents, as well as the high association of human leucocyte antigen and DRB1, a gene complex.

Although the initial trigger of this immunologic disorder is unknown, it produces an influx of CD4-type T cells via the vasa vasorum into the tunica adventitia. These T cells produce interferon γ, which causes obliteration of the vessel lumen. Macrophages also enter via the vasa vasorum and they secrete interleukin (IL)-6 and IL-1β. These macrophages in the media

of the arterial wall secrete metalloproteinases, which are enzymes that can digest arterial wall components. This causes liberation of smooth muscle cells, which migrate toward the lumen causing intimal hyperplasia. Thus, the major process that produces ischemia in GCA is not destruction of the arterial wall but luminal obstruction caused by a hyperplastic reaction of the intima. This hyperplasia of the intima in response to an antigen-driven immune response requires new capillary formation in all three layers (media, adventitia, interna) to support this new tissue. These inflamed arteries produce platelet-derived growth factors (A and B), whose expression correlates with luminal obstruction. These factors are produced by macrophages and giant cells found at the media–intima border. Stenotic lesions also have a higher concentration of vascular endothelial growth factor (VEGF).

Clinical Characteristics

GCA is a disorder that is closely related to the systemic disorder polymyalgia rheumatica (PMR). About 50% of the people who have biopsy-proven GCA will have PMR. A form of GCA termed *occult* presents with sudden visual loss without the patient having any of the systemic signs or symptoms that are normally associated with GCA and PMR. It is estimated that approximately 20% of the patients with biopsy-proven GCA may have the occult form.

Symptoms

• Visual loss: It is sudden and usually profound.

• Diplopia: This is estimated to be the presenting symptom of GCA in approximately 10% to 15% of the patients.

• Transient visual loss: This may be in one or both eyes and can last from minutes to hours.

• Headache: Usually the headache is of new onset.

• Scalp tenderness: Patients may localize this to the area over the superficial temporal artery or it may be more generalized. They will frequently complain of difficulty combing their hair, wearing their glasses, or even resting the side of their head on a pillow.

• Jaw claudication: Chewing produces pain in the masseter muscle because of ischemia. This symptom is highly suggestive of GCA.

• Constitutional symptoms: Patients have loss of appetite, weight loss, night sweats, and general malaise.

• PMR: This is characterized by pain and stiffness in the proximal muscle groups that is worse in the morning and after activity.

Signs

• A variety of ocular problems may occur with GCA, but the most distressing is visual loss, which is estimated to occur in approximately 50% of GCA patients. The causes of visual loss in GCA are as follows:

▪ Arteritic anterior ischemic optic neuropathy (AAION): AAION is an infarction within the prelaminar and laminar portion of the optic nerve because of vaso-obliterative occlusion of the short posterior ciliary arteries. AAION is the most frequent cause of visual loss in GCA patients. The AAION of GCA has a characteristic appearance. The optic disc is infarcted and has a chalky white appearance more commonly involving the whole optic nerve head rather than segmental involvement (Fig. 5-23A). Often, areas of ischemia, such as retinal whitening continuous with the optic disc ischemia (Fig. 5-23B) or isolated cotton wool infarcts in the retina (Fig. 5-23C), may accompany AAION. Retinal ischemia in the presence of AION is overwhelming circumstantial evidence that the cause of the AION is GCA. The visual loss in AAION usually is much more profound than in NAION. Vision can be severely reduced to hand motion and no light perception, levels of visual dysfunction that are infrequently encountered with

NAION. AAION also is not uncommonly bilateral. It can affect the contralateral eye, usually within days or weeks, even if treatment is administered. Thus, the diagnosis of GCA and the institution of the appropriate treatment become critical before the second eye becomes involved. Following resolution of the optic disc edema, the optic disc appearance is different in AAION than in NAION. Although the latter presents with sectoral or total pallor, the AAION disc typically shows excavation of the optic cup (Fig. 5.22E).

▪ Retinal artery occlusion: Central retinal artery occlusion (CRAO) (more rarely, branch retinal artery occlusion) is a less frequent cause of visual loss in GCA. Clinically, it presents in a manner similar to other retinal artery occlusions with sudden visual loss and the appearance of retinal whitening. The appearance of CRAO in an elderly patient who does not have visible embolic material in the retinal arterioles must raise the suspicion of GCA.

▪ Posterior ischemic optic neuropathy: Infarction of the optic disc posterior to the lamina cribrosa may occur in GCA. This will result in sudden visual loss, which may be unilateral or bilateral, and the optic disc will appear normal acutely. Subsequently, the disc will become pale. This is an unusual manifestation of GCA, but overall GCA is one of the more frequent causes of PION.

▪ Choroidal ischemia: At times, the fundus appears normal or minimally involved for the profound degree of visual loss. Fluorescein angiography may reveal marked deficiency of blood flowing to the choroid (Fig. 5-24).

▪ Ocular ischemic syndrome: This is an unusual presentation for GCA, but the diagnosis must be kept in mind in patients who present with decreased vision, ocular hypotony, and anterior segment inflammation. This syndrome is due to involvement of the ophthalmic artery by the arteritic process.

■ Ocular misalignment: Double vision may be caused by infarction of the extraocular muscles, CN III, IV, or VI, or by infarction in the brain stem, causing ocular misalignment as part of the overall stroke syndrome.

■ Abnormal superficial temporal arteries: they may be indurated, prominent, without a pulse, and painful (Fig. 5-25).

● Other systemic problems secondary to arteritis that may be associated with GCA include

■ brain stem strokes

■ dissecting aneurysm

■ aortic incompetence

■ myocardial infarction

■ infarction of other organs: bowel and kidney

Diagnostic Evaluation

● The ESR is the time-honored test for GCA and is usually elevated. It is, however, not specific and may be elevated when GCA is not present or be normal when it is. We prefer the Westergren method because it is more accurate at higher levels. We use the formula of age/2 in men and age +10/2 in women as the normal values for the Westergren ESR. Furthermore, a significant minority of patients have been shown to have biopsy-proven GCA with normal ESR, and therefore, a normal ESR does not exclude a diagnosis of GCA.

● The CRP is a more sensitive indicator for the presence of GCA than is the ESR. It is estimated that fewer than 2% of the patients with AION will have a TAB positive for GCA and have a normal CRP.

● Thrombocytosis: Patients with GCA will often have platelet counts greater than $400 \times 10^3/\mu L$.

● Intravenous fluorescein angiography will often show delayed choroidal filling in patients with GCA.

● Ultrasonic imaging of the superficial temporal artery using color Doppler technology has shown a characteristic dark halo, which was interpreted as being due to edema in the arteriole wall. Ultrasound should not be used as a substitute for TAB to diagnose GCA. Color Doppler will also show decreased blood flow velocity in the involved superficial temporal artery.

● TAB is the gold standard for the diagnosis of GCA. A positive biopsy consists of finding inflammatory mononuclear cells with destruction of the internal elastic lamina. There may be necrosis of the media and multinucleated giant cells may be present, but the diagnosis may be made in their absence (Fig. 5-26). Statistics show that a unilateral negative TAB is excellent evidence that the patient does not have GCA. However, if the clinical suspicion is high, the consequences of missing the diagnosis, even though this is statistically unlikely, are so important that the second, contralateral artery should be biopsied. It matters little whether biopsies are done simultaneously, sequentially, or under frozen-section guidance. All patients suspected of having GCA should undergo TAB even if the clinical picture is compelling. This prevents the premature interruption of treatment when complications of steroid therapy occur. It also avoids the difficult task of trying to diagnose GCA by finding evidence of the so-called healed GCA on TAB months after treatment has begun.

Treatment

There is only one treatment for GCA and that is systemic corticosteroids. The exact dosage of corticosteroids required to prevent visual loss and the duration of the treatment regimen are unknown. The primary goal of treatment in a patient who has GCA is to prevent visual loss in either eye if the diagnosis is made before visual loss occurs or in the fellow eye if the diagnosis is established after unilateral visual loss. The second goal of therapy, that is, reversal of visual loss, is more problematic. There are no prospective randomized studies that have investigated the efficacy of different corticosteroid treatment regimens in reversing visual loss. Recently tocilizumab, a monoclonal antibody against the IL-6 receptor, has been approved as a steroid-sparing agent in the treatment of GCA. It may not be used as a primary treatment to substitute for corticosteroids.

We recommend that patients who have suffered a fixed visual deficit be treated with 1 g of intravenous methylprednisolone per day. During the 3 days of intravenous treatment, TAB should be performed, and if it is positive, the therapy is changed to oral prednisone beginning at 1 mg/kg/day. Patients who do not have visual loss may be treated initially with oral prednisone, pending results of TAB. All patients suspected of having GCA should be treated with corticosteroids while diagnostic information, including the results of the TAB, is being collected.

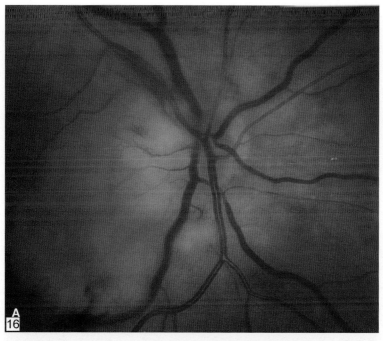

FIGURE 5-23. Giant cell arteritis. A. The optic disc is infarcted. It has a chalk-like color. There are some nerve fiber layer hemorrhages.

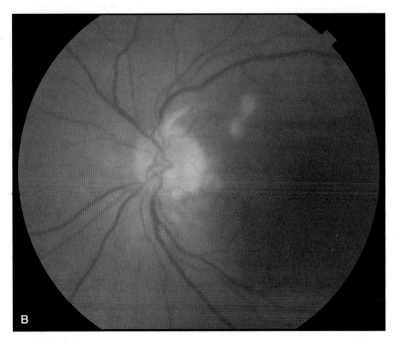

FIGURE 5-23. (*continued*) **B.** Concomitant retinal infarction and anterior ischemic optic neuropathy characteristic of giant cell arteritis.

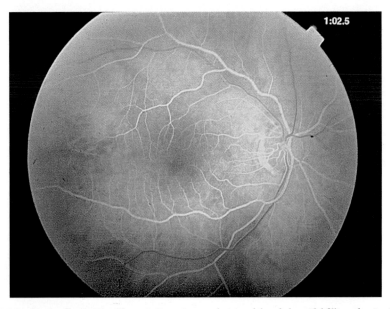

FIGURE 5-24. **Giant cell arteritis.** Fluorescein angiogram showing delayed choroidal filling after 1 minute.

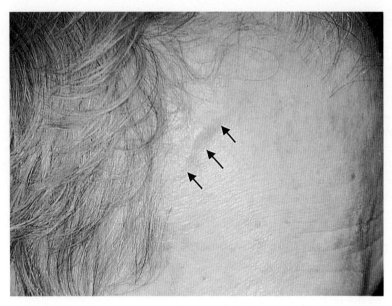

FIGURE 5-25. **Giant cell arteritis.** Patient with giant cell arteritis showing indurated nonpulsatile tender superficial temporal artery (*arrows*)

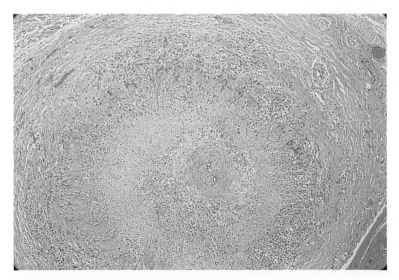

FIGURE 5-26. **Giant cell arteritis.** Temporal artery biopsy specimen shows inflammation with occlusion of the arterial lumen. Multinucleated giant cells also are evident. (Courtesy of Ralph Eagle, M.D.)

PERIOPERATIVE ISCHEMIC OPTIC NEUROPATHY

Nonocular surgeries such as spine, cardiac, or head and neck procedures may precipitate either AION or PION. The most common procedures are coronary artery bypass grafting and prolonged spinal fusion surgery, with the patient in the prone position. The clinical presentation is of bilateral (but can be unilateral) profound visual loss. The definitive cause has not been identified, but may include profound blood loss, hypotension, anemia, or vascular congestion.

HYPERTENSIVE OPTIC NEUROPATHY

Hypertensive optic neuropathy is characterized by bilateral optic disc swelling in hypertensive patients.

Epidemiology and Etiology
• Hypertension is usually significant, with diastolic pressures over 100 mm Hg.

Clinical Characteristics
Symptoms
• Decreased vision is the only symptom. The disc edema may be noted on routine eye or medical evaluation.

Signs
• Decreased acuity may be on the basis of optic nerve or retinal involvement.
• Constricted visual fields
• An RAPD if asymmetric
• Swollen optic discs (Fig. 5-27)
• Fundus changes characteristic of systemic hypertension with arteriolar narrowing, A-V crossing changes, retinal exudates, or retinal/choroidal infarcts

Differential Diagnosis
• Papilledema
• Ischemic optic neuropathy
• Uremic papillopathy

Treatment
• Lowering of blood pressure. It is thought that a too rapid lowering of the blood pressure may cause optic nerve infarction.

Special Comments
Hypertensive optic neuropathy is thought to be a form of ischemic optic neuropathy. However, there are instances where hypertensive optic neuropathy is due to increased ICP. When this is the cause of the optic disc swelling, patients usually have symptoms of diffuse encephalopathy.

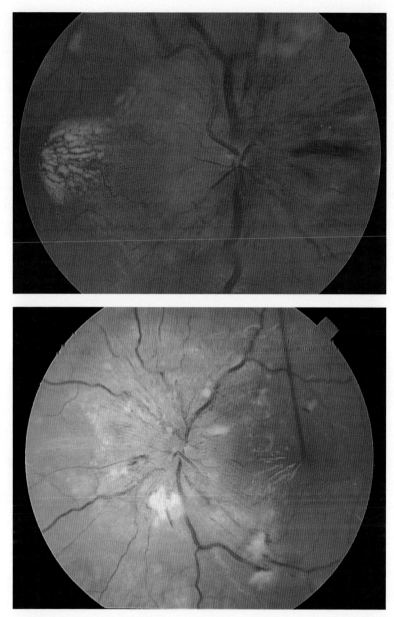

FIGURE 5-27. **Hypertensive optic neuropathy. A, B.** Bilateral swollen optic discs with retinal infarcts and exudates in the form of a hemimacular star figure. The patient's blood pressure was 210/130 mm Hg.

DIABETIC PAPILLOPATHY

Diabetic papillopathy is unilateral or bilateral optic disc swelling that occurs in patients with diabetes mellitus. It is thought to be an atypical form of NAION.

Epidemiology and Etiology

- Diabetic papillopathy was initially described in type 1 diabetes mellitus, but occurs in both type 1 and type 2 diabetes mellitus. The cause of the disc swelling is not known.

Clinical Characteristics

Symptoms

- Visual loss is usually present and is the only symptom.

Signs

- Optic disc swelling, which may be unilateral or bilateral. More peripapillary hemorrhages are present than in NAION (Fig. 5-28).

- An RAPD if visual loss is asymmetric or unilateral

- Visual field defects including central scotomas, arcuate visual field defect

- Diabetic retinopathy is usually present, although rarely it may be absent.

- Macular edema is frequently present.

Natural History

- The clinical course of diabetic papillopathy is usually benign, with many patients experiencing complete recovery of vision. The disc edema may take months to disappear.

Treatment

- None is required other than control of the diabetic state

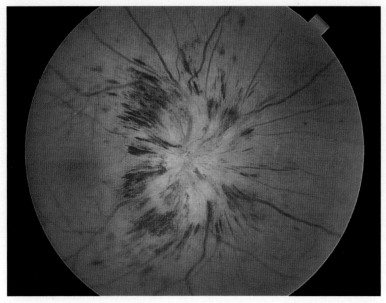

FIGURE 5-28. **Diabetic papillopathy.**   Optic disc is elevated with numerous peripapillary hemorrhages. Diabetic retinopathy and macular edema are also present.

RADIATION OPTIC NEUROPATHY

A unilateral or bilateral optic neuropathy may develop following radiation therapy.

Epidemiology and Etiology

This optic neuropathy usually occurs in patients with intracranial, skull base, or paranasal sinus tumors who have undergone radiation therapy where the optic nerves are included in the radiation field. A dose above 6,000 cGy with daily fractions of about 200 cGy is necessary to produce radiation-induced optic neuropathy. It is also known to occur following radiation for thyroid orbitopathy in patients with preexisting diabetes mellitus. It should be remembered that lower doses of radiation might produce radiation optic neuropathy if given at the same time as chemotherapy, which seems to potentiate the effect of the radiation on the optic nerve.

The exact mechanism is not known but is presumed to be radiation-induced damage to the vascular endothelial cells that subsequently results in vascular occlusion and necrosis. It usually presents as a retrobulbar optic neuropathy, although rarely, it may present as an anterior optic neuropathy with a swollen optic nerve.

Clinical Characteristics

Symptoms

• Visual loss occurs acutely and progresses until most or all vision is lost in one or both eyes. Visual loss usually occurs an average of 18 months following the radiation therapy, but may occur within the first year, and has been reported to occur after 20 years.

Signs

• Decreased visual acuity

• Visual field defects of optic nerve or chiasmal origin

• Initially, the optic discs appear normal, but subsequently become pale.

Differential Diagnosis

• Recurrence of the initial tumor

• Secondary empty sella syndrome with optic nerve and chiasmal prolapsed

• Radiation-induced parasellar tumor

• Arachnoiditis

Diagnostic Evaluation

• The diagnosis is established clinically in a patient who has received the appropriate amount of radiation and in whom other causes of visual loss have been excluded.

• CT scans are normal and there is no enhancement with contrast. However, T1-weighted gadolinium-enhanced MRI will show enhancement of the optic nerves, optic chiasm, and possibly the optic tracts (see Fig. 6-12, p. 251). The enhancement resolves when the visual function stabilizes. Unenhanced T1- and T2-weighted image will show no abnormality.

Treatment

• This is a vascular necrosis that causes visual loss. Various treatments have been championed, including high-dose corticosteroids, alone or combined with hyperbaric oxygen treatment, or intravitreal anti-VEGF injections. Their effectiveness is somewhat doubtful.

• Radiation necrosis of the brain appears to respond to anticoagulation therapy. There are no studies, however, to indicate that this treatment is effective in radiation-induced optic neuropathy.

Prognosis

• Almost half of all patients will have a final visual outcome of no light perception despite various treatment attempts. Those who maintain some vision will have visual acuity worse than 20/200.

AMIODARONE OPTIC NEUROPATHY

Amiodarone optic neuropathy has been attributed to the systemic administration of the cardiac antiarrhythmic drug amiodarone.

Epidemiology and Etiology

- Amiodarone-associated optic neuropathy is thought to occur in approximately 1% to 2% of patients taking the drug.

- The exact cause of the optic neuropathy is not known. Lipid inclusions characteristic of amiodarone have been found in one optic nerve studied histopathologically, but this patient had no history of visual dysfunction.

Clinical Characteristics

Symptoms

- Decreased vision is insidious in onset and is slowly progressive as long as the drug is taken. Some patients may have no visual complaints.

Signs

- Optic disc swelling is bilateral (Fig. 5-29). Cases of unilateral involvement have been reported but these may be instances of NAION in patients who happen to be taking amiodarone.

- Decreased visual acuity which is usually not worse than 20/200

- Visual field deficits of the optic nerve variety
- An RAPD if visual deficits are asymmetric
- Acquired dyschromatopsia
- Vortex keratopathy: Whorl-like opacities in the corneal endothelium that do not produce decreased vision but are present in patients taking amiodarone

Differential Diagnosis

- Papilledema: because of the bilateral disc elevation. However, the loss of vision in the absence of chronic disc changes eliminates papilledema as a possible diagnosis.

- Ischemic optic neuropathy is the entity most often confused with amiodarone optic neuropathy. A comparison of their differentiating characteristics is seen in **Table 5-14**.

Diagnostic Evaluation

- No investigations prove the existence of amiodarone-induced optic neuropathy.

- The presence of optic disc edema in a patient taking amiodarone is grounds to suspect this diagnosis.

Treatment

- In any patient with suspected amiodarone-induced optic neuropathy, the drug should be discontinued if another form of treatment for the cardiac disorder is available. No other treatment to reverse the optic neuropathy exists.

TABLE 5-14. Amiodarone-Induced Optic Neuropathy vs. Nonarteritic Anterior Ischemic Optic Neuropathy (NAION)

	Amiodarone	NAION
Onset of symptoms	Insidious	Acute
Laterality	Bilateral, simultaneous	Unilateral, if bilateral, usually sequential
Resolution of edema	Months	6–8 wk

- We recommend that the prescribing physician discontinue amiodarone if this is medically feasible. The patient is reexamined within 6 to 8 weeks. If the disc edema is still evident, the diagnosis of amiodarone-induced optic neuropathy is made.

Natural History

- After discontinuation of medication, the optic disc edema slowly resolves and in approximately one-third of patients, visual function recovers as the optic disc edema subsides. Vision usually stabilizes in the other patients.

Special Features

There is controversy as to whether amiodarone-induced optic neuropathy exists as a diagnosis *sui generis* or whether these patients actually have NAION and happen to be taking amiodarone. It is difficult at times to make a distinction between the two entities. We believe the major differentiating factor that distinguishes the two is the time to resolution of the optic disc swelling. The disc edema of NAION will resolve within 6 to 8 weeks, whereas the edema of amiodarone-induced optic neuropathy will take many more weeks to months to resolve.

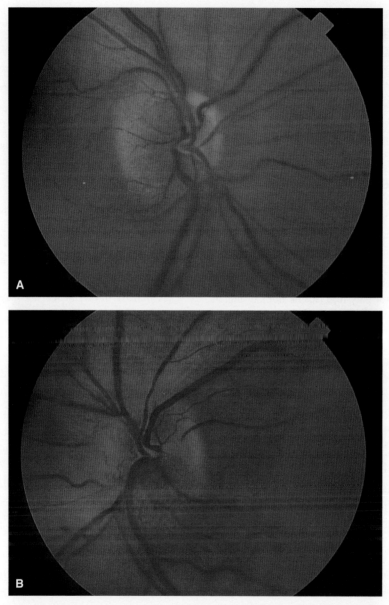

FIGURE 5-29. Amiodarone optic neuropathy. A, B. Bilateral optic disc edema with decreased vision and visual field loss in a patient taking amiodarone. The disc edema subsided with return of visual function 4 months after the medication was discontinued.

NUTRITIONAL DEFICIENCY AND TOXIC OPTIC NEUROPATHIES

Nutritional Optic Neuropathy

In the past, nutritional optic neuropathy was referred to as tobacco alcohol amblyopia because it was believed that the combined toxic effect of those two agents produced this optic neuropathy. It is now accepted that this is a nutritional optic neuropathy. Dietary deficiencies of vitamin B_{12}, folate, copper, and thiamine may cause optic neuropathy.

However, toxic substances may also cause optic neuropathies independent of nutritional abnormalities. Agents that are recognized in this category include ethambutol, methanol, ethylene glycol, organic solvents, lead (in children), disulfiram, ciprofloxacin, antineoplastic drugs (cisplatin and vincristine), and antitumor necrosis factor (TNF)-α agents (etanercept, infliximab, and adalimumab). The TNF-α antagonists may produce an acute optic neuritis. Some toxic optic neuropathies are more commonly associated with disc swelling. Methanol and ethylene glycol toxicity result in a rapid onset of severe bilateral vision loss with prominent disc edema.

Etiology and Epidemiology

- A specific nutritional deficit has not been identified. Causation is likely to be multifactorial.
- These patients ordinarily do smoke and drink to excess and do have a very poor diet, usually lacking in fresh vegetables.
- There is a suspicion that the cyanide contained in tobacco may contribute to the production of this optic neuropathy in smokers.

Clinical Presentation

- The hallmark of the optic neuropathy because of either nutritional deficiencies or toxic exposure is bilateral, simultaneous, painless visual loss.

Symptoms

- Progressive loss of vision
  - Bilateral: Although may be somewhat asymmetric, particularly in the early stages
  - Rate of decline: May be quite rapid
  - Extent of visual loss: Variable, but central acuity is usually better than count fingers
- Acquired dyschromatopsia: Usually presents early and may be the initial symptom

Signs

- Bilateral central or centrocecal scotomas, usually with intact peripheral visual fields, are the hallmark of toxic optic neuropathies.
- Pupillary reaction usually is sluggish.
- Absence of an RAPD: Because of the bilateral and symmetric involvement of the optic nerves
- Optic atrophy, involving mostly the papillomacular area of the disc, appears later in the disease course (Fig. 5-30). Initially, the optic disc may be normal or hyperemic (Fig. 5-31).

Diagnostic Evaluation

- Detailed history: With particular attention to dietary intake, smoking habits, alcohol consumption, and other medical conditions of relevance and medications. Other disorders that may produce bilateral visual loss are listed in Table 5-15.
- Physical examination seeking other signs of nutritional deficiencies

TABLE 5-15. Differential Diagnosis of Bilateral Visual Loss

Macular disease
Compressive or infiltrative lesions of the optic nerve or chiasm
Dominant optic atrophy
Leber optic neuropathy
Conversion disorder or malingering

- Neuroimaging: MRI with intravenous injection of gadolinium diethylenetriamine penta-acetic acid is usually prudent to exclude an underlying compressive lesion of both optic nerves or the optic chiasm.

- Special investigations
  - Vitamin B_{12} level: To exclude pernicious anemia
  - Red blood cell folate level may be normal.
  - Exclusion of subtle maculopathies that may mimic the clinical picture

Treatment

- Discontinue alcohol consumption and use of tobacco.
- Improve dietary intake, specifically with green and yellow vegetables.
- Prescribe thiamine 100 mg po bid and folate 1.0 mg po daily.
- Vitamin B_{12} injections are recommended by some.
- The goal of treatment is usually to prevent further visual loss. Most patients present when their optic discs are atrophic and have well-established visual loss. If patients are diagnosed and treated early, when the optic discs are normal or even hyperemic, there is a possibility of return of some visual function.

Vitamin B_{12} Deficiency

Etiology

- Pernicious anemia is the most common cause.
  - Autoimmune disorder most commonly seen in middle-aged and elderly Caucasians.
  - Vitamin B_{12} is poorly absorbed from the ileum because the parietal cells of the gastric mucosa do not produce intrinsic factor.
  - Megaloblastic anemia
  - Neurologic symptoms: Subacute combined degeneration

- Poor diet: Usually in strict vegans
- Other causes of impaired absorption:
  - gastrointestinal surgery,
  - intestinal disease,
  - diphyllobothriasis, and
  - intestinal tapeworms.

Treatment

- Intramuscular injections of hydroxocobalamin

Thiamine Deficiency

The evidence that thiamine deficiency can produce an optic neuropathy is inconclusive, although patients who have nutritional optic neuropathy may also be thiamine deficient. It is still recommended that patients with nutritional optic neuropathy be screened for thiamine and folic acid deficiency and treated.

Toxic Optic Neuropathies: Methanol

For a detailed list, see **Tables 5-16** and **5-17**.

Clinical Characteristics

- The patient usually has accidentally ingested methanol because it was mistaken for or substituted for ethyl alcohol. Methanol toxicity is an acute event.

Symptoms

- Nausea and vomiting: Occur early after ingestion
- Respiratory distress, abdominal discomfort, and headache: after 18 to 48 hours. The patient also may have confusion, generalized weakness, and drowsiness.
- Metabolic acidosis
- Visual loss is acute and severe most commonly, but visual acuity may be reduced to any level. Central or centrocecal scotomas are characteristic if some vision is preserved.

TABLE 5-16. Toxic Optic Neuropathies

Agent	Usage	Systemic Association	Optic Neuropathy	Other Neuro-ophthalmic Findings
Ethylene glycol	Automobile antifreeze	Nausea, vomiting, abdominal pain, coma	Mild to profound visual loss	Nystagmus, ophthalmoplegia
Halogenated hydroxyquinolines	Amebicidal drugs	Abdominal discomfort, paresthesias, dysesthesias	Dyschromatopsia early finding	Subacute myelooptic neuropathy
Disulfiram	Chronic alcoholism	Sensorimotor peripheral neuropathy	Subacute or chronic visual loss	

TABLE 5-17. Medications Producing Optic Neuropathies

Cisplatin

Isoniazid

Sulfonamides

Vincristine

Chloramphenicol

Disulfiram

Signs

- Ophthalmoscopic findings include (Fig. 5-32) the following:
  - Early: Hyperemia of the optic disc with blurred margins
  - Later: Pallor or cupping of the optic disc; thinning of the retinal arterioles
- Pupils: Usually sluggish response to light, except in total loss of vision when the pupils are dilated and nonreactive

Diagnostic Evaluation

- Serum methanol levels are greater than 20 mg/dL.

Treatment

- Ethanol should be given because it interferes with the metabolism of methanol. Treat the metabolic acidosis.

Prognosis

- Visual loss may be minimized with prompt treatment.

Toxic Optic Neuropathies: Ethambutol

General

- This drug is used as an antituberculous agent.
- The L form of ethambutol is primarily responsible for the toxic optic neuropathy, whereas the D form is responsible for the therapeutic effect.
- Ocular toxicity is dose related, with an optic neuropathy most likely to occur at doses greater than 25 mg/kg/day, although visual loss has been documented to occur at lower doses.

Onset: No earlier than 2 months after starting the medication. Median onset is 7 months.

Greater susceptibility for the development of optic neuropathy in patients with renal tuberculosis as the drug is excreted via the kidneys.

Signs

- Visual field: Central scotoma, bitemporal or peripheral constriction
- Optic nerve: Initially normal, followed by optic atrophy

Prognosis

● Vision usually improves slowly after the drug is discontinued; however, some patients may be left with permanent visual loss.

Toxic Optic Neuropathies: Tobacco (Also Known as Tobacco Alcohol Amblyopia)

The role of tobacco alone in producing optic neuropathy has not been clearly elucidated.

It may be that patients with malnutrition are predisposed to developing tobacco optic neuropathy. Tobacco may impair the absorption of vitamin B_{12}. Some investigators suggest that the cyanide present in tobacco produces a cyanide optic neuropathy, although this has yet to be proven conclusively. The disease is found to be more common in pipe smokers.

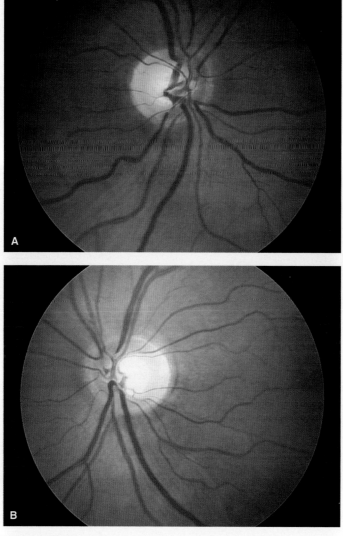

FIGURE 5-30. **Nutritional deficiency optic neuropathy.** **A, B.** Bilateral temporal optic disc pallor with decreased vision and central scotomas in a patient with presumed nutritional deficiency optic neuropathy.

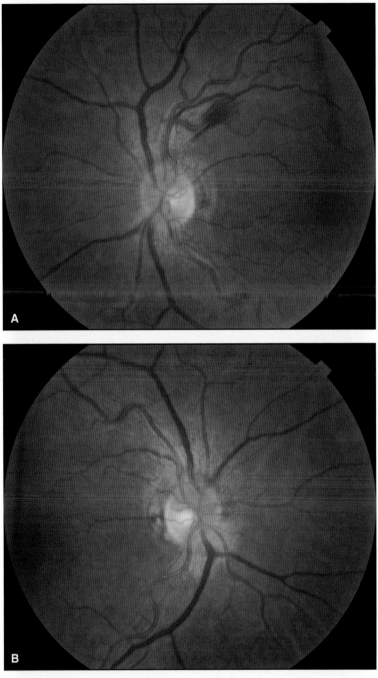

FIGURE 5-31. Toxic optic neuropathy. A, B. Bilateral hyperemia with peripapillary hemorrhage OS in a patient with toxic optic neuropathy due to habitual mouth wash ingestion.

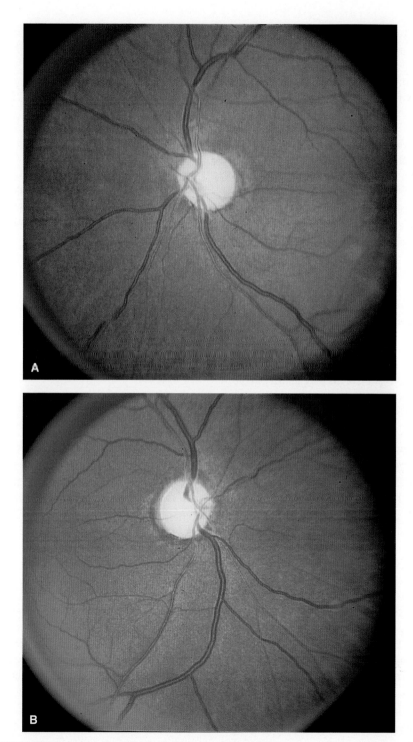

FIGURE 5-32. Toxic optic neuropathy. A, B. Bilateral optic disc pallor in a patient who lost vision after drinking methanol. (Courtesy of Neil R. Miller, MD.)

PAPILLEDEMA

Papilledema is defined as optic disc elevation, almost always bilateral, caused by increased ICP.

Epidemiology and Etiology

- Any condition that produces increased ICP may produce papilledema.

Stages of Papilledema

There are several stages in the development of papilledema that occur over days or weeks depending on the cause. Some publications use the Frisén classification. A blinded evaluation of disc photographs by several neuro-ophthalmologists revealed limited reproducibility and discriminative ability of the classification. Therefore, we prefer the following:

1. *Incipient* (early) papilledema is characterized by mild disc hyperemia and minimal opacification of the peripapillary nerve fiber layer (Fig. 5-33A). Spontaneous venous pulsations may be lost.
2. *Acute* (well-developed) papilledema shows unequivocal opacification of the nerve fiber layer with the presence of nerve fiber layer hemorrhages in the peripapillary area (Fig. 5-33B).
3. *Chronic* papilledema is characterized by an optic disc that appears less hyperemic than in the earlier acute stages and is less likely to have hemorrhages. There may be white concretions in the optic nerve (pseudodrusen), which are presumed accumulations of dammed-up axoplasm because of the papilledema itself. Optociliary shunt vessels may begin to develop at this stage. Visual loss also begins to accelerate at this stage (Fig. 5-33C).
4. *Atrophic* papilledema is the final stage of the disease. This is the process in which the optic nerves are pale, at times flat,

and there is usually marked visual acuity and visual field loss (Fig. 5-33D).

Clinical Characteristics
Symptoms
- The patient may be completely asymptomatic.
- Headaches may be present.
- Transient visual obscurations lasting seconds and occurring mainly when the patient changes position or bends over and then stands up quickly are typical of papilledema.
- Decreased vision occurs from optic nerve involvement when the papilledema is chronic. Acuity may be decreased because of fluid or folds in the macula (Fig. 5-34) even in acute papilledema.
- Diplopia because of unilateral or bilateral CN VI palsy
- Nausea and vomiting

Signs
- Optic disc changes:
  - Bilateral swollen hyperemic optic discs
  - Blurring of disc margin and opacification of the retinal nerve fiber layer that produces obscuration of the peripapillary retinal blood vessels
  - Papillary or peripapillary retinal hemorrhages
  - Loss of venous pulsations
  - Dilated tortuous retinal veins
- Visual field deficits begin with an enlarged blind spot, and as the papilledema becomes chronic, they progress to overall depression of the visual field, then the development of arcuate visual field defects, and only later the involvement of central fixation.
- Visual acuity is lost late in the development of chronic papilledema. Acuity may

be depressed in acute papilledema when the swollen optic disc produces retinal folds, exudates, or hemorrhages in the macula.

- Unilateral or bilateral CN VI palsy

Differential Diagnosis

- Papilledema is not the only cause of an elevated optic disc. Inflammatory, ischemic, or infiltrative processes may cause optic disc edema. Ophthalmoscopically, a congenitally elevated optic disc may be confused with papilledema, thus the term pseudopapilledema (see p. 182).
- The most frequent causes of papilledema are listed in **Table 5-18**.

Diagnostic Evaluation

- All patients who are discovered to have any stage of papilledema constitute a medical emergency. They require immediate imaging to rule out an intracranial mass lesion or hydrocephalus. MRI is the best test to obtain; however, CT scanning is acceptable as

an emergency procedure to rule out a mass lesion.

Treatment

- The treatment of the papilledema is directed primarily at the underlying cause. If this is not possible, treatment of the papilledema itself with a shunting procedure or optic nerve sheath fenestration to preserve vision may be considered.

TABLE 5-18. Frequent Causes of Papilledema

Intracranial tumors: Primary or metastatic
Pseudotumor cerebri
Sagittal sinus thrombosis
Aqueduct stenosis
Subdural or epidural hematoma
Arteriovenous malformation
Subarachnoid hemorrhage
Other: Brain abscess, encephalitis, meningitis

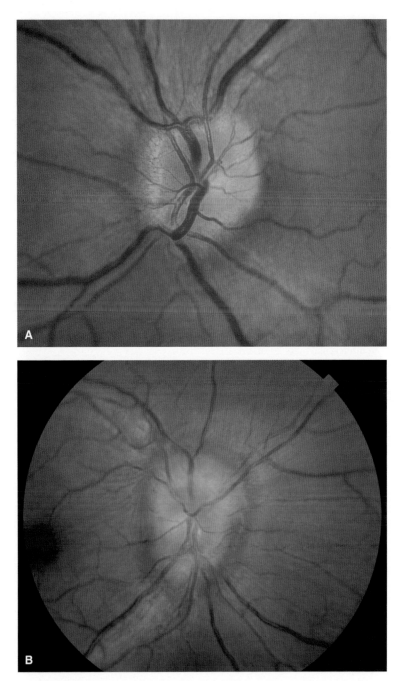

FIGURE 5-33. **Papilledema.** **A.** Incipient papilledema with early nerve fiber layer opacification. **B.** Acute papilledema with more extensive nerve fiber layer opacification and retinal folds.

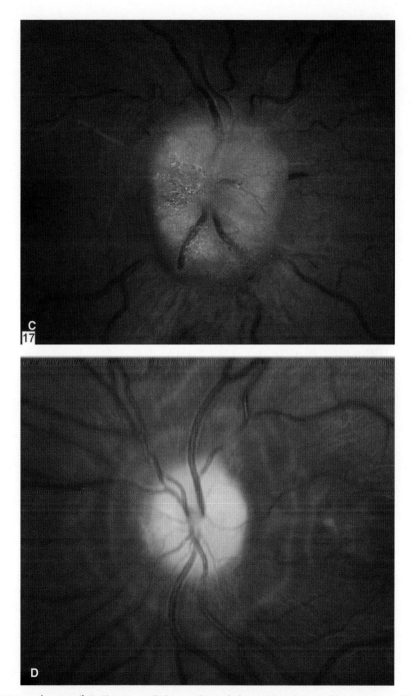

FIGURE 5-33. (*continued*) **C.** Chronic papilledema with pseudodrusen. Note the loss of the retinal nerve fiber layer and concentric peripapillary retinal folds. **D.** Atrophic papilledema with concentric peripapillary rings indicating extent of the previous disc elevation.

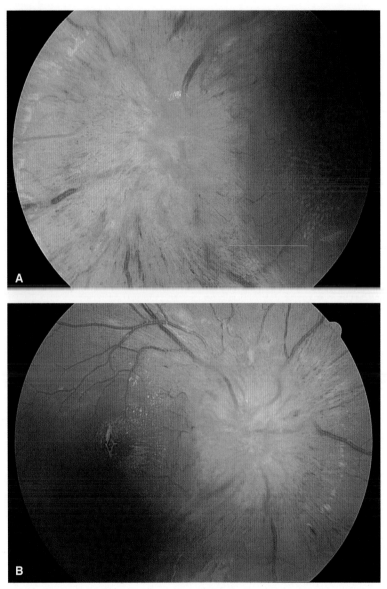

FIGURE 5-34. **Papilledema. A, B.** Papilledema with fluid and exudates in the macula causing decreased acuity.

PSEUDOTUMOR CEREBRI

Pseudotumor cerebri [PTC, or idiopathic intracranial hypertension (IIH)] is the constellation of elevated ICP with normal neuroimaging and normal CSF composition. Although this disorder is most commonly encountered in young, overweight women, it may be seen in men or in thin patients of both genders. Usually, however, patients are overweight or have a history of recent weight gain.

The diagnostic criteria for PTC are:

• normal CT or MRI of the brain,

• increased CSF pressure on lumbar puncture with an otherwise normal CSF composition,

• absence of focal neurologic signs except CN VI palsies.

Etiology

• There are two large categories of PTC.

   ▪ The idiopathic variety of PTC, called by some IIH, but referred to by others as the PTC syndrome. No identifiable cause for the papilledema is ever found in these patients.

   ▪ Several conditions or agents may produce increased ICP including sleep apnea syndrome, chronic anemia, excessive doses of vitamin A, tetracycline, isoretinoids, cyclosporine, and corticosteroids. In addition, patients may have papilledema as a result of intracranial venous sinus thrombosis.

Clinical Characteristics

Symptoms

• Headache is usually present but may be absent

• Transient visual obscurations

• Visual loss if chronic and progressive

• Double vision: because of CN VI palsies (Fig. 5-35)

• Tinnitus

• Dizziness

• Nausea and vomiting

Signs

• Bilateral optic disc edema

• Visual field deficits, which may be mild (enlarged blind spot) to severe. Nerve fiber bundle defects or depression of central acuity occurs with chronic papilledema.

• Unilateral or bilateral CN VI palsy

Diagnostic Evaluation

• Detailed history to identify any medications or toxins that may be producing this syndrome.

• MRI to exclude an intracranial mass or hydrocephalus is performed in all patients, even if they fit the clinical profile of PTC (Fig. 5-36)

• Magnetic resonance venography (MRV) or computed tomography venography (CTV) is the best test to rule out intracranial venous sinus thrombosis. We believe that MRV/CTV should be performed on all patients suspected of having PTC (Fig. 5-37).

• Lumbar puncture should be performed in all patients who do not have a mass lesion or hydrocephalus. This will document that the CSF pressure is elevated but is otherwise normal in its composition.

Treatment

• In the event of an identifiable medicinal cause, for example, tetracycline or excessive vitamin A ingestion, immediate discontinuation of the agent is indicated.

• In intracranial venous sinus thrombosis, there is some debate about the treatment, but most authorities prefer aggressive anticoagulation. These patients should also be investigated for coagulopathies. Stenting of the venous sinus is sometimes performed.

• In PTC patients who are losing vision from the papilledema, the treatment options include the following:

■ Weight loss (approximately 10% to 15% of body weight in overweight patients) is effective.

■ Acetazolamide beginning at 1 g/day and increasing as tolerated. There is no firm evidence that any other diuretic is effective in the treatment of PTC. Topiramate, approved for the treatment of epilepsy and migraine prophylaxis, has also been shown to be a carbonic anhydrase inhibitor and hence has been used in patients intolerant to acetazolamide. It also produces anorexia which may be helpful in this condition.

■ Optic nerve sheath fenestration, if visual loss is profound at presentation or is progressing in the presence of chronic papilledema and headache is not a prominent symptom.

■ Lumboperitoneal or ventriculoperitoneal shunt is the procedure of choice if headache is severe.

■ Repeat spinal taps should not be used as a routine treatment in PTC. There are only rare instances in which we believe they should be employed, for example, in a pregnant woman who is losing vision, in whom medication is inadvisable and optic nerve sheath fenestration or shunting is contraindicated.

■ Bariatric surgery is a treatment option in patients refractory to other treatments.

■ Systemic corticosteroid administration is to be avoided except to lower ICP for a short period of time prior to surgical intervention for progressive visual loss.

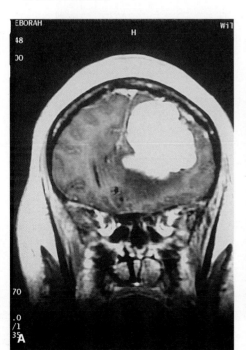 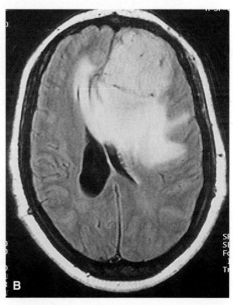

FIGURE 5-35. **Young, obese woman, with chronic papilledema,** who on axial (**A**) and coronal (**B**) MRI was found to have a large meningioma and not pseudotumor cerebri as the cause of the papilledema.

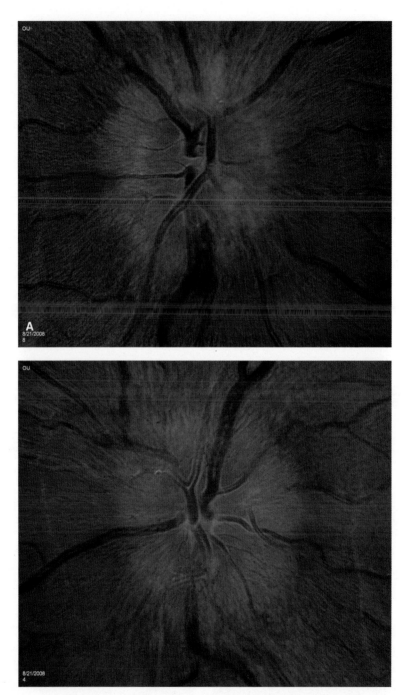

FIGURE 5-36. Pseudotumor cerebri patient with papilledema (**A**) and esotropia (**B**) in primary position (top) and bilateral abduction defects because of bilateral VI palsies. (Pupils dilated pharmacologically.)

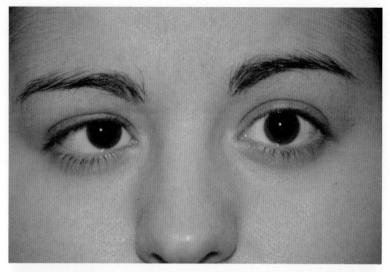

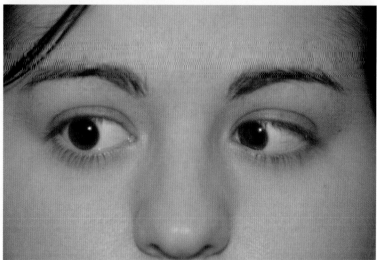

FIGURE 5-36. (*continued*)

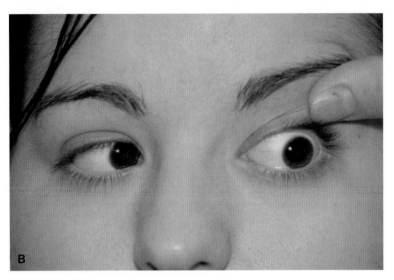

FIGURE 5-36. (*continued*)

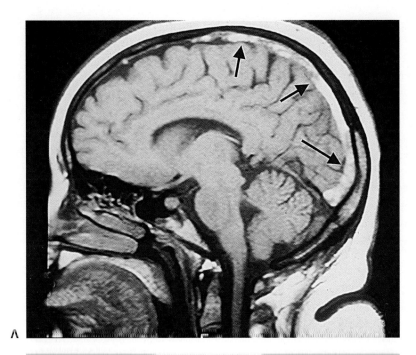

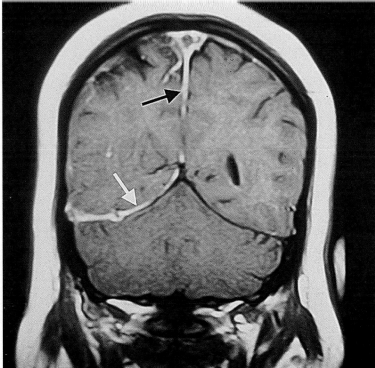

FIGURE 5-37. **Sinus thrombosis.** Patient with papilledema shows increased signal because of thrombosis in the sagittal (**A**, *black arrows*) and transverse sinuses (**B**, *white arrow*).

OPTIC NERVE GLIOMA

This benign tumor of the optic nerve usually occurs in children and is often found in association with neurofibromatosis type 1 (NF-1).

Etiology and Epidemiology

• These tumors are true neoplasms of the optic nerve and are most often juvenile pilocytic astrocytomas. They are commonly (30%) associated with NF-1.

• Optic nerve gliomas are the most common infiltrative tumor of the optic nerve.

Clinical Characteristics

Symptoms

• Decreased vision: the majority of patients with optic nerve gliomas develop symptoms and signs within the first decade of life, and over 90% will present before the second decade.

• Proptosis is the presenting characteristic if the bulk of the tumor is in the orbit. The proptosis is associated with features of an anterior optic neuropathy.

Signs

• An RAPD if asymmetric or unilateral
• Optic nerve–type visual field defects
• Proptosis that may be progressive
• Ocular motility disturbances: usually a sensory exotropia
• Optic disc may show (Fig. 5-38):
  ▪ Swelling
  ▪ Pallor: The most common optic disc finding
  ▪ Optociliary shunt vessels: Occasionally seen
• Associated signs and symptoms of NF-1 (Table 5-19)

Diagnostic Evaluation

• MRI scan of the optic nerve and the brain is the diagnostic procedure of choice. It will characterize the tumor as being isolated or as part of a more extensive intracranial disease.

• The typical MRI characteristics of an optic glioma are as follows (Fig. 5-39):
  ▪ Fusiform enlargement of optic nerve with or without associated enlargement of optic canal
  ▪ Hypointense or isointense on T1
  ▪ May show enhancement after injection of gadolinium, but the enhancement is not as pronounced as that produced by meningioma
  ▪ "Kinking" of optic nerve within orbit: Seen exclusively in patients with NF-1
  ▪ Increased T2 signal around the nerve (pseudo-CSF signal)

• All patients diagnosed with optic nerve glioma should be investigated for evidence of NF-1. Conversely, all patients diagnosed with NF-1 should be screened for the presence of optic nerve gliomas because 30% of gliomas occur in patients with NF-1.

Treatment

• The treatment of optic nerve gliomas remains controversial.

• Surgical resection may be considered if
  ▪ the glioma is extending intracranially but has not yet reached the optic chiasm,
  ▪ there is severe proptosis causing corneal ulceration,
  ▪ no light perception vision at presentation is not universally accepted as an indication for surgical excision of the optic nerve.

• If vision is poor or vision is progressively getting worse, treatment will depend on the patient's age.
  ▪ Under 5 years, radiation therapy is not used, but chemotherapy may be administered. Chemotherapy may halt or retard growth of the tumor until the child reaches the age when radiation therapy may be administered safely.
  ▪ Over 5 years, radiation to the optic glioma is the treatment of choice. However, it should be remembered that radiation therapy might produce side effects (Table 5-20).

TABLE 5-19. Features of Neurofibromatosis Type 1

Cutaneous

    Café au lait spots: Flat light brown patches

        Adults usually have more than six

        Appear during the first year of life and increase in size and number

    Axillary freckling: Becomes obvious around the age of 10 y

    Fibroma molluscum: Pedunculated flabby pigmented nodules that may be widely distributed throughout the body

    Plexiform neurofibroma: Larger and less well defined than fibroma molluscum

Skeletal

    Congenital bone defects: Aplasia of greater wing of sphenoid (may produce pulsating enophthalmos or exophthalmos)

    Acquired scoliosis

    Facial hemiatrophy

    Short stature

    Mild macrocephaly

Ocular features

    Eyelid and anterior segment

        Eyelid plexiform neuroma

        Prominent corneal nerves

        Lisch iris nodules: Present in 95% of patients

        Congenital ectropion uveae

Other

    Glaucoma: Rare, but if present it is usually unilateral and congenital; approximately half will have ipsilateral facial hemiatrophy and upper eyelid neurofibroma

    Choroidal hamartoma

Other features

    Neural tumors: May develop in the brain, spinal cord, and the cranial, peripheral, and sympathetic nerves

    Malignancies

        Embryonal tumors of childhood or neurofibrosarcoma (5%)

        Pheochromocytoma

    Hypertension: Secondary to renal artery stenosis or pheochromocytoma

TABLE 5-20. Side Effects of Radiotherapy in Children with Optic Nerve Glioma

Induction of secondary malignancies, endocrinopathies

Developmental delay

Vasculitis

Moyamoya disease

Radionecrosis of the temporal lobes

Leukoencephalopathy

Prognosis

● The prognosis of isolated optic nerve gliomas is reasonably good for vision, with most
patients maintaining stable visual acuity for
years. Most optic nerve gliomas remain confined to one optic nerve. In our experience,
it is rare for an isolated optic nerve glioma to
spread to the optic chiasm or to the contralateral optic nerve.

● Patients with more extensive intracranial
gliomas, particularly those involving the hypothalamus, have a more progressive disorder
and the process may progress to blindness
and/or death.

● If the glioma involves the optic tracts and
chiasm, vision may deteriorate, but survival is
usually not affected.

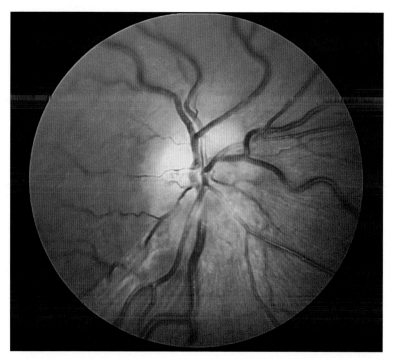

FIGURE 5-38. **Optic nerve glioma.** The optic disc is elevated and hyperemic in the inferior two-thirds, with the
superior one-third being paler. Optociliary shunt vessels are forming at the 9 o'clock position on the optic disc.

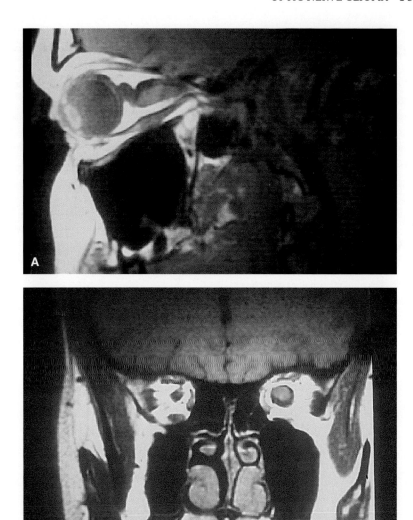

FIGURE 5-39. **Optic nerve glioma.**   Coronal (**A**) and sagittal (**B**) MRIs of the left optic nerve glioma.

MALIGNANT GLIOMA OF ADULTHOOD

This unusual tumor is a malignant glioma that involves the optic nerve. Malignant gliomas can be an isolated lesion or be multicentric. This disorder usually affects older patients and is characterized by rapid progressive visual loss.

Etiology and Epidemiology
● Malignant glioma of the brain

Clinical Characteristics

Symptoms
● Visual loss in one or both eyes, which is rapidly progressive over a period of weeks or months.

Signs
● Decreased vision that is progressive.

● An RAPD, if asymmetric or unilateral

● Optic nerve–type visual field deficits, which rapidly progress to no light perception vision.

● Patients may present initially with a swollen optic disc and are often diagnosed as having AION or with a normal fundus (diagnosed erroneously as PION). Subsequently, a central retinal vein occlusion often develops and frequently progresses to CRAO (Fig. 5-40).

Diagnostic Evaluation
● MRI scan that shows an enhancing lesion. The lesions are characteristic of malignant glioma of the optic nerve and possibly other parts of the brain if the lesion is multicentric (Fig. 5-41).

Treatment
● Radiation therapy and chemotherapy are treatments that can be tried; however, the prognosis for vision and life is uniformly dismal. Most patients die within 1 year of diagnosis.

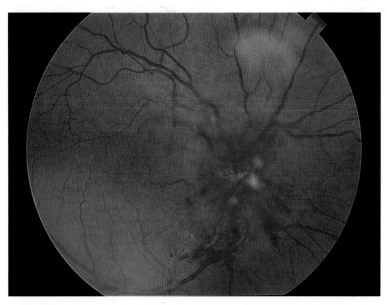

FIGURE 5-40. **Malignant glioma of adulthood.** Patient with malignant glioma of adulthood shows fundus picture of venous congestion, nerve fiber layer hemorrhages, and ischemia of the optic nerve head, consistent with combined retinal artery and vein occlusion. (Courtesy of Robert C. Sergott, MD.)

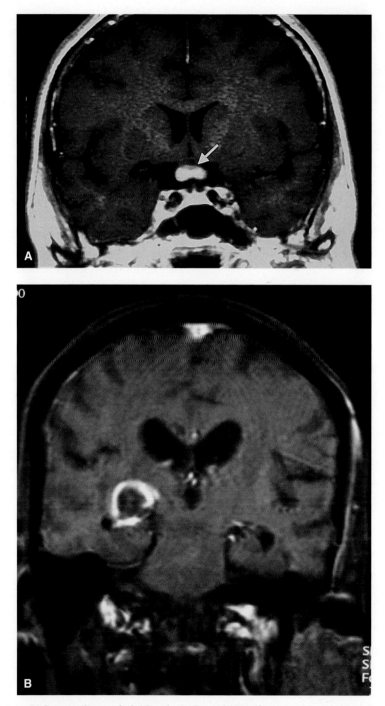

FIGURE 5-41. Malignant glioma of adulthood. A. Coronal MRI of patient with malignant glioma that has extended to the optic chiasm, which is enlarged and enhanced (*arrow*). **B.** There is a second ring enhancing tumor in the area of the right lateral geniculate body.

OPTIC NERVE SHEATH (PERIOPTIC) MENINGIOMA

Optic nerve sheath meningiomas are benign tumors that surround the optic nerve causing progressive visual loss.

Etiology and Epidemiology

- Optic nerve sheath meningiomas are primary tumors that arise from meningoendothelial cells of the arachnoid. They usually involve the optic nerve in the orbit but may extend into the optic canal and through it to occupy the intracranial space.

- Meningiomas typically affect women over the age of 40 years and are a cause of progressive visual loss.

Clinical Characteristics

Symptoms

- Slow, progressive visual loss, which may be unilateral or bilateral, is the only symptom of this disorder.

- The tumors usually do not produce proptosis or ocular motility disturbances until very late in their course.

Signs

- Decreased acuity
- Acquired dyschromatopsia

- Central visual field defects, central scotomas, or nerve fiber bundle defects

- An RAPD, if asymmetric or unilateral

- The optic disc is usually swollen, with characteristic changes in the vasculature of the optic nerve head (optociliary/optic choroidal shunt vessels) (Fig. 5-42). As the tumor grows, the edema resolves and optic atrophy supervenes.

Diagnostic Evaluation

- CT scan shows the "tram-track" sign from calcifications along the optic nerve and tubular thickening of the nerve (Fig. 5-43A).

- A meningioma usually appears as a thickened optic nerve (Fig. 5-43B) that enhances with gadolinium on MRI.

Treatment

- Many patients may be observed without treatment if visual loss is not progressing. If vision is deteriorating, the preferred treatment is radiation therapy with conformal three-dimensional technology.

- There is no alternative therapy that appears to be effective.

- Surgery with attempted extirpation of the meningioma will result in blindness.

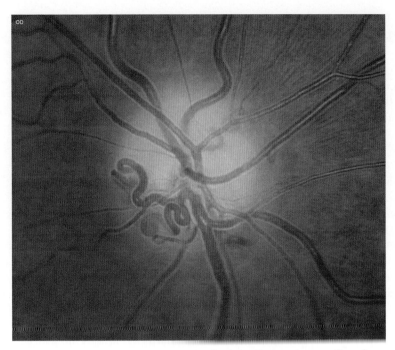

FIGURE 5-42. **Optic nerve sheath meningioma.** Pale, elevated optic disc with optociliary shunt vessels in a blind eye. These are the typical findings of an optic nerve meningioma.

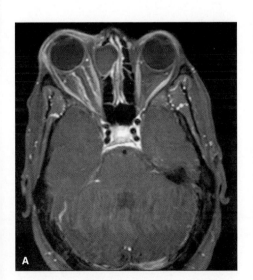
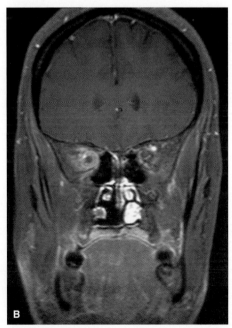

FIGURE 5-43. **Optic nerve sheath meningioma. A.** Axial MRI scan after contrast with typical enhancement of the optic nerve sheath. There is an incidental ethmoidal opacification. **B.** Coronal MRI with contrast shows thickening around the optic nerve in the orbit. (Courtesy of Jennifer Hall, MD.)

LEBER HEREDITARY OPTIC NEUROPATHY

Leber hereditary optic neuropathy (LHON) is a maternally inherited mitochondrial disease that presents as a bilateral sequential or simultaneous optic neuropathy.

Etiology

• LHON is a disorder of mitochondrial (mt) DNA. There are several mutation sites in the (mt) DNA that are deemed to be primary mutations in that their presence alone can produce the disease. These sites are 11778, 3460, and 14484. It is estimated that approximately 90% of all cases of LHON are due to one of these three mutations. A number of secondary mutations have also been identified.

• Inheritance pattern: All of the children of the mother will receive the trait, but only the female children are able to transmit the trait to the next generation. Both men and women can be afflicted with the optic neuropathy; however, the incidence is 9:1 men over women. The age of involvement is usually quite young, with most patients being involved in their teens or early twenties. It is unusual, but not unheard of, for patients to experience visual loss later in life.

Clinical Characteristics

Symptoms

• Visual loss is the only ocular symptom of LHON. The visual loss is usually sequential, the second eye being affected within weeks to months of the first. Rarely, both the eyes may be involved simultaneously or there will be only one eye involved.

Signs

• Decreased visual acuity, usually 20/200 or worse. Vision may be lost abruptly or may progressively worsen over days.

• An RAPD if unilateral or asymmetric

• Dyschromatopsia

• Optic disc changes are characteristic of this disorder (Fig. 5-44).

• Visual field defect, which is usually a central or cecocentral scotoma, with relative sparing of the peripheral vision (Fig. 5-45A).

• *Acute phase:* The optic disc is usually swollen and hyperemic. There are often circumpapillary telangiectasias that are characteristic of LHON. The nerve fiber layer appears opacified, but there is no leakage from the optic disc on fluorescein angiography.

• *Chronic phase:* Optic nerve pallor often localized to the papillomacular bundle area

Differential Diagnosis

• Optic neuritis: Most patients are initially misdiagnosed as having optic neuritis because of the unilateral visual loss, swollen optic nerve, and very young age. Involvement of the second eye in a short period of time would be unusual for optic neuritis.

• Ischemic optic neuropathy: This is an unusual finding in the age range that is usually affected by LHON.

• Papilledema: This diagnosis is usually considered when both optic nerves are swollen. However, the profound loss of vision in the presence of optic disc edema that is not chronic papilledema establishes that this is not the correct diagnosis.

Diagnostic Evaluation

• Determination of genetic mutation. Laboratory testing is available for the primary and secondary mutations. Screening for the three primary mutations in the mitochondrial DNA (positions 11778, 14484, 3460). The 11778 mutation is the most common.

• Fluorescein angiography is employed to demonstrate the peripapillary telangiectasias

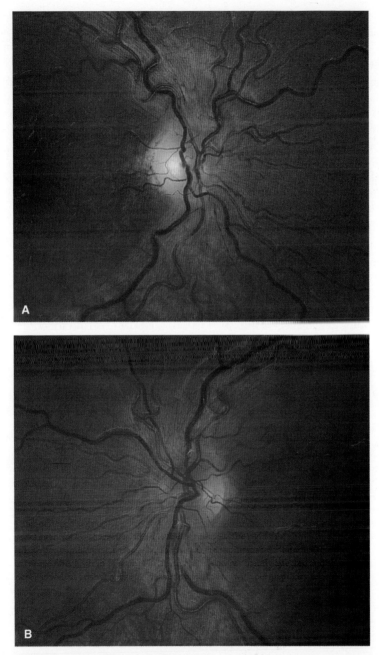

FIGURE 5-44. Leber hereditary optic neuropathy.   A 17-year-old man with visual loss with central scotoma first in OD then 2 weeks later in OS. There is bilateral disc elevation. **A.** The right disc shows opacification of the retinal nerve fiber layer with peripapillary telangiectasia. The area of the papillomacular bundle (temporal disc) is pale with loss of the retinal nerve fiber layer in this area. **B.** The left eye is more recently affected and shows hyperemia in the papillomacular area as well as retinal nerve fiber layer opacification with peripapillary telangiectasia.

and the absence of leakage from the optic disc.

● MRI scan may show subtle enhancement of the affected optic nerve, but neuroimaging is unnecessary in this disorder.

Associated Clinical Features

● Cardiac conduction defects, usually preexcitation syndromes, are seen in some patients with LHON.

● An MS-like disorder may appear in some patients.

Prognosis

● Usually the vision remains poor once LHON has occurred. Some patients, however, may experience spontaneous recovery of visual acuity months to years later. This can occur by a gradual fading of the central scotoma or by the development of a small, clear area in the midst of the central scotoma, allowing the patient better visual acuity (Fig. 5-45B). Patients with the primary mutation 14484 tend to have the best chance of visual recovery (60%), whereas those with the 11778 (4%) mutation have the poorest. Patients who are afflicted at a younger age appear to have a higher chance of visual recovery.

● Not all those who test positive for a mutation will develop visual loss but visual loss occurs in 20% to 60% of men and 4% to 32% of women.

Treatment

● No treatment is available for LHON. A randomized trial investigating idebenone, a potent antioxidant and inhibitor of lipid peroxidation, suggested there may be some mild benefit in patients with recent attacks.

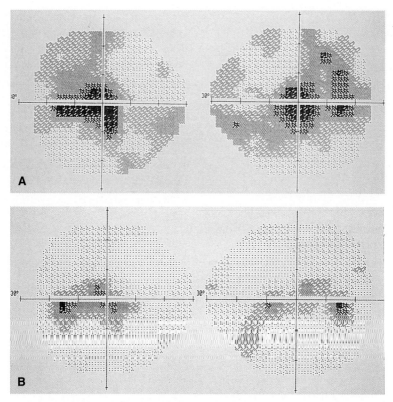

FIGURE 5-45. **Leber hereditary optic neuropathy. A.** Visual fields of a patient with Leber hereditary optic neuropathy with dense central scotomas and vision of 20/400 bilaterally. **B.** Vision improved to 20/25 OD and 20/40 OS 2.5 years later. The central scotomas are much less dense bilaterally.

DOMINANT OPTIC ATROPHY

Dominant optic atrophy (DOA) is statistically the most frequently inherited optic neuropathy. Visual acuity loss is usually moderate and hence diagnosis is often delayed. It is characterized by symmetrical, slowly progressive visual loss.

Epidemiology and Etiology

• The estimated prevalence of DOA is approximately 1:50,000. It is inherited in a dominant fashion. Genetic analysis has isolated one of the DOA genes (OPA1) on chromosome 3q28 to 29. However, visual loss is variable within families. It affects men and women equally.

Clinical Characteristics

Symptoms

• Decreased acuity usually occurs by the age of 10 years but may be minimal and go unnoticed by the patient for years.

• Acquired dyschromatopsia, with many patients having tritanopia (blue/yellow) as the predominant color vision anomaly, as opposed to other optic neuropathies that have deuteranopia (red/green)-type color defects. Some patients with DOA will have nonspecific color confusion.

Signs

• The acuity loss is bilateral and progressive but does not usually fall below 20/200.

• Pallor of the optic disc temporally affecting the papillomacular bundle area (Fig. 5-46A-D)

• Bilateral central or cecocentral scotomas (Fig. 5-46E & F)

Differential Diagnosis

• Other bilateral optic neuropathies, mainly toxic or nutritional

Diagnostic Evaluation

• A D-15 or Farnsworth–Munsell 100 Hue test may be used to document the tritanopia (Fig. 5-46G). Genetic testing now is available commercially.

Treatment

• Genetic counseling. No therapy is effective.

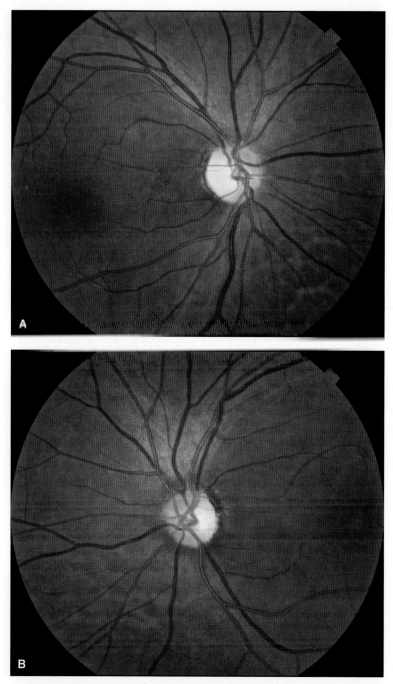

FIGURE 5-46. Dominant optic atrophy.   A, B. Optic discs pale sectorally in the papillomacular bundle area with visible loss of this bundle. Retinal pigment abnormalities are seen in the macula.

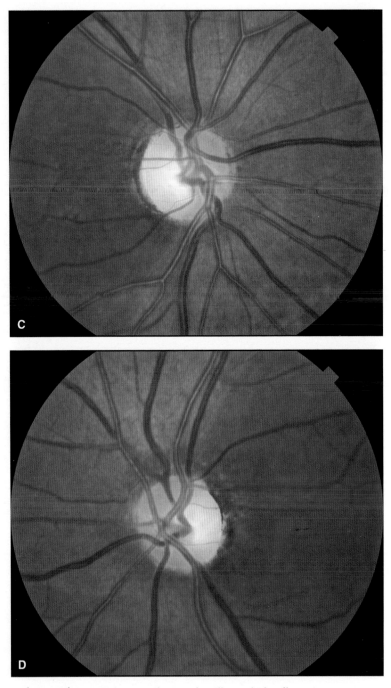

FIGURE 5-46. (*continued*) **C, D.** Higher magnification of papillomacular bundle area.

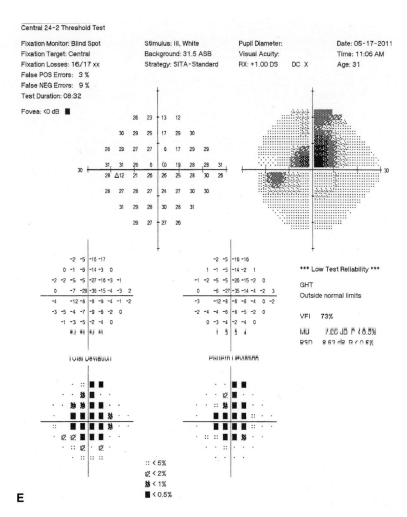

Central 24-2 Threshold Test

Fixation Monitor: Blind Spot
Fixation Target: Central
Fixation Losses: 16/17 xx
False POS Errors: 3 %
False NEG Errors: 9 %
Test Duration: 08:32

Fovea: <0 dB ■

Stimulus: III, White
Background: 31.5 ASB
Strategy: SITA-Standard

Pupil Diameter:
Visual Acuity:
RX: +1.00 DS   DC X

Date: 05-17-2011
Time: 11:06 AM
Age: 31

```
              26  23   13  12
          30  29  25  17  29  30
      28  29  27  27   6  17  29  29
      31  31  26   6  <0  19  28 ,28  31
  30                 
      28 Δ12  21  26  26  25  28  30  26
      28  27  28  27  24  27  30  30
          31  29  28  30  28  31
              29  27   27  26
```

```
     -2  -5 |-16 -17
   0  -1  -6|-14 -3  0
 -2 -2 -2  -5|-27 -16 -3 -1
  0    -7 -28|-39 -15 -4 -3  2
 -4    -12 -8|-8  -9 -4 -1 -2
 -3 -5 -4 -7|-9 -6  -2  0
 -1 -3 -5|-2 -4  0
```

Total Deviation

```
     -2  -5 |-16 -16
   1  -1  -5|-14 -2  1
 -1 -2 -2  -5|-26 -15 -2  0
  0    -6 -27|-35 -14 -4 -2  3
 -3    -12 -8|-8  -8 -4  0 -2
 -2 -4 -4 -6|-8 -5  -2  0
  0 -3 -4|-2 -4  0
```

Pattern Deviation

*** Low Test Reliability ***

GHT
Outside normal limits

VFI   73%

MD   7.00 dB P <0.5%
PSD   8.62 dB P <0.5%

:: < 5%
✗ < 2%
✗✗ < 1%
■ < 0.5%

E

FIGURE 5-46. (*continued*) **E, F.** Visual fields show bilateral central scotomas. (© 2007 Carl Zeiss Meditec.)

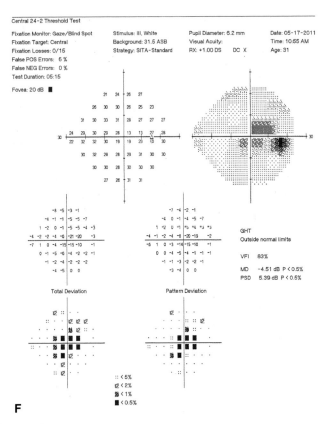

Central 24-2 Threshold Test

Fixation Monitor: Gaze/Blind Spot   Stimulus: III, White   Pupil Diameter: 6.2 mm   Date: 05-17-2011
Fixation Target: Central   Background: 31.5 ASB   Visual Acuity: Time: 10:55 AM
Fixation Losses: 0/15   Strategy: SITA-Standard   RX: +1.00 DS   DC   X   Age: 31
False POS Errors: 6 %
False NEG Errors: 0 %
Test Duration: 05:15

Fovea: 20 dB

GHT
Outside normal limits

VFI   83%

MD   −4.51 dB P < 0.5%
PSD   5.39 dB P < 0.5%

Total Deviation

Pattern Deviation

:: < 5%
🟦 < 2%
🔷 < 1%
■ < 0.5%

F

FIGURE 5-46. (*continued*)

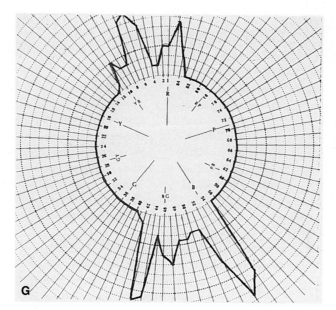

FIGURE 5-46. (*continued*) **G.** The Farnsworth–Munsell 100 Hue axis is a blue–yellow deficiency, characteristic of DOA. A 30-year-old man with decreased vision since childhood.

CONGENITALLY ANOMALOUS DISCS (PSEUDOPAPILLEDEMA)

The normal optic disc is a rounded structure in the fundus and usually consists of a central cup. The disc is relatively flat to the retinal surface. Elevation of the optic disc above the retinal surface may be an acquired phenomenon (papillitis, papilledema) but may also be congenital. This condition may be bilateral and may be confused with papilledema because of increased ICP, thus the term "pseudopapilledema."

Etiology

● This is a congenital phenomenon and may be familial.

Clinical Characteristics

● The characteristics of a typical congenitally anomalous optic disc (Fig. 5-47A, B) are as follows:

   ▪ Is devoid of a physiologic cup

   ▪ Has the blood vessels originating at the center of the disc

   ▪ Is yellow or gray in color, not hyperemic

   ▪ Has abnormalities of the large blood vessels including loops, coils, and multiple branching patterns

   ▪ Is obliquely inserted into the globe (Fig. 47C, D).

   ▪ Some congenitally anomalous discs contain hyaline bodies (drusen) (Fig. 5-48; see p. 185).

   ▪ Normally the retinal nerve fiber layer is devoid of myelin. Occasionally, myelin does extend from the retrolaminar optic nerve into the retina appearing as opacified white areas of nerve fibers (Fig. 5-49). They may cause confusion with papilledema when they are in the immediate peripapillary area.

Differential Diagnosis

● Congenitally anomalous discs may be confused with the acquired disc elevation of papilledema. Table 5-21 contrasts the appearance of a congenitally anomalous disc with that of true papilledema.

Diagnostic Evaluation

● If the ophthalmoscopic appearance is typical of a congenitally anomalous disc, and/or the presence of hyaline bodies or myelinated nerve fibers has been documented, no further investigations are required.

TABLE 5-21. Clinical Appearance of Congenitally Anomalous Disc vs. Papilledema

	Congenitally Anomalous Disc	Papilledema
Laterality	Unilateral in one-third of patients	Bilateral
Disc color	Yellowish white	Hyperemic
Vessels	Anomalous large vessels with loops, coils, and multiple branching patterns	Increased capillaries on the disc surface
Cup	Absent	Present until late in the course
Hemorrhage	Unusual	Frequent
Other	Drusen (hyaline bodies) may be visible in the disc	Small concretions (pseudodrusen) are a sign of chronic disc edema
Retinal nerve fiber layer	Clear	Opacified

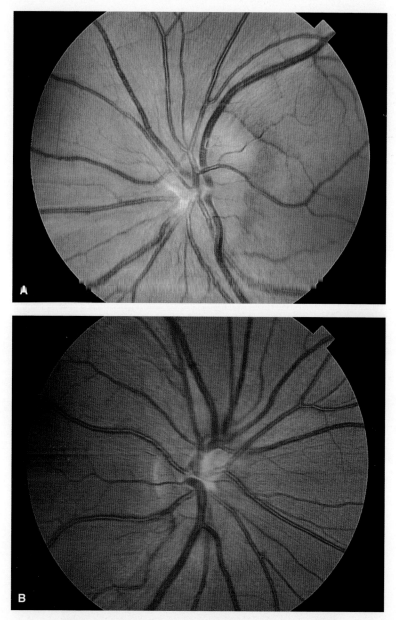

FIGURE 5-47. **Congenitally anomalous disc. A, B.** Congenitally anomalous disc. Optic discs are elevated with no physiologic cup. There is a remnant of glial tissue centrally on each disc. The retinal nerve fiber layer is not opacified.

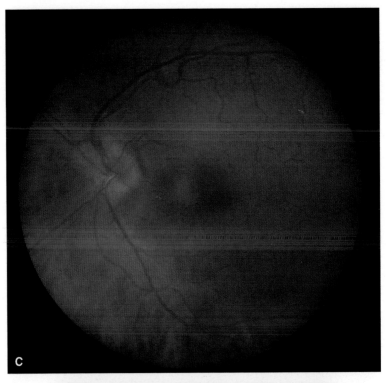

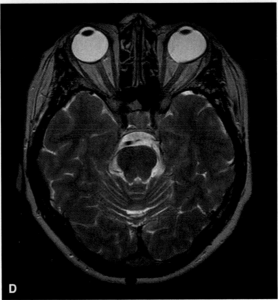

FIGURE 5-47. (*continued*) **C.** Obliquely inserted optic disc simulating disc edema. **D.** MRI shows misshapen left globe with oblique entry of the optic nerve into the globe.

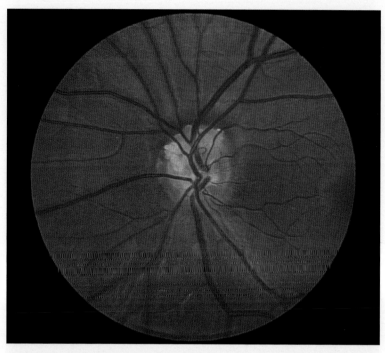

FIGURE 5-48. Congenitally anomalous optic disc with visible drusen superiorly. Note absence of retinal nerve fiber layer striations superiorly and their presence inferiorly, where there are no drusen.

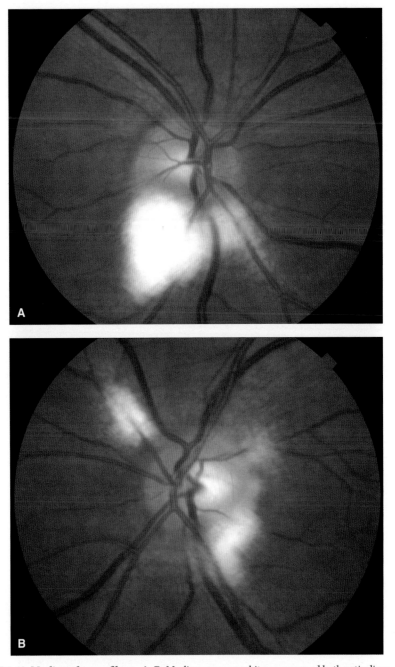

FIGURE 5-49. **Myelinated nerve fibers. A, B.** Myelin appears as white areas around both optic discs.

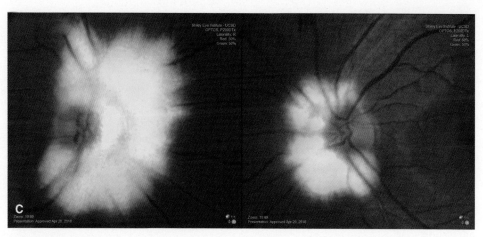

FIGURE 5-49. (*continued*) **C.** A 25-year-old woman with bilateral myelinated nerve fibers investigated in ER for papilledema.

OPTIC DISC DRUSEN

These are accumulations of a *hyaline* material within the optic nerve. The drusen become progressively larger as the patient ages.

Epidemiology and Etiology

• Inherited: The exact pattern is not known, although it has been suggested to be an irregular dominant trait with incomplete penetrance.

• Drusen tend to occur almost exclusively in Caucasians and are present in about 1% of the population.

• They are bilateral in approximately 70% of the cases.

Clinical Characteristics

Symptoms

• Usually the patient is asymptomatic. The disorder is usually detected on a routine ophthalmologic examination. However, occasionally, the associated visual field defects may be symptomatic.

Signs

• Acuity is usually intact

• An RAPD if unilateral or asymmetric

• Visual field defects are usually arcuate defects, especially inferiorly. They can slowly progress. It is rare, however, for central acuity to be decreased by drusen of the optic disc.

• Characteristic appearance of glistening material within the optic disc (Fig. 5-50). In children, drusen usually remain "buried" in small, pink optic disc and become more apparent in the succeeding decades (Fig. 5-51). These discs have indistinct margins and anomalous branching of the central retinal vessels may occur (see congenitally anomalous disc).

• Several types of hemorrhage may be associated with disc drusen:

■ Peripapillary nerve fiber layer (splinter) hemorrhages

■ Hemorrhages on the optic disc overlying the drusen (Fig. 5-51 middle right)

■ Peripapillary, crescent-shaped hemorrhages that may be subretinal or beneath the RPE. The typical alterations of the peripapillary RPE occur on resolution of these sub-RPE hemorrhages (Fig. 5-52).

■ Vitreous hemorrhage

■ Bleeding from a subretinal neovascular membrane that may be adjacent to or distant from the optic disc (Fig. 5-53)

■ Peripapillary hemorrhage from AION that can occur on the background of drusen

Differential Diagnosis

• Papilledema is bilateral and the optic disc drusen are buried within the substance of the disc and not visible ophthalmoscopically.

Diagnostic Evaluation

• Visualization of the drusen ophthalmoscopically establishes the diagnosis and no further testing is necessary.

• If the drusen are not obvious, B-scan ultrasonography will establish their presence (Fig. 5-54).

• CT scan may also detect the presence of optic disc drusen (Fig. 5-55).

• Drusen will autofluoresce before the injection of dye during fluorescein angiography. Modern retinal autofluorescence is also effective in demonstrating drusen (Fig. 5-56).

• Optical coherence tomography is a useful tool to show the extent of the buried drusen (Figs. 5-57 and 5-58).

Treatment

• No therapy is effective.

Special Comment

• If the patient has elevated intraocular pressures, it is often impossible to tell if the progressive visual field loss is due to drusen or glaucoma, because in glaucoma, discs with drusen often do not develop typical cupping.

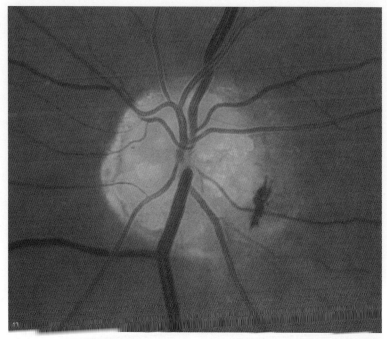

FIGURE 5-50. **Optic nerve drusen.** The optic disc contains drusen appearing as glistening masses throughout the disc. There is peripapillary pigment atrophy and hypertrophy frequently noted in drusen.

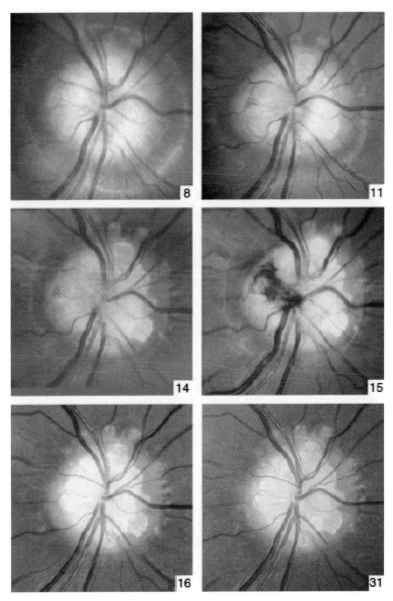

FIGURE 5-51. **Optic nerve drusen.** Progression of optic disc drusen over time in a single patient. The patient's age at each stage is in the photo inset.

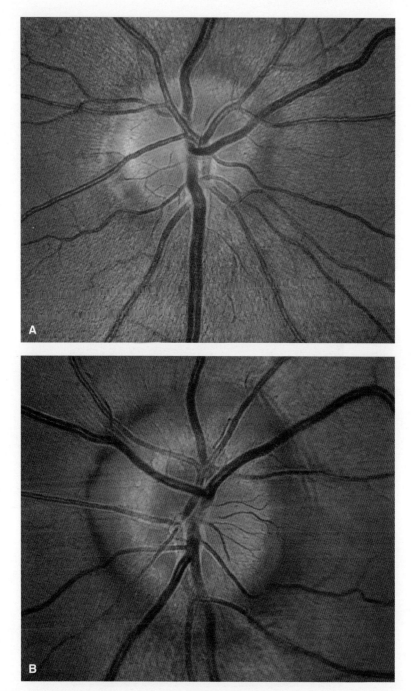

FIGURE 5-52. Optic nerve drusen. The top disc (**A**) has peripapillary pigment atrophy. Bottom optic disc (**B**) has circumpapillary subretinal hemorrhage.

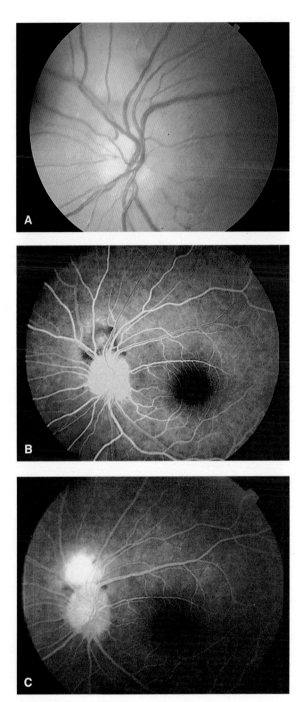

FIGURE 5-53. Optic nerve drusen. A. Congenitally anomalous disc with visible drusen. There is a crescent-shaped hemorrhage at the superior pole with retinal nerve fiber layer edema. **B, C.** Fluorescein angiography shows early blockage of background fluorescence by the hemorrhage and edema at 12 o'clock (0.21.8 seconds). Leakage of dye with late straining is typical of a subretinal neovascular membrane.

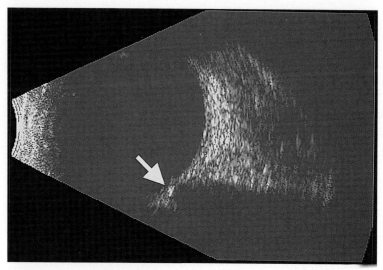

FIGURE 5-54. **Optic nerve drusen.** Ultrasonogram in B-scan mode illustrating calcified disc drusen (*arrow*).

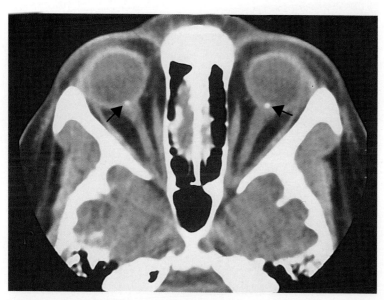

FIGURE 5-55. **Optic nerve drusen.** Unenhanced axial CT scan with drusen appearing as a white spot in the area of each optic disc (*arrows*).

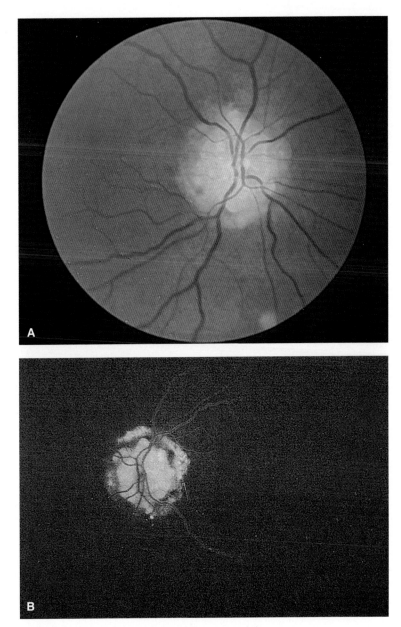

FIGURE 5-56. **Optic disc drusen** (**A**) showing autofluorescence (**B**).

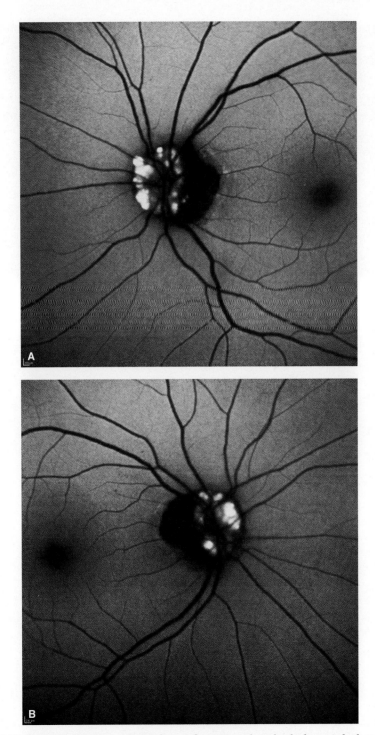

FIGURE 5-57. Optic nerve drusen. A, B. Fundus autofluorescence shows bright drusen in both optic discs.

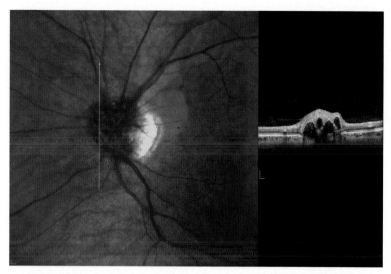

FIGURE 5-58. Optic nerve drusen. Optical coherence tomography showing typical appearance of buried drusen nasally, in the area of the cursor.

OPTIC NERVE HYPOPLASIA

Optic nerve hypoplasia is a congenital anomaly in which the optic nerve is smaller than usual. This phenomenon is present from birth and does not progress. It is frequently associated with other CNS abnormalities. Complete absence of the optic disc (aplasia) is very rarely encountered.

Etiology and Epidemiology

● Several risk factors are associated with the development of optic nerve hypoplasia. These include a young maternal age, primaparity, and maternal insulin-dependent diabetes mellitus.

● Some but not all studies implicate the use of alcohol (fetal alcohol syndrome) and various drugs (illicit drugs, quinine, and some anticonvulsants) during pregnancy have been implicated as causes of optic nerve hypoplasia.

● Maternal weight loss and early gestational vaginal bleeding have also been implicated as etiologic correlates.

Clinical Characteristics

Symptoms

● Decreased vision in one or both eyes.

● Vision may vary from normal acuity with a constricted visual field to no light perception.

● Patients may experience growth retardation and hormonal imbalances.

Signs

● An RAPD if unilateral or asymmetric

● Strabismus is often present

● The optic disc is smaller than normal and often surrounded by a ring of choroid (double ring sign) (Fig. 5-59). Histopathologically, the outer ring corresponds to the normal junction between the lamina cribrosa and the sclera. The inner ring represents the termination of retina and RPE over the lamina cribrosa.

■ Astigmatism is frequently associated with hypoplasia.

Diagnostic Evaluation

● The primary investigation in patients with optic nerve hypoplasia is endocrinologic. These patients will often have growth retardation and corticotropin deficiency; therefore, they should be referred to a pediatric endocrinologist.

● MRI scanning might be considered given that the optic nerve hypoplasia may be associated with intracranial developmental abnormalities which include

■ hemispheric migration anomalies (schizencephaly, cortical heterotopia),

■ intrauterine or perinatal injury (periventricular leukomalacia, encephalomalacia, porencephaly), and

■ posterior pituitary ectopia.

Treatment

● The only treatment is occlusion therapy to combat any amblyopia that might have developed as a result of the optic nerve hypoplasia and/or strabismus.

Special Forms

Hemihypoplasia: Topless Disc Syndrome

● A special form of optic nerve hypoplasia occurs in children of insulin-dependent diabetic mothers. This form is characterized by hypoplasia of the superior portion of one or both optic nerves (Fig. 5-60A) and rather dense inferior arcuate or altitudinal visual field defects (Fig. 5-60B).

● Often, the patients are unaware of these visual field defects because they exist from birth.

Septo-optic Dysplasia: de Morsier Syndrome

- Septo-optic dysplasia refers to:
  - Small anterior visual pathways (Fig. 5-61)
  - Agenesis of corpus callosum
  - Absence of septum pellucidum

- Other associated features may include:
  - Pituitary dwarfism
  - Diabetes insipidus
- This may not be as specific a syndrome as previously believed.

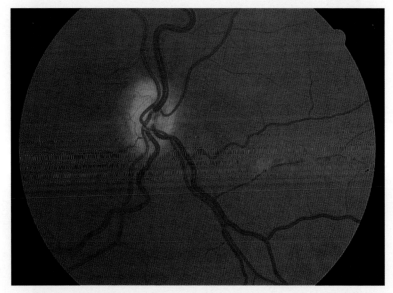

FIGURE 5-59. **Optic nerve hypoplasia.** There is almost no disc tissue. The central white area is sclera. Note that the retinal nerve fiber layer is absent and the retinal blood vessels are of normal size.

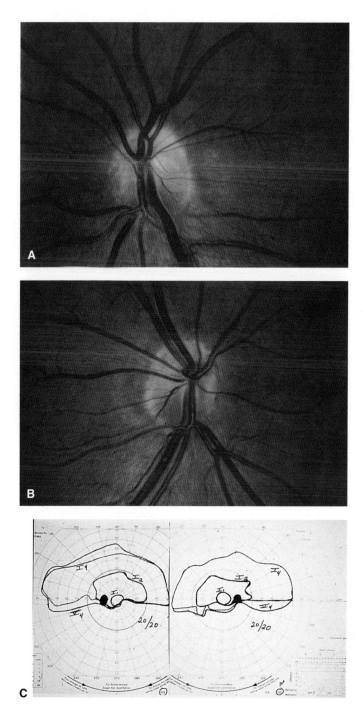

FIGURE 5-60. Optic nerve hemihypoplasia. A, B. The optic discs are hypoplastic superiorly. The central vessels, which are of normal caliber, exit at the very top (not the center) of the disc. **C.** Kinetic perimetry shows bilateral inferior altitudinal defects with preserved central acuity.

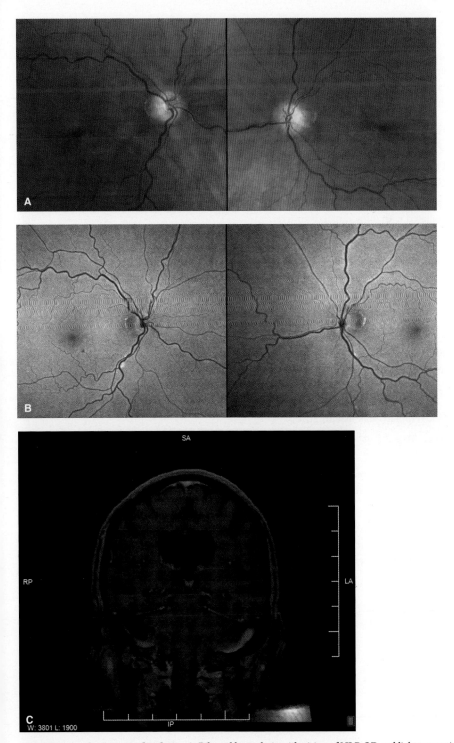

FIGURE 5-61. Septo-optic dysplasia. A. Bilateral hypoplasia with vision of NLP OD and light perception (LP) OS in a patient with septo-optic dysplasia. **B.** Fundus autofluorescence shows small size of the discs. **C.** MRI shows absences of the septum pellucidum.

OPTIC DISC COLOBOMAS

Colobomas of the optic disc are congenital anomalies in which the optic disc is dysplastic and may be larger than normal or has other defects that are visible ophthalmoscopically.

Etiology and Epidemiology

● Colobomas are the result of the failure of fusion of the embryonic fissure during the fifth to sixth weeks of gestation.

● They are usually isolated findings and are rarely associated with intracranial disorders, such as transsphenoidal encephaloceles and other signs of a midline cleft syndrome.

● They commonly occur bilaterally.

Clinical Characteristics

Symptoms

● Decreased vision to a variable extent in one or both eyes or the patients may be asymptomatic.

Signs

● An RAPD if unilateral or asymmetric

● Optic nerve–type visual field defects that are not progressive

● Usually, they are positioned inferiorly and can affect the optic disc, retina, choroid, inferior iris, and lens.

● Common ophthalmoscopic findings (Fig. 5-62):

  ▪ Enlarged disc that may be partially or completely excavated

  ▪ Peripapillary pigmentary changes are common (either hyper- or hypopigmentation)

  ▪ The coloboma has a glistening white appearance.

  ▪ The retinal blood vessels are normal.

● Serous retinal detachments: Nonrhegmatogenous

● A variety of ocular anomalies may be associated with colobomas (Table 5-22).

Diagnostic Evaluation

● An MRI scan is not required because transsphenoidal encephaloceles are rarely encountered with colobomas but more frequently with the so-called morning glory disc anomaly (Fig. 5-63).

Treatment

● No treatment is effective, except for occlusion therapy for amblyopia that may have developed as a result of these dysplastic lesions of the optic disc.

TABLE 5-22. Associated Ocular Features of Colobomas

Posterior lenticonus
Congenital optic disc pit
Hyaloid artery remnant
Posterior embryotoxon
Myopia
Strabismus (in children)

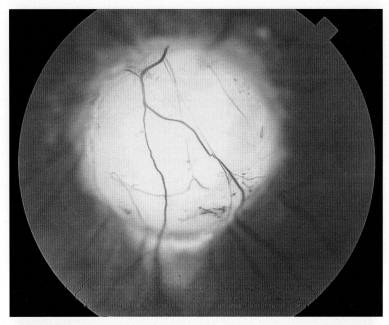

FIGURE 5-62. **Optic disc coloboma.** The optic disc is enlarged, but there is disc tissue superiorly. There is minimal retinal pigment epithelium pigmentation change and the defect extends inferiorly in the area of the embryonic fissure. The retinal vasculature is normal.

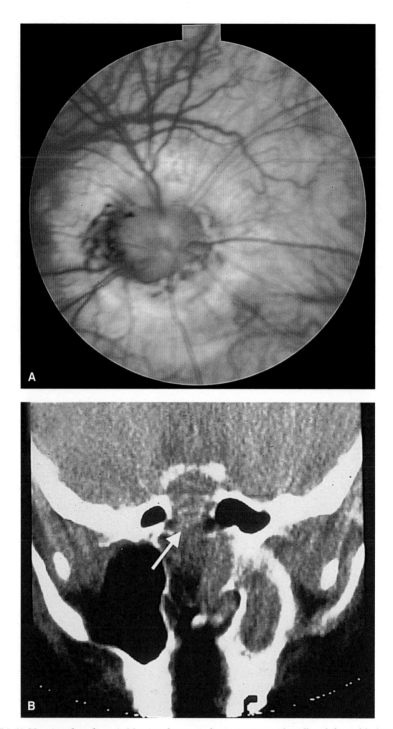

FIGURE 5-63. **Morning glory disc.** **A.** Morning glory optic disc in a patient with midline defects of the lip and palate. **B.** Coronal CT scan shows midline defect in the sphenoid bone with herniation of tissue into the nasopharynx (*arrow*).

OPTIC PIT

Optic pits appear as dark depressions in the optic nerve. They are typically located inferotemporally on the optic disc. They may communicate with the subarachnoid space.

Etiology and Epidemiology

• The optic pit is a form of optic disc dysplasia that is thought to occur during development prior to the differentiation of the neural retina and the optic nerve head. It is actually a defect in the lamina cribrosa into which grow areas of dysplastic retina.

• The exact cause of the pit formation is unknown.

Clinical Characteristics

• Unilateral in 85%.

• Round or oval depression that may be pigmented in a normal size optic disc (Fig. 5-64).

◼ Vary in size: Quarter to half disc diameter

◼ Rarely, more than one pit may be present (Fig. 5-65).

• Located most frequently in the inferior temporal region of the disc.

• Does not affect the disc margin (unlike coloboma) and the physiologic optic cup remains distinct.

• Peripapillary chorioretinal atrophy with changes in the pigment epithelium where the pit is situated.

• Abnormal vascular pattern:

◼ Cilioretinal artery can be identified arising from the periphery of the pit.

◼ Retinal vessels cross the optic pit.

• Retinal elevation: develops in 30% of the cases and may cause (Fig. 5-66) visual field defects and metamorphopsia.

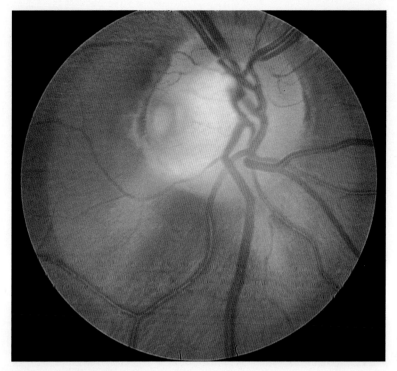

FIGURE 5-64. **Optic pit of right disc in the typical location.** Note pigmentation of pit and adjacent chorioretinal and retinal pigment epithelium defects.

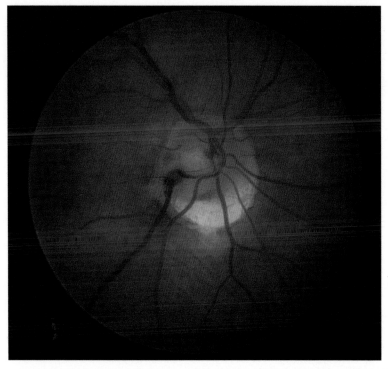

FIGURE 5-65. **Three pits in the right optic disc.** The largest pit has a large artery and vein. The smaller pits are at 6 and 10 o'clock.

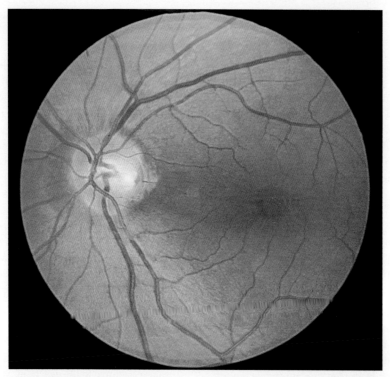

FIGURE 5-66. **Optic pit of the left eye** at 3 o'clock with apparent cilioretinal artery. Macula edema is the cause of decreased vision.

TRAUMATIC OPTIC NEUROPATHY

Jurij R. Bilyk ■

Traumatic optic neuropathy (TON) occurs by a variety of mechanisms, typically in the setting of closed head trauma. The most frequent cause of TON is compressive optic neuropathy from an orbital compartment syndrome from orbital hemorrhage.

Epidemiology and Etiology

● TON occurs most frequently in young men, the population that is most frequently involved in both penetrating and nonpenetrating trauma.

● Mechanisms by which TON may be produced include the following:

■ Blunt head trauma, usually to the forehead, producing a *deceleration injury*. Upon striking a hard object, the bones of the skull and face stop suddenly while the soft tissues (brain, globe, optic nerve, etc.) continue to move forward up to their points of tethering. The optic nerve sheath is fused to the dura of the optic canal, creating a tether to the optic nerve and causing shearing of the nutrient pial vessels during a deceleration injury. A second mechanism may also play a role. One cadaveric study reported that the force of impact on the forehead is propagated and focused at the orbital apex in the area of the optic canal as a shock wave, also producing optic nerve injury. Posterior indirect TON (PITON) is the most common form of TON if orbital hemorrhage is excluded.

■ Patients may develop a TON from *compression* by a bony fragment as a result of fracture of the optic canal (Fig. 5-67) or from an active hemorrhage that is developing in a closed tight compartment (e.g., the orbit). Orbital compartment syndrome is an ophthalmic emergency that necessitates immediate management. It is also the most common form of TON.

■ *Penetrating injury* is a less frequent cause of direct TON because of the relative laxity of the intraorbital optic nerve, which allows for absorption of the impact of the penetrating object. In addition, because the dural tissue of the optic nerve sheath is thick, it resists laceration. If penetration of the dura of the optic nerve does occur, then TON can present by several mechanisms, including transection of nerve fibers or compression from hemorrhage, edema, or impingement on the nerve by a foreign body (Fig. 5-68). This final mechanism must be considered if the foreign body is localized at the orbital apex, where the optic nerve is inflexible because of tethering by the annulus of Zinn.

■ Complete or partial *avulsion* of the optic nerve can occur, usually from a direct rotational force to the eye. In most cases of optic nerve head avulsion, prepapillary vitreous hemorrhage occurs relatively quickly, obscuring the view of the optic nerve head and making definitive diagnosis difficult. Posterior avulsion of the optic nerve at or beyond the orbital apex is also possible and may be associated with significant skull base or intracranial injuries (Fig. 5-69).

■ A rare cause of direct TON is *optic nerve sheath hematoma*. This typically presents with signs of progressive visual loss and optic neuropathy and necessitates the presence of venous congestion or occlusion on funduscopic examination. Arterial compromise may also be noted. CT imaging may show expansion of the optic nerve sheath, but this finding may also be seen in cases of intraconal orbital hemorrhage, where blood within the fat compartment around the optic nerve sheath may give the false impression of a true nerve sheath hematoma.

Clinical Characteristics

Symptoms

- The primary symptom of TON is visual loss (either unilateral or bilateral). The visual loss may be total or partial and subtle.

- Visual field defects should be performed bilaterally when possible.

- The tempo of loss of vision is important in determining its cause. The shearing force injury of posterior indirect TON results in immediate visual loss. The compressive TON from hemorrhage develops more slowly, with the patient initially having preserved vision, but then losing vision over a period of hours. Avulsions result in sudden visual loss.

Signs

- Decreased visual acuity
- Impaired color vision
- An RAPD if unilateral or asymmetric bilateral optic neuropathy

- Orbital hemorrhage presents as ecchymosis and eyelid edema. Proptosis and external ophthalmoplegia are usually present (Fig. 5-70). The orbit will be tight to palpation and lid opening may require the use of retractors. Intraocular pressure may be elevated and signs of vascular compromise may be seen on funduscopic examination.

- Ophthalmoscopy may reveal a partial or complete avulsion of the optic nerve with a ring of hemorrhages at the site of injury. Prepapillary vitreous hemorrhage in the setting of profound visual loss is also suggestive of optic nerve head avulsion.

Diagnostic Evaluation

- In blunt head trauma, the patient should undergo a CT scan, with adequate views of the optic canal, to detect any impinging fractures (Fig. 5-71). CT of the head should also be included to rule out intracranial injury (note that dedicated CT of the head and orbits should be performed. A head CT alone does not provide adequate views of the orbit, and vice versa). If no metallic foreign bodies are seen, an MRI may be considered to look for hematomas that might be causing compression, but is usually unnecessary. These two tests are most important to perform in a situation where the patient had preserved or relatively preserved vision after the trauma and then begins to lose vision. Note that TON from an orbital compartment syndrome requires *immediate* treatment that should not be delayed while awaiting a CT.

- Although a case can be made for an intracranial injury in a patient who suffers immediate loss of vision with head trauma, because this is most likely due to shearing force injury, we recommend at the very least a CT to rule out intracranial injury and impingement of the optic nerve by a bone fragment.

Treatment

- There is no effective treatment for optic nerve head avulsion. If external ophthalmoplegia is present or significant vitreous hemorrhage obscures the view, B-scan ultrasonography may be helpful in ruling out other globe rupture or avulsion of the extraocular muscles. Surgical exploration of the globe and extraocular muscles may be necessary if ultrasonography is equivocal.

- Suspected posterior optic nerve avulsion necessitates urgent imaging of the skull base and head to rule out pituitary, carotid artery, or brain injury, including intracranial hemorrhage.

- The treatment of PITON is limited. No clear benefit to megadose intravenous corticosteroids has been proven, and a large, prospective study of corticosteroid use in traumatic brain injury (TBI) showed an increased long-term morbidity and mortality in patients with TBI who received corticosteroids when compared to controls. Therefore, no patient with PITON and TBI should be given corticosteroids. A study of acute spinal cord injury concluded that megadose corticosteroids may be beneficial if given within the initial 8-hour window following trauma. This finding has been extrapolated by some for the treatment of acute TON. However, limited animal models for TON have also suggested that corticosteroids may result in more axonal injury than no treatment alone. Therefore, at this juncture it is safest NOT to offer megadose corticosteroids (or, for that matter, any dose of corticosteroids) in the management of PITON.

• There have been reports of optic canal decompression in patients with PITON even in patients with normal CT scans, resulting in improvement of vision. These results are controversial and most neuro-ophthalmologists and orbital surgeons in the United States do not employ this method of treatment. In addition, surgical decompression of the optic canal requires intimate knowledge of skull base anatomy and an experienced skull base surgeon because of the inherent morbidity and mortality of the procedure. A meta-analysis by the Cochrane Collaboration failed to find any definitive efficacy for this procedure. Furthermore, a recent cadaveric study concluded that attmepted surgical decompression of the optic canal may result in additional injury to the optic nerve.

• Orbital compartment syndrome from orbital hemorrhage is treated effectively with inferior cantholysis (Fig. 5-72). Lateral canthotomy alone is ineffective therapy. Cantholysis should be performed expeditiously in cases of optic neuropathy to maximize the potential for visual recovery. Intravenous corticosteroid therapy may also help to soften the orbital soft tissues but should only be used in patients without concomitant TBI. A recent study has also found that intravenous mannitol can effectively (albeit temporarily) decrease intraorbital pressure and should be considered if there is any delay in cantholysis (e.g., patient transfer to another facility). Any contraindications to intravenous mannitol and corticosteroids should be discussed first with the primary team.

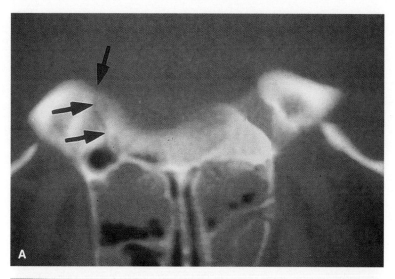

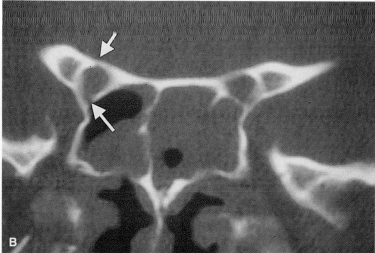

FIGURE 5-67. **Fracture of the optic canal** (*arrows*) shown in axial (**A**) and coronal (**B**) views.

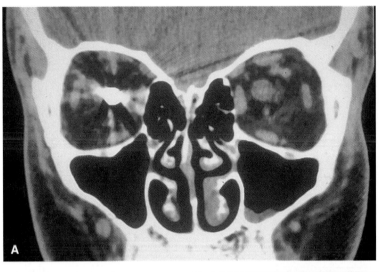

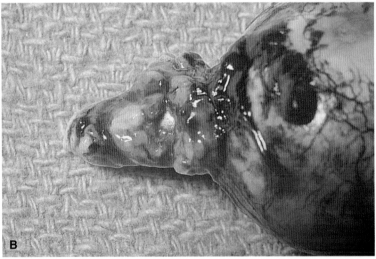

FIGURE 5-68. **Immediate visual loss from a perforating globe injury by a BB pellet. A.** Coronal CT shows proximity of the BB to the optic nerve. **B.** Enucleation specimen demonstrates the BB lodged in the optic nerve.

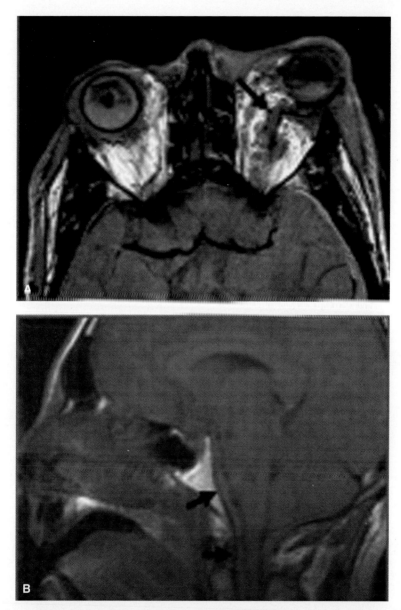

FIGURE 5-69. Optic nerve avulsion with intracranial bleeding and stroke. A. Axial MR fluid-attenuated inversion recovery image shows an abnormal curvature to the left intraorbital optic nerve (*arrow*) consistent with avulsion. **B.** Parasagittal T1-weighted image without contrast reveals a large amount of blood (*arrows*) tracking subdurally along the brain stem.

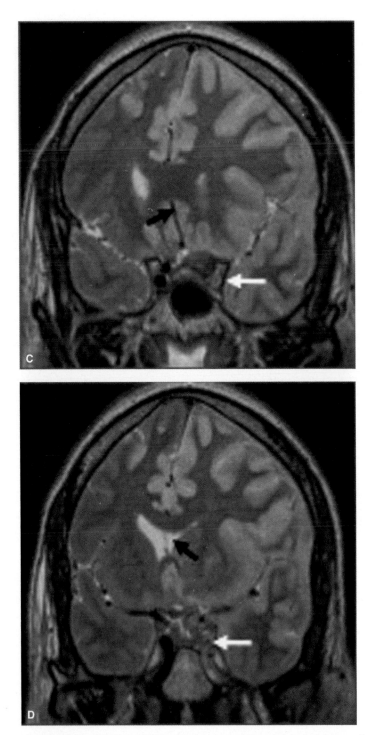

FIGURE 5-69. (*continued*) **C** and **D**. Coronal T2 images demonstrate thrombus in the left internal carotid artery (*white arrows*) at and below the cavernous sinus. Marked left cerebral edema with midline shift and compression of the lateral ventricle (*black arrows*) is present.

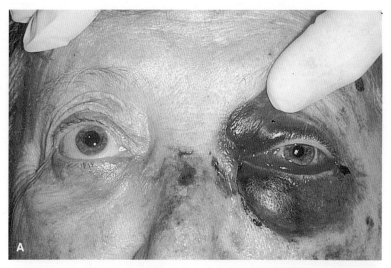

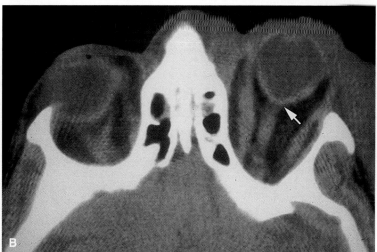

FIGURE 5-70. **Orbital hemorrhage with optic neuropathy. A.** Note the ecchymotic, tense eyelids along with proptosis and external ophthalmoplegia. **B.** Axial CT reveals a "tenting sign" of the globe: distortion of the eyeball by a combination of proptosis and tethering by the optic nerve (*arrow*).

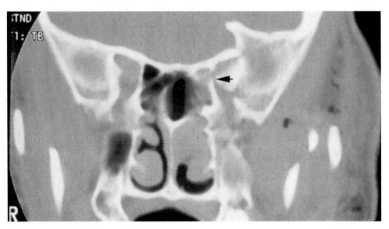

FIGURE 5-71. **Orbital wall fracture.** A lateral wall fracture is displaced medially and compresses the optic nerve between it and the medial orbital wall (*arrow*) at the orbital apex.

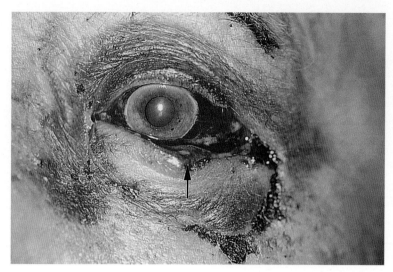

FIGURE 9.7. **Orbital hemorrhage with successful inferior cantholysis.** Note the marked medial migration of the lateral canthus (*arrow*). When performed expeditiously, visual recovery is often complete.

Optic Chiasm

INTRODUCTION

The optic nerves elevate and move medially as they extend intracranially to form the optic chiasm. The optic chiasm, which is the confluence of the optic nerves, sits approximately 10 mm above the dorsum sellae. At the chiasm, the nasal fibers of each optic nerve that represent the temporal visual field cross to the contralateral optic tract. Temporal optic nerve fibers which represent the nasal visual fields proceed posteriorly along the ipsilateral portion of the optic chiasm to join the crossing nasal fibers to form the ipsilateral optic tract. Posterior to the optic chiasm, the optic tracts comprise ipsilateral temporal fibers and contralateral nasal fibers.

Several anatomic features of the chiasm contribute to the specific types and patterns of visual field defects that occur with lesions in this region. Given that optic chiasm lies 10 mm above the roof of the pituitary fossa, pituitary microadenomas or small macroadenomas (Fig. 6-1) do not produce visual field defects. The macular fibers, which comprise 90% of the optic fibers, cross in the posterior aspect of the chiasm. Inferior retinal fibers that represent the superior visual field are located in the inferior portion of the optic chiasm.

The position of the chiasm influences the pattern of visual field loss produced by lesions in the parachiasmal area. The most common position (approximately 80%) for the chiasm is on the diaphragm sellae projecting onto the dorsum sellae. In a prefixed chiasm (15%), the chiasm lies upon the tuberculum sellae or diaphragma sellae, whereas in a postfixed chiasm (5%), the chiasm lies on the dorsum sella posterior to the fossa. The other important structure in the parachiasmal area is the cavernous sinus. The cavernous sinus comprises the venous space situated between the meningeal and periosteal layers of the dura mater on either side of the sphenoid bone. It extends from the end of the superior orbital fissure to the apex of the petrous bone. The cavernous sinus contains the carotid artery and the cranial nerves (CNs) III, IV, and VI. Parachiasmal tumors may cause visual field defects as well as ocular motility disturbances.

Disorders of the optic chiasm initially may present with visual acuity loss. The clinical demonstration of a chiasmal pattern of visual loss enables the physician to order the appropriate tests and to establish the correct diagnosis. The single most important nonradiologic test in determining if the optic chiasm is the involved site producing visual loss is the visual field. The confluence of the optic nerves and the crossing of the nasal fibers at the chiasm, combined with the 90-degree rotation that the visual fibers undergo en route to the chiasm from the retina, orient the nerve fibers along the vertical meridian. Therefore, visual field defects at the optic chiasm and posteriorly will characteristically respect the vertical meridian on perimetric testing.

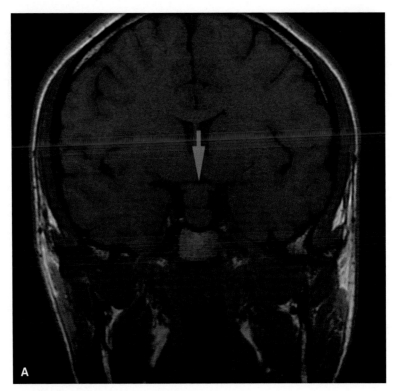

A

FIGURE 6-1. **Small pituitary adenoma.** A 25-year-old man in an auto accident found to have an incidental pituitary tumor in ER. **A.** Adenoma extends to the optic chiasm (*arrow*) but does not elevate or distort it.

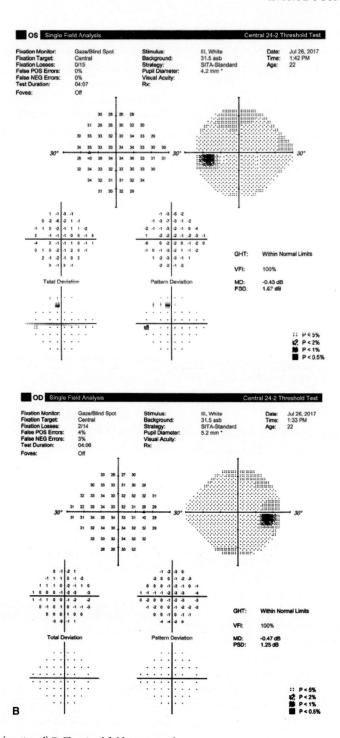

FIGURE 6-1. (*continued*) **B.** The visual fields are normal.

TYPES OF VISUAL FIELD ABNORMALITIES IN CHIASMAL DISEASE

Junction Scotoma

Classically, this is a combination of a central scotoma, or another optic nerve visual field defect, in one eye and a temporal hemianopic defect in the other (Fig. 6-2). The localization of this visual field defect is the junction of the optic nerve, on the side of the central scotoma, and the optic chiasm. The classically accepted cause for this pattern of visual loss is the existence of Wilbrand knee, which is the anterior extension of the inferior nasal crossing fibers from one eye into the opposite optic nerve. Therefore, a lesion of the right optic nerve will produce a right central scotoma and a left superior temporal defect. However, studies in monkeys have failed to show the anatomic existence of Wilbrand knee, despite the fact that the junctional scotoma remains a valid sign that localizes lesions to the junction of the optic nerve and chiasm.

A lesion may involve only the crossing visual fibers at the anterior angle of the optic chiasm. This produces a monocular temporal hemianopic defect with no visual field loss in the contralateral eye.

Bitemporal Hemianopia

It is described in textbooks as the classic visual field abnormality produced by lesions of the body of the optic chiasm. The visual field defects may be complete (Fig. 6-3A) or incomplete (Fig. 6-3B), but always obey the vertical meridian. In most cases, however, pure bitemporal hemianopic defects are infrequent. Usually, there is decreased acuity in one or both eyes. A central bitemporal defect may occur in patients with prefixed chiasm or posterior growing tumors because the macular fibers are located posteriorly in the chiasm.

Homonymous Hemianopia

A parasellar lesion may produce an incongruous homonymous hemianopia by involving the optic tracts. This may occur with mass lesions that are directed posteriorly or because the optic chiasm is prefixed. The homonymous hemianopia often is associated with a central scotoma and a relative afferent pupillary defect (RAPD) on the side of the mass lesion. This is known as the *optic tract syndrome* (see page 256).

Binasal Visual Field Defect

This is said to occur in a patient with a postfixed chiasm in which the lesion is located between both optic nerves along the anterior aspect of the chiasm displacing the optic nerves laterally against the supraclinoid internal carotid arteries or A1 segments of the anterior cerebral arteries. This is such an extraordinarily uncommon visual field defect that we have never encountered.

Any patient with decreased vision of unknown etiology requires a visual field. When the visual field shows one of the defects associated with chiasmal involvement, the next test to perform is an MRI scan.

Etiology

- Approximately 90% of the disorders that produce chiasmal syndromes are mass lesions. The most frequent of these are listed in Table 6-1.

TABLE 6-1. Frequency of Pituitary Mass Lesions*

Type	Percentage
Pituitary adenoma	50–55
Craniopharyngioma	20–25
Meningioma	10
Glioma	7

*Other causes of chiasmal syndrome such as aneurysm and other compressive lesions are relatively uncommon.

Clinical Characteristics

Symptoms

● Visual loss is the most frequent and most important symptom of parachiasmal disorders; other symptoms may be associated with it but are infrequent in the absence of visual loss.

● Headache may be seen with pituitary tumors and implies a stretching of the meninges in the area.

● Diplopia: parachiasmal lesions may cause double vision in several ways:

  ▪ Extension of a mass into one or both cavernous sinuses with involvement of CN III, IV, or VI (Fig. 6-4). This produces a variety of diplopia patterns depending on which CNs are affected.

  ▪ A form of diplopia without presumed ocular misalignment is the so-called *hemifield slide phenomenon*. This phenomenon occurs when patients lose the ability to fuse because the bitemporal hemianopia produces a situation where there is no binocular area of overlapping or interlocking visual field. Thus, the eyes can slide in a vertical plane. These patients have difficulty adding a column of numbers because the numbers from one line suddenly appear on the line above or below. It is difficult, however, to explain how this could occur without ocular misalignment.

● Postfixation blindness: This is a peculiar type of visual disability that afflicts patients with chiasmal disease. The bitemporal hemianopia causes patients to have an area of blindness immediately beyond the point of fixation when viewing something at near (Fig. 6-5). This occurs because when converging on a point, the area beyond the point of regard falls within the blind bitemporal fields.

● Depth perception problems: Patients may complain of difficulty with depth perception, near tasks, or using precision tools.

● Photophobia may occur in patients with parasellar tumors. Possible mechanisms postulated include hypersensitivity of trigeminal nerve endings, chemical meningitis, or a "central dazzle" because of damage to the hypothalamic–thalamic axis.

Signs

● Decreased acuity is usually present, although infrequently a bitemporal hemianopia or other visual field defect may be present with normal acuity.

● Acquired dyschromatopsia in one or both eyes

● Visual field defect (see the previous discussion)

● An RAPD is usually present with asymmetric or unilateral visual loss.

● The optic disc may be normal or pale. Disc edema, or papilledema, is unusual but may be seen, especially with craniopharyngiomas. With bitemporal visual field defects, there is compression of the fibers subserving the nasal retinal. These fibers insert along a horizontal band into the optic nerve head. Hence, a bitemporal visual field defect produces a characteristic band atrophy of the optic disc (Fig. 6-6).

● Ocular misalignment is usually the result of involvement of the CN (III, IV, VI) in the cavernous sinus.

● Endocrinologic signs and symptoms are often seen with chiasmal disorders and include pituitary insufficiency, amenorrhea galactorrhea syndrome in women and impotence in men, acromegaly, precocious puberty, diabetes insipidus, etc.

● Proptosis may occur secondary to vascular obstruction within the cavernous sinus but is unusual.

● See-saw nystagmus occurs rarely and is associated with parasellar lesions. In see-saw nystagmus, one eye elevates and intorts, whereas the other eye depresses and extorts. See-saw nystagmus most commonly occurs with craniopharyngiomas.

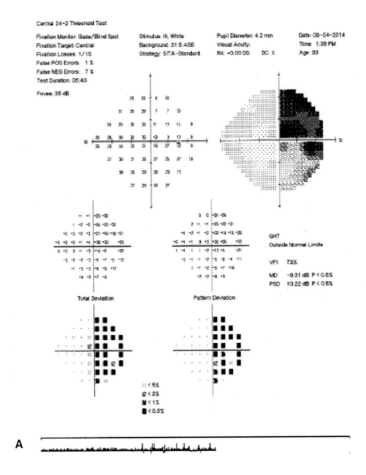

FIGURE 6-2. Junction scotoma. A. Temporal hemianopic defect in the right eye, the left eye vision is no light perception (NLP).

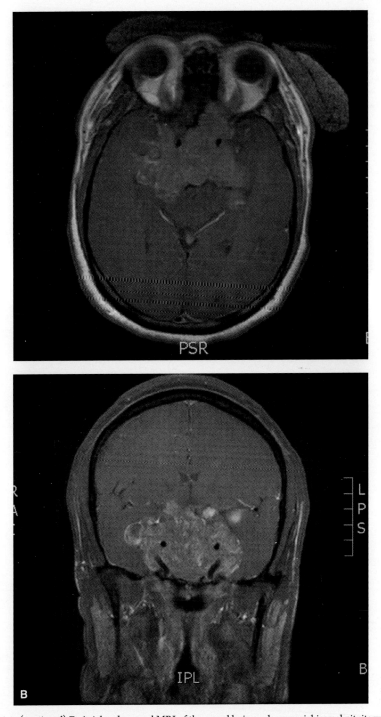

FIGURE 6-2. (*continued*) **B.** Axial and coronal MRI of the causal lesion, a large perichiasmal pituitary tumor.

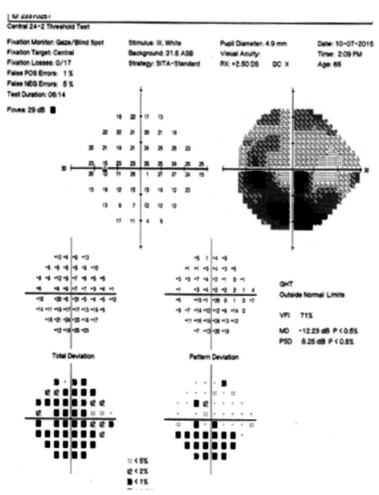

FIGURE 6-2. (*continued*) **C.** Left optic nerve visual field defect (inferior arcuate scotoma) and a temporal hemi-anopic defect in the right eye.

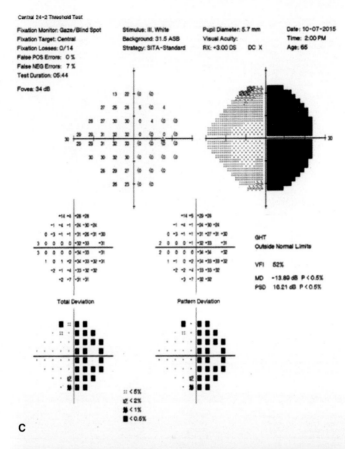

C

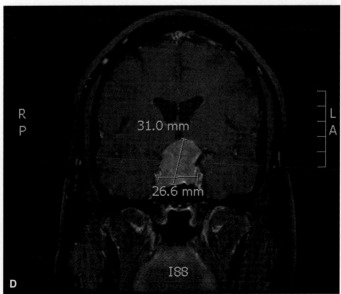

D

FIGURE 6-2. (*continued*) **D.** Coronal MRI showing causative pituitary tumor.

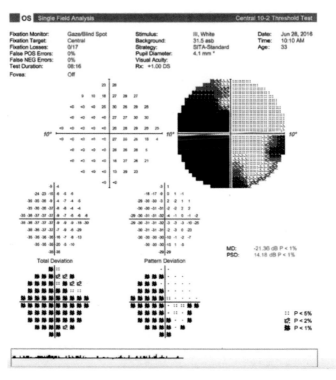

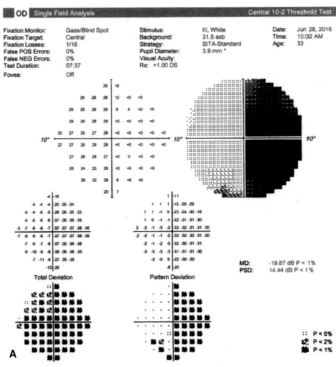

FIGURE 6-3. Bitemporal hemianopia. A. Complete bitemporal hemianopia (Central 10-2).

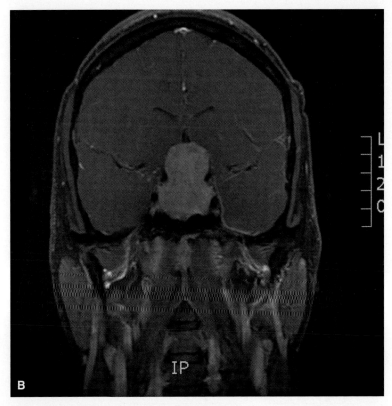

FIGURE 6-3. (*continued*) **B.** Coronal MRI of large pituitary tumor.

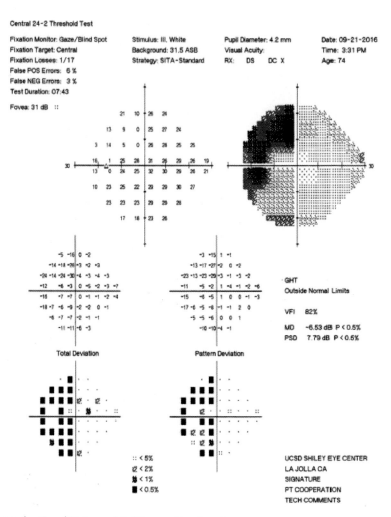

FIGURE 6-3. (*continued*) **C.** Incomplete bitemporal hemianopia.

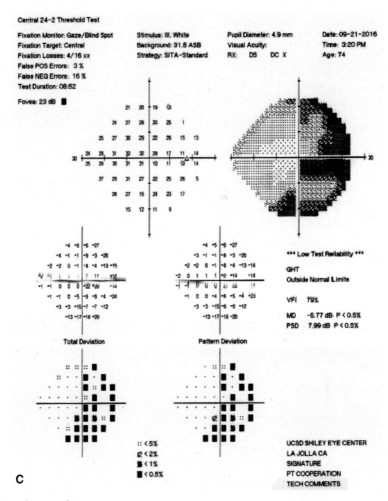

C

FIGURE 6-3. (*continued*)

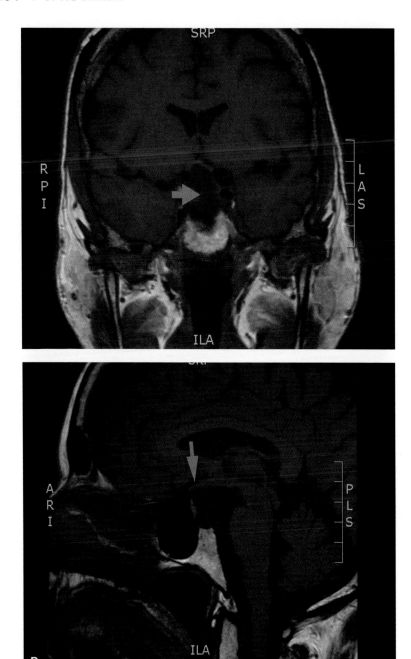

FIGURE 6-3. (*continued*) **D.** Coronal and sagittal MRI show cystic lesion (*arrow*) elevating the optic chiasm (*vertical arrow*).

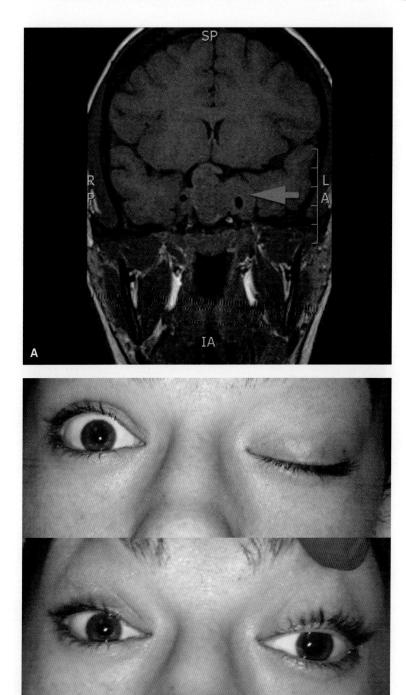

FIGURE 6-4. **Large pituitary tumor.** **A.** Axial MRI shows large pituitary tumor extending into the left cavernous sinus (*arrow*). **B.** The patient presented with a pupil involving left cranial nerve III palsy.

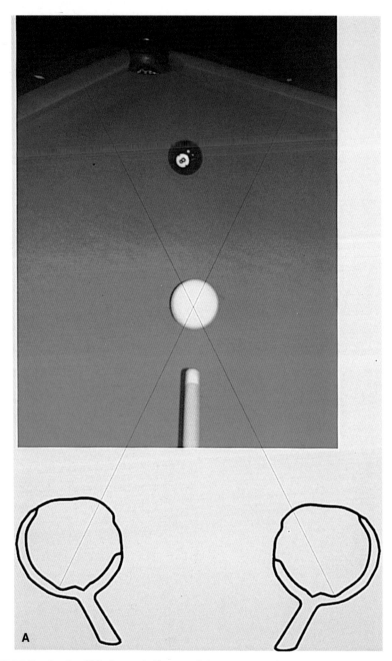

FIGURE 6-5. **Postfixational blindness. A.** The normal view.

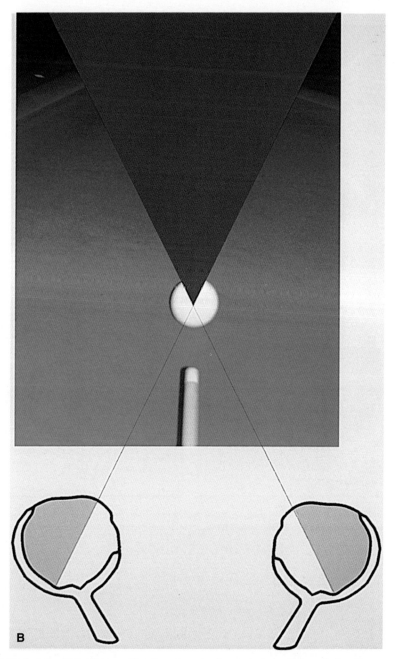

FIGURE 6-5. (*continued*) **B.** Bitemporal hemianopia causes the area in front of the cue ball to disappear.

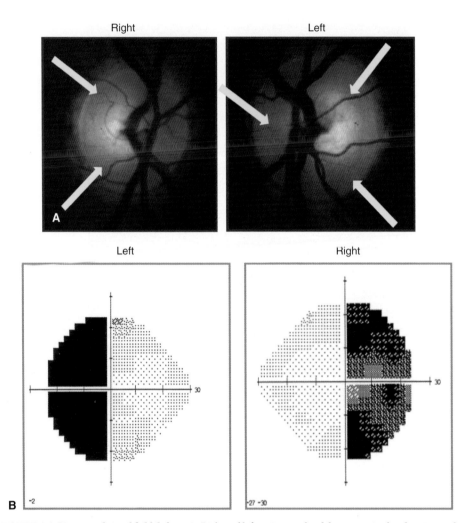

FIGURE 6-6. **Bitemporal visual field defect. A.** Right and left optic nerve head demonstrating band optic atrophy of a patient with a bitemporal visual field defect (**B**).

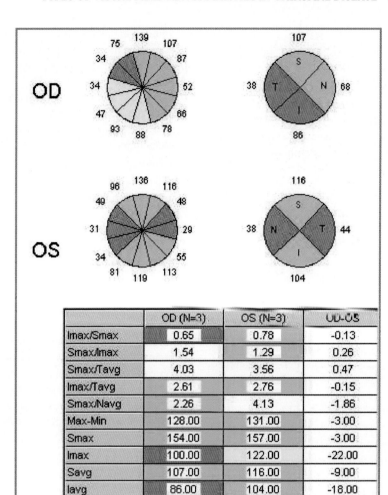

	OD (N=3)	OS (N=3)	OD-OS
Imax/Smax	0.65	0.78	-0.13
Smax/Imax	1.54	1.29	0.26
Smax/Tavg	4.03	3.56	0.47
Imax/Tavg	2.61	2.76	-0.15
Smax/Navg	2.26	4.13	-1.86
Max-Min	128.00	131.00	-3.00
Smax	154.00	157.00	-3.00
Imax	100.00	122.00	-22.00
Savg	107.00	116.00	-9.00
Iavg	86.00	104.00	-18.00
Avg.Thickness	74.92	75.55	-0.62

FIGURE 6-6. (*continued*) **C.** Corresponding optical coherence tomography demonstrating thinning of the retinal nerve fiber layer corresponding to the areas of optic nerve pallor in (**A**). Note the increased thinning of nasal and temporal sectors.

SPECIFIC CAUSES

Pituitary Tumors

Pituitary tumors are the most frequent cause of the chiasmal syndrome. They may be endocrinologically inactive or may secrete a variety of hormones, which produce symptoms other than those produced by compression of the optic chiasm.

- Tumors that secrete prolactin will produce amenorrhea galactorrhea syndrome in women and impotence in men.
- Acromegaly occurs when tumors produce an excessive amount of growth hormone.
- Nelson syndrome is characterized by acquired cutaneous hyperpigmentation and increased adrenocorticotropin levels following a total adrenalectomy for Cushing disease.

The diagnosis of the various forms of pituitary tumors is made by a combination of imaging and endocrinologic findings. The typical MR finding is one of a large mass lesion that displaces and distorts the optic chiasm. Because of its location 10 mm above the dorsum sellae, small pituitary tumors never produce visual field deficits. Tumors must extend out of the sella turcica and become quite large before they produce disturbances of visual acuity or visual field. This makes these tumors readily diagnosable by neuroimaging (Fig. 6-7A).

- Several types of pituitary tumors are important to identify:
    - Prolactin-secreting tumors produce high levels of prolactin and, because of this, are amenable to medical treatment. Prolactin-secreting pituitary tumors that produce visual loss usually produce prolactin levels over 1,000 ng/mL (normal <100 ng/mL). These tumors may dramatically decrease in size with dopamine agonist therapy. The visual field defects may disappear within weeks of instituting bromocriptine or cabergoline (see Fig. 6-7B–D).
    - Endocrinologically inactive pituitary tumors are the most frequent pituitary tumors and produce endocrine abnormalities such as hypothyroidism and hypopituitarism. These tumors are not amenable to medical treatment. In order to decompress the visual pathway, surgery and/or radiation is required.
    - Pituitary apoplexy is a special manifestation of pituitary tumors. Although pituitary tumors produce slowly progressive, almost insidious visual loss, pituitary apoplexy is a dramatic event. The patient experiences *headache* (often as bad as the headache experienced in subarachnoid hemorrhage) and may suddenly develop *blindness* and/or *ophthalmoplegia* in one or both eyes. Pituitary apoplexy is due to a rapid expansion of a preexisting pituitary tumor because of swelling produced by hemorrhage into the tumor (Fig. 6-8). This is an emergency. Patients often are suffering from hypopituitarism and hypocortisolism that should be treated medically to restore normal hormonal levels before invasive procedures are performed.

The role of the ophthalmologist following any treatment for pituitary tumor is to perform sequential visual fields in conjunction with sequential MRIs, and to document as early as possible any recurrence of these tumors.

- A typical schedule for follow-up perimetry is as follows:
    - Every 3 months for the first year, then annually for 5 years
    - After 5 years, every 2 years

Craniopharyngioma

Craniopharyngiomas arise from Rathke pouch, which is located between the anterior and posterior lobes of the pituitary gland. They are seen in children as well as adults. They may be solid or cystic, with the cysts filled with a viscous fluid that contains cholesterol-like flecks.

- The signs and symptoms of craniopharyngioma include the following:
  - Visual acuity loss in one or both eyes
  - Visual field abnormalities
  - Papilledema (may be present but is not common)
  - Endocrinologic abnormalities
  - Adults may become demented or confused

- The diagnosis of craniopharyngioma is based on visual field evaluation, indicating a chiasmal localization and the MR that is characteristic (Fig. 6-9).

- The treatment for craniopharyngioma is surgery. Most often, the tumor cannot be removed in toto; therefore, postoperative radiation or chemotherapy to the tumor bed may be indicated. Close follow-up with visual fields and MRI scan is required because of the propensity of the craniopharyngioma to regrow.

Meningioma

Parachiasmal meningiomas may be suprasellar or located in the area of the tuberculum sellae or planum sphenoidale (Fig. 6-10). They are also slow-growing tumors that often produce visual loss as the only sign. Endocrine abnormalities are much less likely to occur in meningiomas than in pituitary adenomas or craniopharyngiomas.

- The treatment for parachiasmal meningiomas is surgery. Overaggressive surgical removal is to be discouraged, because this will often result in further loss of vision.

- The ophthalmologist's role is to perform visual fields in the postoperative period.

Glioma

Optic gliomas are intrinsic lesions of the optic chiasm that are relatively uncommon. They also produce a chiasmal syndrome with visual acuity and visual field loss and often are associated with neurofibromatosis (NF). Approximately one-third of patients with NF type 1 (NF1) have gliomas of the anterior visual pathways on MRI (Fig. 6-11).

- The symptoms of chiasmal glioma are again those of visual loss and chiasmal visual field abnormalities. The association of NF1 must raise the real possibility of chiasmal glioma.

- Glioma may involve the optic chiasm also in adults. This is a more aggressive glioma, known as malignant glioma of adulthood, and is actually a glioblastoma of the anterior visual pathways. It progresses rapidly, and patients usually expire within 1 year (see Chapter 5).

- The treatment of gliomas is controversial. Some clinicians recommend radiation therapy; chemotherapy is used in some patients, especially children under 5 years of age, where radiation therapy may produce long-term mental deficits.

Other Mass Lesions

Any mass lesion in and around the optic chiasm may produce the same spectrum of clinical signs and symptoms. These include aneurysms, dermoid tumors, and metastatic lesions. The exact diagnosis is arrived at through neuroimaging and, at times, biopsy.

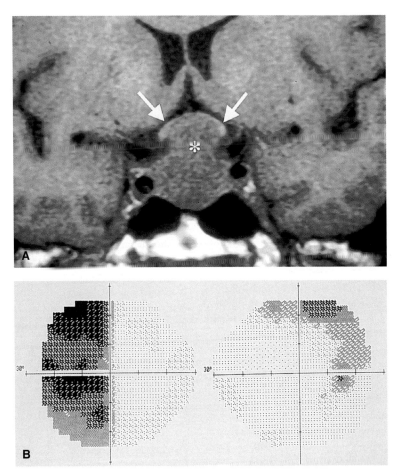

FIGURE 6-7. Pituitary tumor.   Coronal MRI scan showing a large prolactin-secreting pituitary tumor (asterisk) capped by a distorted optic chiasm (*arrows*) (**A**) and corresponding visual fields (**B**).

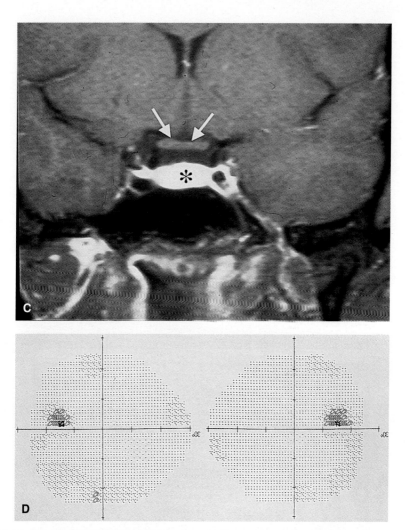

FIGURE 6-7. (*continued*) **C.** Following the administration of bromocriptine, the pituitary tumor shrunk and the optic chiasm is in its normal position (*arrows*) without compression. **D.** Visual fields postbromocriptine therapy show disappearance of the bitemporal hemianopia.

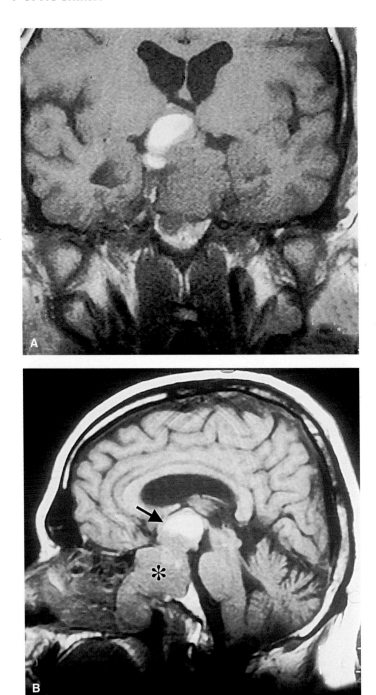

FIGURE 6-8. **Large pituitary tumor.** Coronal (**A**) and sagittal (**B**) MRI of a large pituitary tumor (*asterisk*) capped by a crescent of hyperintense blood (*arrow*), which caused rapid expansion of the tumor.

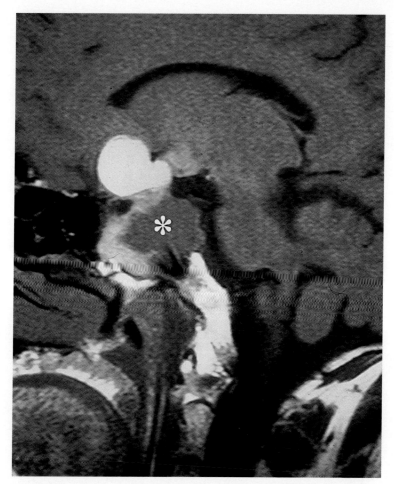

FIGURE 6-9. Craniopharyngioma with a solid component (asterisk) capped by a hyperintense cyst filled with colloid material.

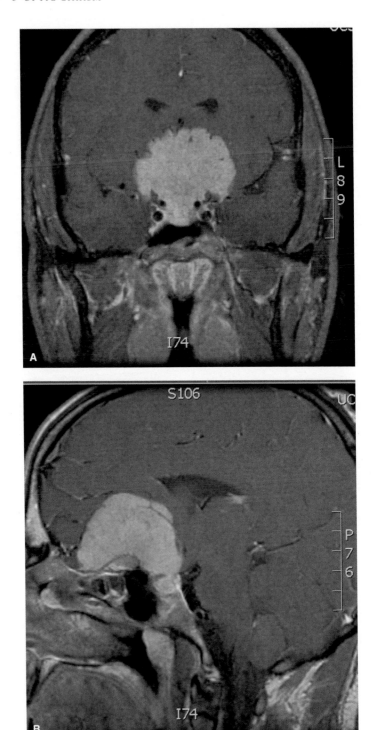

FIGURE 6-10. **Parasellar meningioma.** Coronal (**A**) and sagittal (**B**) MRI showing parasellar meningioma.

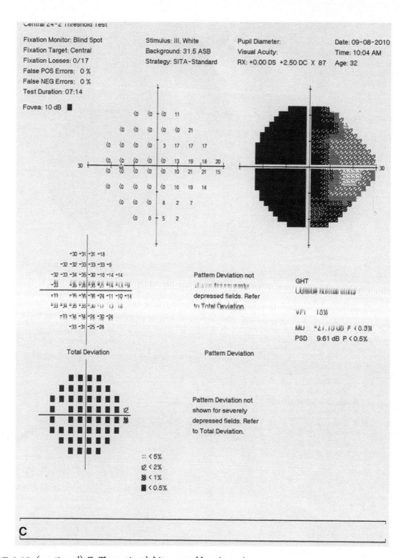

FIGURE 6-10. (*continued*) **C.** The patient's bitemporal hemianopia.

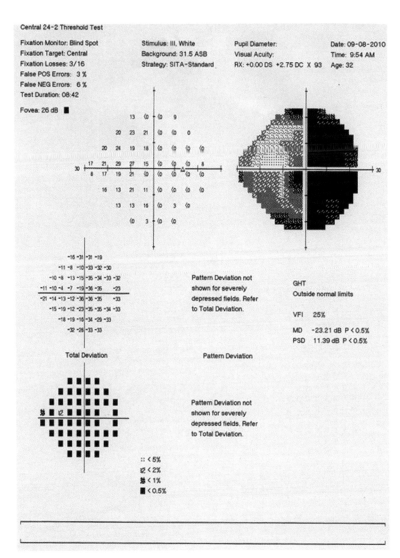

Central 24-2 Threshold Test

Fixation Monitor: Blind Spot
Fixation Target: Central
Fixation Losses: 3/16
False POS Errors: 3 %
False NEG Errors: 6 %
Test Duration: 08:42

Fovea: 26 dB

Stimulus: III, White
Background: 31.5 ASB
Strategy: SITA-Standard

Pupil Diameter:
Visual Acuity:
RX: +0.00 DS +2.75 DC X 93

Date: 09-08-2010
Time: 9:54 AM
Age: 32

Total Deviation

Pattern Deviation

Pattern Deviation not
shown for severely
depressed fields. Refer
to Total Deviation.

Pattern Deviation not
shown for severely
depressed fields. Refer
to Total Deviation.

GHT
Outside normal limits

VFI   25%

MD   -23.21 dB P < 0.5%
PSD   11.39 dB P < 0.5%

:: < 5%
⦂ < 2%
▨ < 1%
■ < 0.5%

FIGURE 6-10. (*continued*)

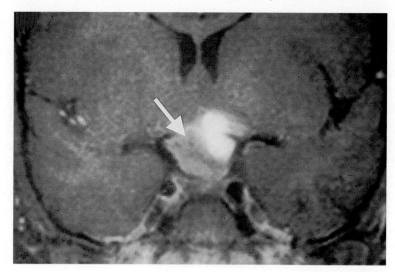

FIGURE 6-11. **Coronal MRI reveals a thickened optic chiasm** (*arrow*) with enhancement of the glioma.

FOLLOW-UP OF PARACHIASMAL TUMORS

- During the follow-up of treated parachiasmal tumors, the visual field may deteriorate. The causes are as follows:
  - Regrowth of tumor
  - Radiation necrosis of the optic chiasm if radiation has been administered (Fig. 6-12)
  - Chiasmal prolapse into an empty sella (Fig. 6-13)
  - Arachnoiditis is a rare cause of visual loss following surgery

Visual Recovery Following Treatment

A significant proportion of patients with parachiasmal tumors show recovery of vision following chiasmal decompression. When visual recovery occurs, it tends to do so in a certain pattern. Within the first 24 hours after surgery, there is often a dramatic and rapid improvement. There is continued improvement, especially over the first 6 weeks, but may continue at a slower rate for a year. Until recently, predicting recovery of visual function following surgery was not possible because neither the history, size of tumor, nor the appearance of the optic nerves reliably predicted recovery. However, measurement of the retinal nerve fiber layer preoperatively with optical coherence tomography has provided a means of predicting the recovery of visual field. Thickness of the retinal nerve fiber layer greater than 76 to 85 μm is associated with dramatic visual field improvement (greater than 10 dB) (Fig. 6-14).

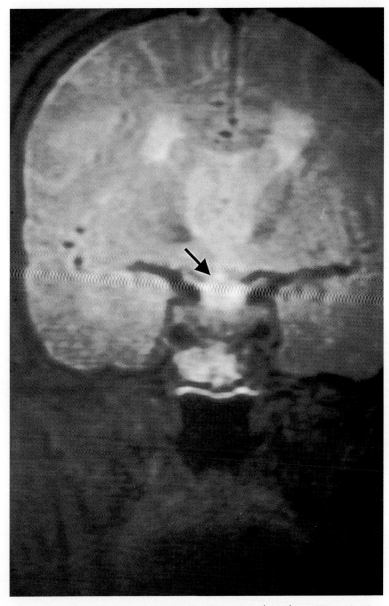

FIGURE 6-12. **Coronal MRI showing enhancement of the optic chiasm** (*arrow*) consistent with radiation necrosis.

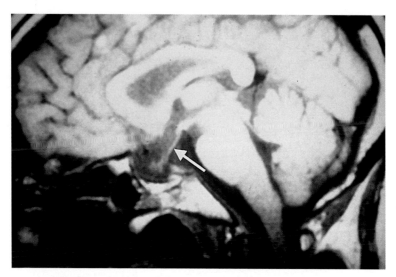

FIGURE 6-13. **Sagittal MRI with prolapse of optic chiasm** (*arrow*) into an enlarged sella turcica following pituitary apoplexy.

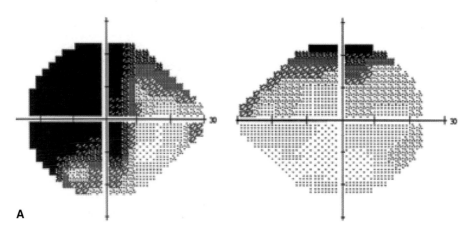

A

FIGURE 6-14. **Pituitary tumor. A.** Visual field defect of a patient with pituitary tumor.

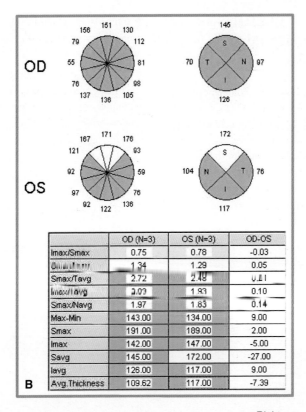

	OD (N=3)	OS (N=3)	OD-OS
Imax/Smax	0.75	0.78	-0.03
Smax/Imax	1.34	1.29	0.05
Smax/Tavg	2.72	2.48	0.11
Imax/Tavg	2.03	1.93	0.10
Smax/Navg	1.97	1.83	0.14
Max-Min	143.00	134.00	9.00
Smax	191.00	189.00	2.00
Imax	142.00	147.00	-5.00
Savg	145.00	172.00	-27.00
Iavg	126.00	117.00	9.00
Avg.Thickness	109.62	117.00	-7.39

B

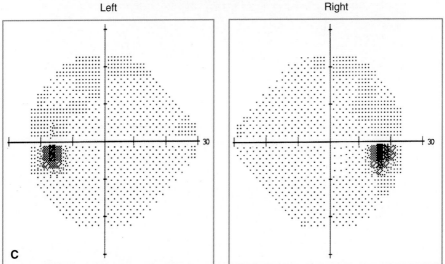

C

FIGURE 6-14. (*continued*) **B.** Optical coherence tomography demonstrating retinal nerve fiber layer thickness in normal range. **C.** Postoperative visual field at 1 month.

NONTUMOR LESIONS CAUSING CHIASMAL SYNDROME

Inflammatory lesions [lymphoid hypophysitis, demyelinating disease (Fig. 6-15), sarcoidosis (Fig. 6-16), etc.] may produce a chiasmal syndrome with typical visual field and acuity loss. Thus, the responsibility of the ophthalmologist in evaluating a patient with unexplained visual loss is as follows:

• Perform a visual field.

• If the visual field indicates a lesion that potentially involves the optic chiasm, perform an MRI scan.

• If the MRI scan identifies a lesion involving the optic chiasm (tumors or nontumors), the patient should be referred to a neurologist or a neurosurgeon.

• Following the treatment of chiasmal disorders (especially tumors), the role of the ophthalmologist is to perform sequential visual field testing to document any possible recurrence of the mass lesion.

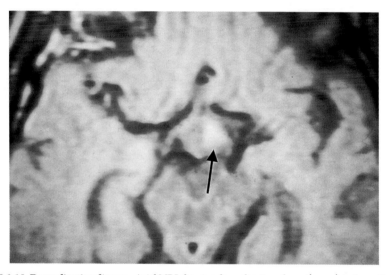

FIGURE 6-15. **Demyelinating disease.** Axial MRI showing demyelinating plaque (*arrow*) in the optic chiasm.

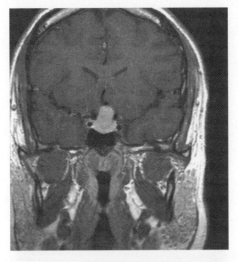

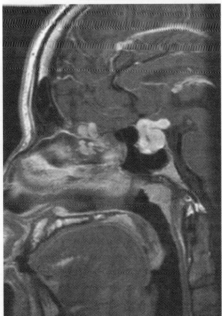

FIGURE 6-16. Sarcoidosis. Enhancing mass diagnosed as pituitary tumor but on histologic examination demonstrated to be a noncaseating granuloma consistent with sarcoidosis.

CHAPTER 7

Retrochiasmal Disorders

INTRODUCTION

The predominant visual sign of any lesion involving the postchiasmal visual pathway is *homonymous hemianopia*.

The form of the homonymous hemianopia differs depending on what portion of the retrochiasmal visual pathway is involved. Incomplete homonymous hemianopias are described as congruous or incongruous. Congruity refers to defects that are identical in shape, location, size, depth, and slope of margins. As the visual fibers course toward the occipital lobe, corresponding retinal points lie adjacent to one another and hence visual field defects because of posterior lesions are more congruous. Incomplete homonymous hemianopias of occipital origin are, therefore, exquisitely congruous. Visual field deficits caused by lesions anterior to the occipital lobe do not produce this degree of congruity. Complete homonymous hemianopias cannot be categorized as congruous and are nonlocalizing in terms of which part of the retrochiasmal pathway is affected.

RETROCHIASMAL VISUAL PATHWAY INVOLVEMENT

Optic Tract

This portion of the visual system is immediately behind the optic chiasm. In the optic tract, nerve fibers of corresponding points do not lie adjacent to one another and consequently incomplete homonymous hemianopias are incongruous in this location.

- Lesions in this area may produce one of two syndromes:

  - Optic tract syndrome type I is the combination of ipsilateral decreased acuity, an incongruous homonymous hemianopia, and an ipsilateral relative afferent pupillary defect (RAPD) (Fig. 7-1). It is caused by large mass lesions that involve the optic tract, optic chiasm, or even the optic nerve. The decreased visual acuity is due to the involvement of the ipsilateral optic nerve or chiasm. The most frequent lesion that causes this form of the optic tract syndrome is craniopharyngioma.

■ Optic tract syndrome type II involves intrinsic lesions of the optic tract, usually produced by demyelinating disease or infarction. Visual acuity is intact, the RAPD is on the side *opposite* the lesion, and the homonymous hemianopia is complete or nearly so.

● Other findings associated with optic tract lesions are as follows:

■ Optic disc changes: Bow-tie atrophy on the side contralateral to the side of lesion (side with temporal field loss) and temporal pallor on the ipsilateral side.

■ Wernickes hemianopic pupil: Projecting light onto the retinal elements that subserve the "blind" hemifield produces a reduced or no pupillary response, but a normal pupillary response is elicited from testing the retinal elements that subserve the normal hemifield. Clinically, this phenomenon is difficult to produce.

Lateral Geniculate Nucleus

Lateral geniculate nucleus (LGN) lesions are very uncommon. The afferent fibers are organized into alternating layers: uncrossed fibers are in layers 2, 3, and 5 and crossed fibers in layers 1, 4, and 6. As the LGN is highly organized, lesions generally produce localizing visual field defects. A congruous horizontal sectoranopia results from damage in the distribution of the posterolateral choroidal artery, which is a branch of the posterior cerebral artery. However, if the disruption is in the distribution of the anterior choroidal artery (a branch of the middle cerebral artery), there is a loss of the upper and lower homonymous quadrants called "quadruple sectoranopia" with preservation of a horizontal wedge.

Temporal Lobe

Lesions of the temporal lobe produce a homonymous hemianopia denser superiorly (Fig. 7-2A).

The most frequent causes are tumors (Fig. 7-2B) or following temporal lobectomy for seizures. Nonvisual manifestations of lesions of the temporal lobe include the following:

● Headache

● Auditory hallucinations or illusions

● Disturbance of language (if dominant temporal lobe is involved)

● Disturbance of memory

● Seizures manifested as transient changes in mood, emotions, and behavior

● Uncinate fits: Aura of unusual taste or smell followed by abnormal motor activity of the mouth and lips

● A sensation of déjà vu

Parietal Lobe

Lesions of the parietal lobe produce a homonymous hemianopia that is denser inferiorly.

● Associated neuro-ophthalmic features may include the following:

■ Conjugate movement of the eyes to the side opposite of the lesion on forced lid closure

■ Abnormal optokinetic response with evoked nystagmus dampened when targets are moved in the direction of the lesion

■ Deficient pursuit eye movements to the side of the lesion

● Neurologic features are as follows:

■ Neglect of contralateral space, inattention (nondominant parietal lobe)

■ Impairment of complex sensory integration

■ Gerstmann syndrome: A lesion in the dominant parietal lobe may result in contralateral homonymous hemianopia, finger agnosia, right–left confusion, agraphia, and acalculia.

Occipital Lobe

Patients with occipital lobe visual field defects are most likely to seek care first from the ophthalmologist because their only symptom or sign is visual. These patients often complain of difficulty reading and are frequently the recipients of multiple pairs of reading glasses before it is recognized that their difficulty is due to inability to see the next letter or word because of a right homonymous hemianopia or the inability to find the next line because of a left homonymous hemianopia (Fig. 7-3).

- There are several hallmarks of occipital lobe visual field defects:

  ▪ Temporal crescent sparing or involvement: The temporal crescent area lies anteriorly in the visual cortex. It represents a portion of nasal retina from one eye that has no shared associated (temporal retinal) fibers from the contralateral eye. Therefore, it is the one place in the visual radiations where a lesion may produce a unilateral visual field defect. The field defect is crescent shaped and its widest extent is in the horizontal meridian, where it extends from 60 to 90 degrees. It is worth remembering that the most used automated static perimetry programs will fail to detect this abnormality because it is further in the peripheral field than these tests measure. The most frequent type of visual field defect associated with this area is sparing of this temporal crescent. The homonymous hemianopia will appear incongruous because there is a rim of preserved vision capping the outermost portion of the temporal visual field defect. MRI scan shows a lesion sparing the anterior portion of the medial surface of the occipital lobe along the calcarine fissure (Fig. 7-4). Rarely is this area involved in a manner to produce loss of the crescent alone. Representation of the temporal crescent occupies less than 10% of total surface area of striate cortex.

  ▪ Macular sparing: A homonymous hemianopia of occipital origin may split fixation or may skirt around fixation (macular sparing) (Fig. 7-5). This is true sparing and is seen only with occipital lobe lesions and is at least 5 degrees. Macular splitting may be seen with homonymous hemianopias from any area of the visual radiations. Macular sparing may at times be an artifact of testing as a result of shifting fixation. True macular sparing occurs because the "macular" area of visual cortex is supplied by terminal branches of posterior and middle cerebral arteries. The macular area of the visual cortex lies in this watershed area. Therefore, with a stroke of the posterior cerebral circulation, blood supply may be provided by the terminal branches of the middle cerebral artery.

  ▪ Paracentral homonymous scotomas: Lesions of the tip of the occipital lobe produce homonymous scotomas that are exquisitely congruous (Fig. 7-6). During generalized hypoperfusion, such as intraoperative hypotension, the first area to be affected is the watershed zone of the occipital cortex with a consequent central homonymous hemianopia.

  ▪ Bilateral occipital lobe disease: Various patterns of visual field loss can be seen with bilateral occipital lobe disease. These include the following:

    ▶ Bilateral homonymous scotomas: May look like bilateral central scotomas

    ▶ "Ring" scotoma: A small island of central vision remains as a result of bilateral, congruous homonymous scotomas with macular sparing. The differential diagnosis of such constricted visual fields includes glaucoma, optic disc drusen, postpapilledema optic atrophy, retinitis pigmentosa, and nonorganic visual loss.

▶ Bilateral altitudinal field defects (usually inferior): Lesions that actually produce bilateral homonymous quadrantic defects

▶ "Checkerboard" field defect (Fig. 7-7): Crossed quadrantanopia. This is caused by lesions, usually consecutive events, that affect the superior occipital lobe above the calcarine fissure on one side and the inferior occipital lobe below the calcarine fissure on the other side.

● The other characteristics of occipital lobe disease that are important to the ophthalmologist include the following:

▪ Cortical blindness: Bilateral occipital lobe disease can produce blindness. These patients are often diagnosed initially as malingerers or hysterics because they complain of very poor or no vision, yet their pupils react briskly and their fundus is normal. At times, the patient will deny the blindness and fabricate a visual environment (Anton syndrome). In any patient with these signs and symptoms, bilateral lesions of the occipital lobe must be ruled out by MRI. The most frequent cause of cortical blindness is stroke in the older age group, although it may be seen after arteriography and in the peripartum period associated with pregnancy-induced hypertension. Cortical blindness may also be seen following chiropractic manipulation of the neck, carbon monoxide poisoning, cyclosporine A toxicity, and occipital lobe seizures.

▪ Dyschromatopsia: Acquired dyschromatopsia is usually an anterior visual pathway phenomenon (optic nerve or chiasm). There is a form of acquired dyschromatopsia (cerebral dyschromatopsia) that is produced by bilateral occipital lobe lesions.

▪ Palinopsia: This phenomenon consists of a persistent or recurrent visual image after the stimulus has been removed. The images are brief and recur periodically in a hemifield. This is typical of a parietal and occipital lesion in the nondominant hemisphere and is usually associated with a homonymous hemianopia. It may be produced, however, by the ingestion of hallucinogens, specifically lysergic acid diethylamide (LSD).

▪ Hallucinations: Occipital lobe hallucinations are not rare. They are unformed as opposed to formed hallucinations produced by lesions of the temporal lobe.

▪ Polyopia: This can occur with occipital lobe disease (Fig. 7-8). There can be any number of images and the diplopia/polyopia does not resolve by closing either eye or with pinhole.

▪ Visual allesthesia: This occurs when visual stimuli are transposed from one hemifield to another and occurs most commonly with parieto-occipital lesions.

In summary, any patient who has a homonymous hemianopia, be it complete or incomplete, congruous or incongruous, requires an MRI scan as the next test.

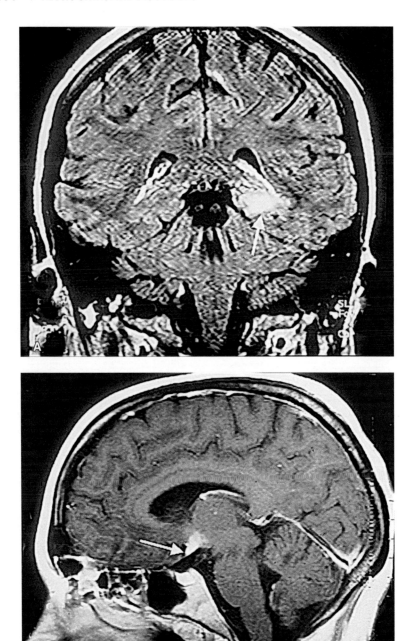

FIGURE 7-1. Neurosarcoidosis. A. Coronal and **B.** Sagittal MRI scans show enhancement of the area of the left optic tract (*arrows*) in a patient with neurosarcoidosis.

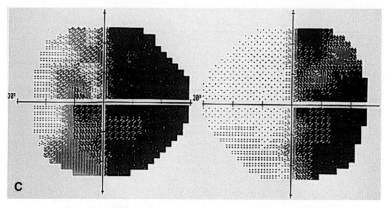

FIGURE 7-1. (*continued*) **C.** Visual fields show a right homonymous hemianopia with involvement of central fixation causing decreased visual acuity in the left eye.

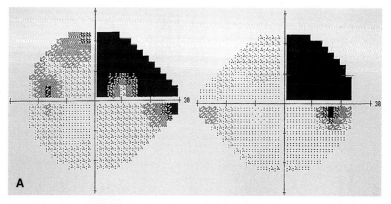

FIGURE 7-2. **Temporal lobe glioblastoma. A.** Following temporal lobectomy for seizures, the patient had a right superior homonymous quadrantanopia characteristic of a temporal lobe lesion.

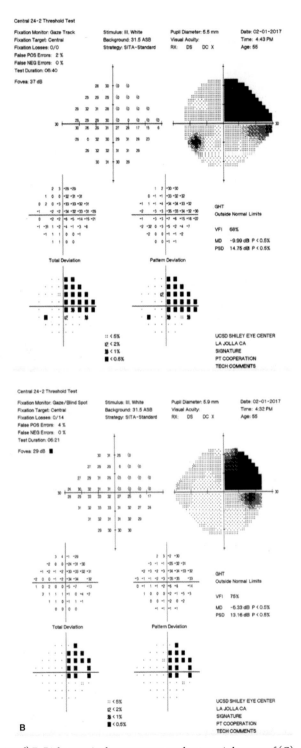

FIGURE 7-2. (*continued*) **B.** Right superior homonymous quadrantanopia because of (**C**).

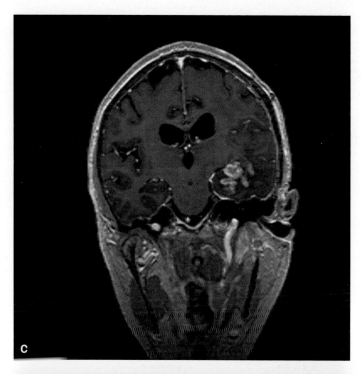

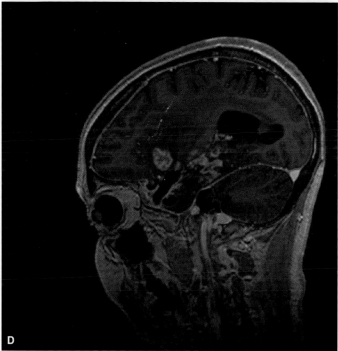

FIGURE 7-2. (*continued*) **D.** Coronal and sagittal MRI of temporal lobe glioblastoma.

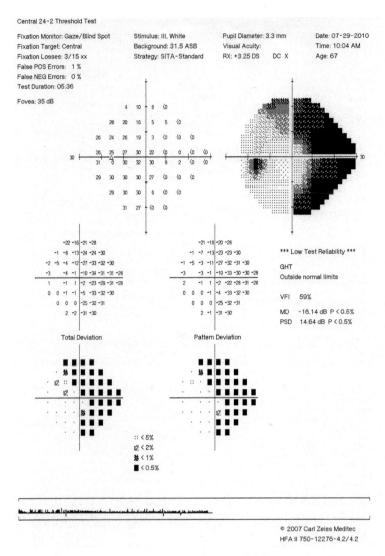

FIGURE 7-3. **Occipital lobe meningioma.** A 67-year-old man with difficulty reading. Upon questioning he also complained of driving difficulties, specifically not seeing autos on the right side. **A.** Right homonymous hemianopia.

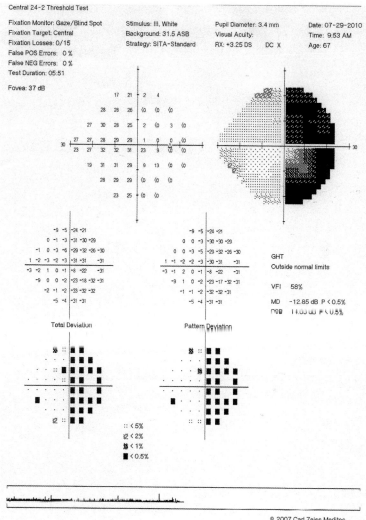

A

FIGURE 7-3. (*continued*)

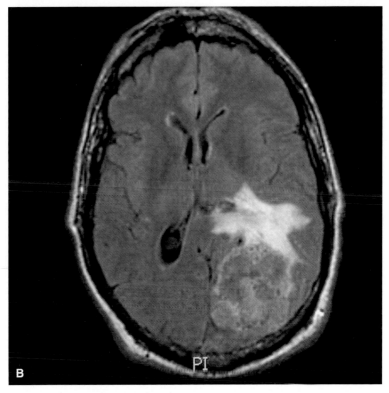

FIGURE 7-3. (*continued*) **B.** MRI shows occipital lobe meningioma.

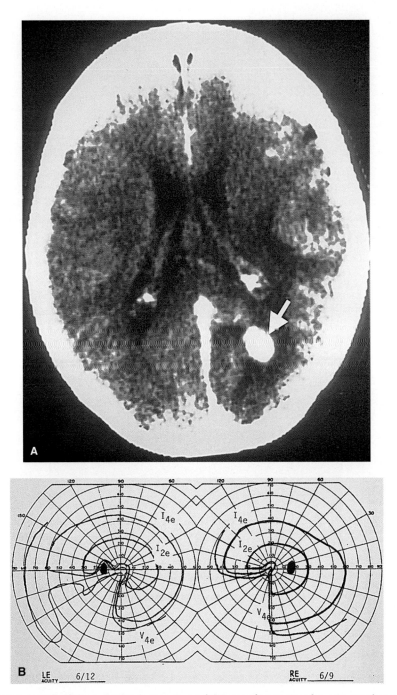

FIGURE 7-4. **Occipital lobe metastatic lesion. A.** Axial CT scan of a patient with a metastatic lesion to right occipital lobe. **B.** Perimetry shows left inferior quadrantanopia with temporal crescent sparing in the temporal portion of the left visual field.

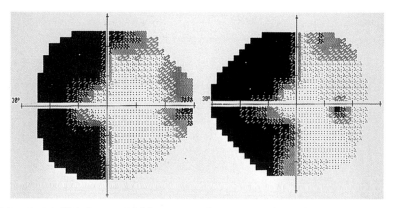

FIGURE 7-5. **Occipital lobe lesion.** A left homonymous hemianopia with macular sparing in a patient with an occipital lobe lesion.

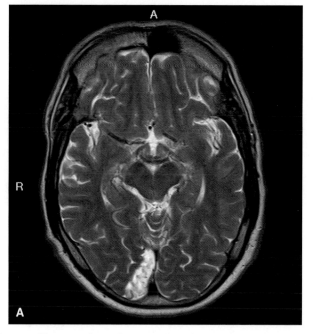

FIGURE 7-6. **A 65-year-old man with a right occipital stroke.** **A.** Axial MRI scan demonstrating a right occipital stroke

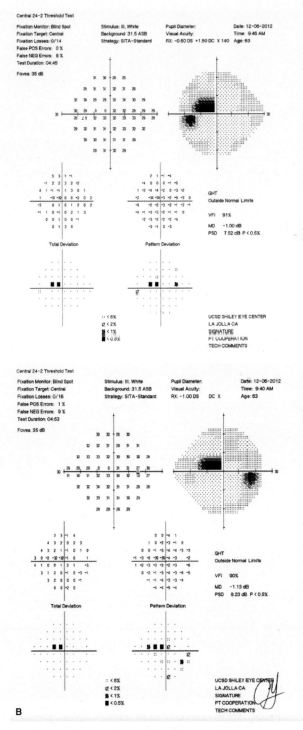

FIGURE 7-6. (*continued*) **B.** Visual fields showed a left homonymous paracentral scotoma.

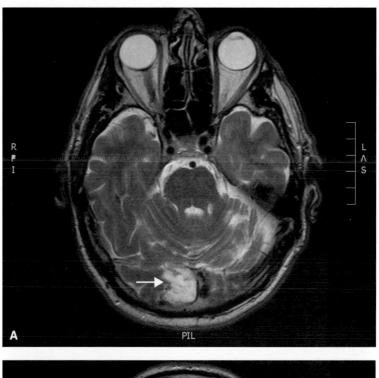

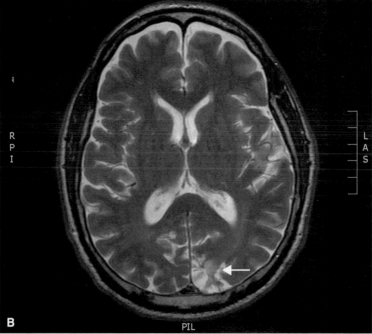

FIGURE 7-7. **Bilateral occipital lobe infarcts.** **A** and **B.** Axial MRI scans show infarcts in both occipital lobes (*arrows*).

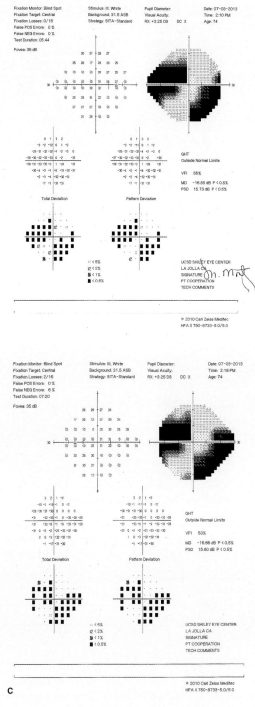

FIGURE 7-7. (*continued*) **C.** There are bilateral relatively congruous visual field defects that correspond to the occipital lobe lesions.

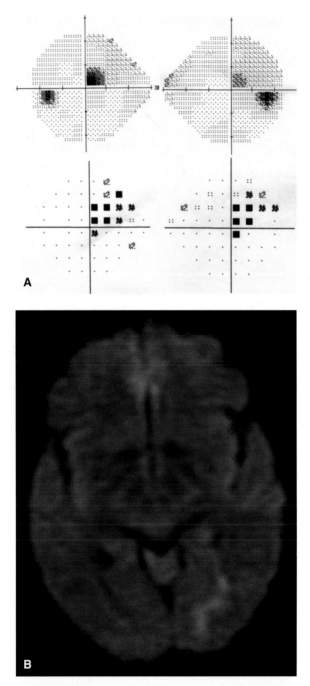

FIGURE 7-8. Left occipital lobe stroke. A 59-year-old woman complained of bilateral monocular oblique diplopia that did not resolve with pinhole. **A.** Visual fields showed a right homonymous scotoma. **B.** MRI showed an occipital stroke.

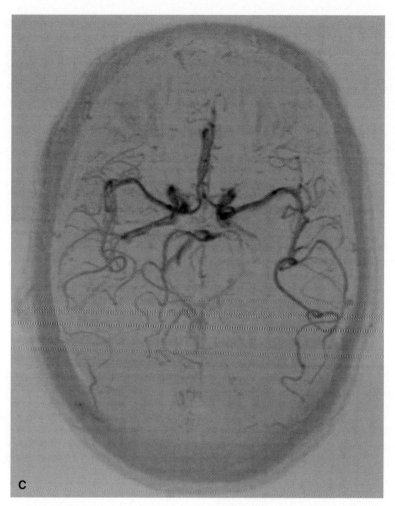

C

FIGURE 7-8. (*continued*) **C.** Catheter angiography showed paucity of vessels to the left occipital area compared to the right.

MIGRAINE

Migraine is the most frequent cause of homonymous visual field loss. The hemianopia is transient but infrequently may become permanent.

Epidemiology

• Migraine is a very frequent phenomenon that can present in various forms. The exact prevalence of migraine is difficult to calculate because of different classifications and descriptions of headaches.

Classification

• The International Headache Society classification of migraine is as follows:

▪ Migraine without aura

▪ Migraine with aura

▪ Typical aura without headache (acephalgic migraine)

▪ Ophthalmoplegic migraine (now considered a cranial neuralgia)

▪ Retinal migraine

▪ Childhood periodic syndromes that may be precursors to or associated with migraine

▪ Complicated migraine

▪ Migrainous disorder not fulfilling above criteria

▪ Patients with migraine with aura will often consult the ophthalmologist first.

Clinical Characteristics

Symptoms

• The patient may experience a *prodrome* with a sense of uneasiness, drowsiness, or depression.

• The *aura* of migraine varies, but the typical visual aura is that of a positive (although it may be negative) scotoma with jagged, often shimmering edges. The scotoma usually expands in size and tends to move across the visual field. The aura is usually in the form of jagged lines—the classic fortification scotoma (Fig. 7-9), but also may be bright lights. The aura typically lasts for 20 to 30 minutes and may be followed by a headache, or the end of the aura may terminate the attack (acephalgic migraine).

• The *headache* phase of migraine with aura occurs immediately after the aura or within 60 minutes, but if the aura is particularly long, there may be some overlap and the headache may begin while the aura is still present. It is distinctly unusual, but possible, for the aura to occur after the headache. The quality of the headache varies from severe and incapacitating to relatively minor. It may last for hours.

Signs

• Between attacks, the patient has a normal examination.

• If examined during the attack, the patient may have a homonymous hemianopia if the origin of the migraine is cortical. Following the attack, no visual field defect is detectable. Patients suspected of having migraine should have formal visual field testing and the presence of a defect requires investigation.

Differential Diagnosis

• Vitreous traction is usually distinguishable from migraine because photopsias produced by vitreous traction last seconds to only a few minutes, whereas the visual aspect of migraine lasts much longer.

• Occipital lobe lesions (Fig. 7-10)

• Arteriovenous malformations (AVMs) (Fig. 7-11) usually cause the most concern as being migraine mimickers. The visual phenomenon of AVMs is usually more short lived than those of migraine and may occur after the headache has already begun.

Diagnostic Evaluation

- We do not routinely image patients who present with typical migraine:
  - Onset before age 50, although migraine may occur de novo after that
  - Family history of migraine or migraine equivalents as a child
  - Classical description of the aura and/or headache, which lasts the appropriate length of time
  - The visual aura alternates sides
  - There is no fixed neurologic or ocular deficit following the migraine
- However, patients who present with the following characteristics receive further investigation.
  - The visual aura is inevitably in the same location in visible space.
  - The headache precedes the visual aura. Although this is sometimes seen in

migraine, it is uncommon and suspicious for an AVM.
- A fixed neurologic (including visual) deficit is noted following termination of the event.
- Any other circumstance that would render the episode atypical for migraine
- MRI is the first test to do in any patient who is going to be evaluated for atypical migraine.s

Treatment

- Treatment of migraine involves a variety of factors:
  - Elimination of precipitators, such as foods (wine, cheese, chocolate), stress modification
  - If behavior modification does not prevent migraine, a series of medications are available that may be used at the appearance of the aura to prevent the headache phase, during the headache phase to shorten it, and prophylactically in the interheadache phase to prevent migraines from recurring.

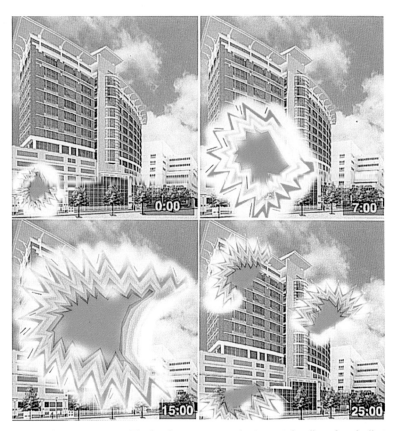

FIGURE 7-9. **Fortification scotoma.** The fortification scotoma begins peripherally and gradually involves the entire visual field. It usually clears without producing a permanent defect.

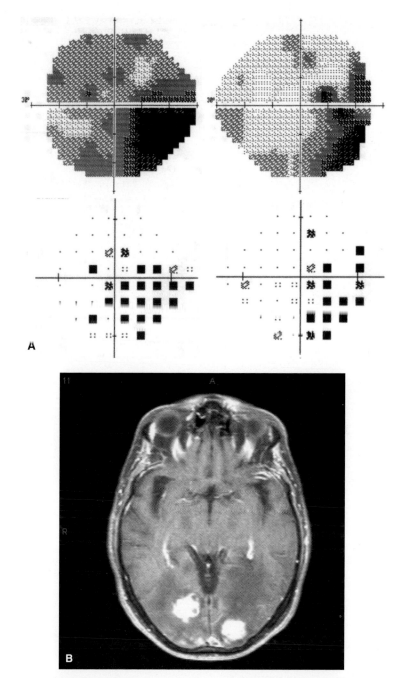

FIGURE 7-10. Occipital lobe lesions. A 67-year-old man complained of flashing lights lasting 15 minutes for 2 months. **A.** Visual fields show a right homonymous defect with some involvement of the left homonymous field. **B.** MRI shows bilateral occipital lung metastasis with surrounding edema.

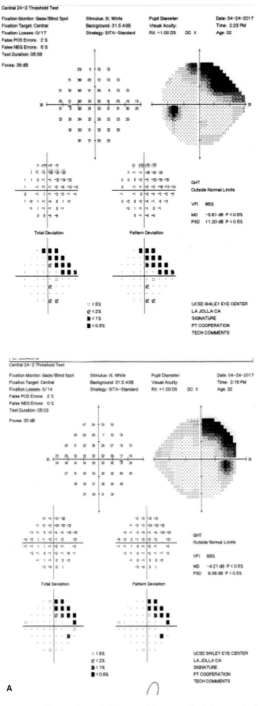

FIGURE 7-11. Arteriovenous malformation. A 32-year-old woman had three episodes of visual fortification in the right upper visual field followed by headache. **A.** Visual field shows an incomplete right superior quadrantanopia.

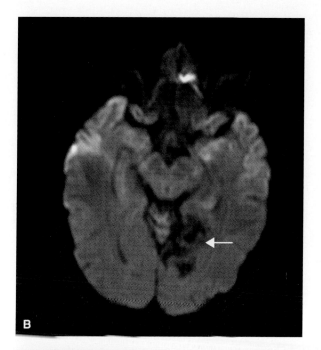

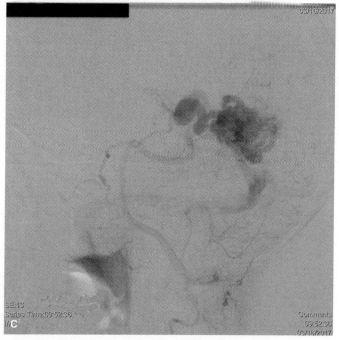

FIGURE 7-11. (*continued*) **B.** MRI shows an arteriovenous malformation of the left occipital/parietal lobes (*arrow*).
C. Arteriography confirms arteriovenous malformation.

Nonphysiologic Visual Loss

INTRODUCTION

Patients may present with complaints that mimic organic disease but are factitious. There is a spectrum of such abnormalities and the terms *nonphysiologic, nonorganic, or functional* are often used. The diagnosis requires demonstrating and documenting normal or better than stated visual function. Furthermore, it is important to perform the relevant investigations to exclude serious organic diseases. Several diseases are often misdiagnosed as nonphysiologic and should be kept in mind when considering this diagnosis, including

- early cone dystrophy or Stargardt disease
- other subtle macular disorders (e.g., acute macular neuroretinopathy)
- bilateral occipital lobe infarcts
- pituitary tumors
- keratoconus
- retinitis pigmentosa, especially sine pigmento
- cancer-associated retinopathy/melanoma-associated retinopathy

The most frequently encountered forms of these disorders involve the afferent visual system and consist of the following:

- No vision (one or both eyes)
- Decreased vision (one or both eyes)
- Visual field loss (one or both eyes)

NO VISION

Nonphysiologic total visual loss is often the easiest to detect. The examiner has to prove that any vision exists in the purported blind eye(s). This can be accomplished by one of several methods:

- Mobility testing: Watch the patient enter the room and perform manual tasks. Patients with nonphysiologic visual loss often claim to be unable to perform any tasks of mobility but can navigate around obstacles placed in their path.
- Functional tests: A blind person will be able to sign his or her name without difficulty. A patient with feigned visual loss may claim to have difficulty doing this.

• Outstretch arm-to-nose test: A blind person will be able to easily touch their nose after the arm has been extended, whereas a person with feigned visual loss, not realizing this is a proprioceptive and not a visual test, may miss his or her nose completely.

• Threat: A sudden threatening movement toward the patient's face that causes him or her to react appropriately proves the existence of vision.

• Mirror test: Hold a mirror up to the blind eye(s) and ask the patient to concentrate on focusing straight ahead. Then, tilt the mirror horizontally and vertically. The more the patient tries to steady the eye, the more it will move in concert with the mirror tilt.

• Optokinetic nystagmus response: The development of an optokinetic response to an appropriate target in a blind eye is evidence of preserved vision. To perform the test, the optokinetic nystagmus drum is slowly rotated in front of the patient. If the eyes move with the drum and beat back in a typical optokinetic response but the patient claims not to see the drum, a nonorganic component has been established. Patients may try to purposely look around the drum or focus past the drum if the nonphysiologic visual loss is intentional.

• Pupillary response: In the setting of one blind eye with no light perception, and one normal eye, an amaurotic pupil must be demonstrated. Pupillary reaction to light is proof that the problem is factitious. This is not necessarily true with bilateral blindness. It is important to remember that patients who are blind from bilateral occipital lobe (or posterior to the lateral geniculate nucleus) disease will have normal reacting pupils.

• Diplopia test (for monocular blindness): The suspected eye is occluded. Use a strong prism with the apex bisecting the pupil of the good eye to produce monocular diplopia. The patient will usually admit to this diplopia. As the suspected eye is uncovered, move the entire prism before the good eye

now to produce binocular diplopia. If the patient still reports diplopia, the visual loss is functional.

• Ten-diopter prism test: When a 10-diopter base-out prism is placed in front of a normal eye, there is a shift of both eyes with a refixation movement of the contralateral eye to avoid diplopia. A blind eye will not refixate and a prism placed before this eye will not produce a movement in either eye.

• Binocular visual field test. True monocular blindness produces a visual field of approximately 150 degrees with the blind spot of the normal eye and loss of the temporal crescent of the blind eye.

• **Electrophysiologic testing** visual evoked potentials (VEPs) have a role in assessing a possible nonphysiologic disorder. Normal VEP results for a patient who reports severe monocular or binocular vision loss and has a normal clinical examination support the diagnosis of nonorganic disturbance of vision. However, both false-negative and false-positive results are possible.

DECREASED VISION

Patients with nonphysiologic incomplete visual loss are often more difficult to diagnose. The examiner must (by any means available) have the patient read better than the claimed defect. The technique must be tailored to the patient and to whether the patient is claiming unilateral or bilateral decreased vision. Techniques include the following:

• Encouragement: Start at 20/10 line and slowly proceed up chart.

• Fogging: Confusing the patient so they read with the "bad" eye when believing they are reading with the "good" one. Fog the patient by adding plus spheres in front of the good eye so that the patient is actually being tested with the eye in which poor vision is claimed. Fogging may also be performed using two strong cylinders of equal power but one plus and the other minus in front of the good eye in a trial lens. Initially, the lenses are placed on the same axis in the trial frame. Then one is rotated 45 degrees fogging the good eye.

- Retest the visual acuity (VA) at half the distance from the chart. The VA should be twice as good.

- Near vision: With appropriate near correction, this should be equivalent to distance vision.

- Worth 4-dot test: If all four dots are seen, vision is better than hand motions.

- Stereopsis: Patients with 60 seconds of arc must have 20/20 in one eye and at least 20/40 in the other.

- A series of devices, including stereoscopic and red-green projectors, can be used to confuse the patient so that they read with the "bad" eye when they believe they are reading with the "good" one. All methods are legitimate tactics.

- **Red-green test**: Duochrome glasses are placed over the patient's eyes. The red-green filter is then placed over the Snellen chart, presenting the letters simultaneously either on a green or a red background. If the letters are read with the background color the same as the lens in front of the "nonseeing" eye, there is confirmation of nonphysiologic visual loss.

VISUAL FIELD LOSS

Feigned visual field loss may be claimed either with preserved or decreased acuity. Formal perimetry, either automated-static or kinetic, will produce typical patterns of factitious visual field loss (Fig. 8-1).

Examination of the patient using confrontation techniques and varying the distance between the patient and the target will often uncover the dissembler. As the distance from the patient increases, the normal visual field expands. Constriction (funnel vision) or nonexpansion (tunnel vision) of the visual field under these conditions is a nonphysiologic response. Remember that when the distance from the test surface is doubled, the size of the test object must also be doubled.

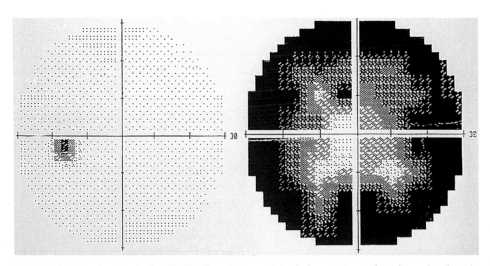

FIGURE 8-1. **Nonphysiologic visual field.** The patient complained of poor vision in the right eye, but the right visual field showed a "clover-leaf" pattern consistent with nonphysiologic visual loss. The left visual field was normal and there was no relative afferent pupillary defect.

CHAPTER

9

Neuro-ophthalmologic Examination—Efferent System

INTRODUCTION

Disorders of the efferent visual system result in either ocular misalignment or abnormalities in ocular motility without ocular misalignment. The most frequent symptom that prompts a neuro-ophthalmologic examination of the efferent system is **diplopia**. Other symptoms such as head tilts, face turns, etc., also require that evaluation of the efferent system be performed looking for disorders of ocular motility even when the patient does not appreciate double vision.

The patient who presents with the symptom of diplopia should be approached in a systematic way to most efficiently identify the cause of diplopia and whether the diplopia has a potentially neuro-ophthalmic cause. There are several steps to follow to arrive at the correct diagnosis.

IDENTIFY MONOCULAR DIPLOPIA

The most important initial aspect of the diplopia evaluation is for the examiner to understand if the double vision is present only with both eyes open or is appreciated monocularly.

Monocular diplopia is almost invariably due to an ocular disorder and is very rarely a manifestation of neuro-ophthalmologic disease. Patients with monocular diplopia therefore need not be subjected to intensive neurologic and neuroradiologic investigations. If the patient has not cross-covered his or her eyes and does not know if the double vision persists when either eye is occluded, that is the first maneuver the examiner should perform. If the patient perceives double vision with one eye occluded, this is monocular diplopia. Monocular diplopia is most often produced by an ocular disorder that will disrupt the incoming parallel rays of light, preventing them from coming to a point focus on the retina. Instead, a blur circle is formed on the retina and a *ghost image* that is often described as diplopia results. The most frequent causes of monocular diplopia are as follows:

- Refractive error, especially astigmatism
- Cataract, usually of the nuclear sclerotic variety
- Corneal scarring
- Iris abnormalities, such as atrophy or generous peripheral iridotomies
- Subluxated lens or implant
- Nonphysiologic causes

The easiest way to document that monocular diplopia is due to a refractive or an anterior segment problem is to use the pinhole. An occluder with multiple pinhole openings from 2 to 2.5 mm each is placed in front of the patient's symptomatic eye (Fig. 9-1A, B). The patient is then asked if the monocular diplopia is improved or has disappeared. An affirmative answer establishes the anterior segment or a refractive error as the cause of the problem. A negative response is suggestive of nonphysiologic diplopia or cerebral polyopia. This syndrome presents with bilateral monocular diplopia that is usually oblique and is the same in each eye. It is invariably associated with other neurologic signs or symptoms.

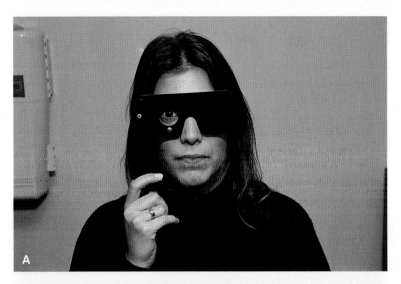

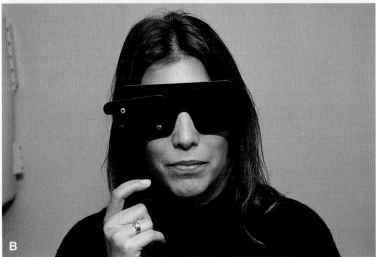

FIGURE 9-1. **Pinhole test.** Patient complains of diplopia in the right eye (**A**) that disappears when the pinhole occluder is placed before the eye (**B**).

DETERMINE WHETHER MISALIGNMENT IS COMITANT OR INCOMITANT

If the patient indicates that diplopia is present only with both eyes open, the patient has true **binocular diplopia**. This symptom is almost always due to ocular misalignment. The purpose of this step and the next several steps is to identify the pattern of the misalignment to see if it corresponds to isolated or combined cranial nerve (CN) palsies.

A *comitant* strabismus is one in which the amount of deviation is the same in all directions of gaze, irrespective of which eye is fixating. A strabismus is *incomitant* when the angle of deviation varies with the direction of gaze or depending on which eye is fixating. Comitant ocular misalignments are usually decompensated congenital deviations. Incomitant misalignments are usually acquired disorders and caused by paralytic or mechanical processes. Certain congenital decompensated phorias, for example, congenital CN IV palsies, may produce incomitant misalignments. The presence of a comitant deviation, particularly when ocular ductions and versions are full, usually indicates a non-neurologic cause for the diplopia.

There are several ways to measure the pattern of the ocular misalignment.

Prism Cover Test

By introducing prism in front of one eye and utilizing a cover/uncover or alternate cover test, the amount of ocular misalignment is measured in prism diopters. All measurements should be performed in at least six directions of gaze: primary position, right, left, up, down, and near. Oblique gaze and measurements on head tilt are employed under special circumstances. The measurement is then recorded on a chart, which signifies these directions of gaze (Fig. 9-2). In the appropriate clinical setting, the ocular misalignment is measured on right and left head

tilt. This is usually used when either a CN IV palsy or an ocular tilt reaction is suspected. The patient is seated in the upright position; the head is tilted to the right and then to the left, and the vertical misalignment is measured in the right and left head tilt positions. In CN IV palsies, the vertical misalignment will be greater when the head is tilted toward the side of the palsy.

The *primary deviation* refers to the amount of ocular misalignment measured when the patient is fixating with the nonparetic eye. The *secondary deviation* is the measured angle of deviation when the patient is fixating with the paretic eye. Patients with nonparalytic strabismus do not measure the difference between the primary and secondary deviations; the ocular misalignment is the same when they fix with either eye. The patient with a paralytic strabismus, however, will have a much larger ocular misalignment when the paretic eye is fixing (secondary deviation) and less of a misalignment when the nonparetic eye is fixing (primary deviation) (Fig. 9-3). In patients with paralytic strabismus, the secondary deviation is always greater than the primary deviation. This is due to Hering's law of equal innervation to yoke muscles because an increase in innervations is needed when the paralytic eye is fixating. Consequently, the contralateral yoke muscle also receives more innervations, resulting in a larger deviation. The deviation is also greatest when the eyes turn in the direction of the paralytic muscle.

Red Lens or Maddox Rod

In this method of measurement, the eyes are dissociated by introducing a red lens or rod in front of one (by convention the right) eye and asking the patient to look at a white fixation light at distance. The patient, therefore, will see the image (point of light) from each eye as different colors in the case of the red lens test and as different shapes (a red line and a white point of light) when the Maddox rod is employed (Fig. 9-4A, B). If two separate images are perceived, the patient is asked if the red image is to the right or left of the fixation light being viewed at distance. Esotropia will have the red image on the same side as the eye that has the red occluder (uncrossed diplopia). Exotropia, on the other hand, will have the red image on the side opposite to the red occluder (crossed diplopia). In vertical misalignments, the red lens or rod in front of the higher (hypertropic) eye projects the red image as being lower, whereas the red image is seen above the fixation light when the eye behind the red occluder is lower (hypotropia).

The Maddox rod may also be used to measure torsion. This may be done behind the phoropter or by placing the Maddox rod in trial frames. Double Maddox rods (white in front of the left eye, red in front of the right eye) may be employed. The patient (or examiner) turns the adjustment knob on the trial frame or appropriate dial on the phoropter until the two lines are parallel. The amount of torsion is read in degrees directly from the apparatus holding the Maddox rods (Fig. 9-5).

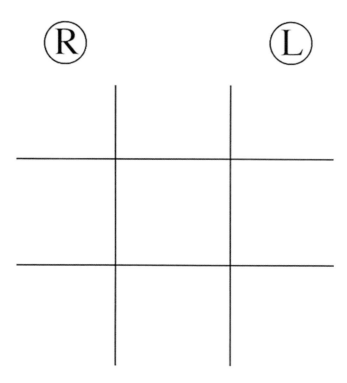

FIGURE 9-2. **Ocular misalignment chart.** Chart for recording the ocular misalignment in prism diopters in the cardinal positions of gaze.

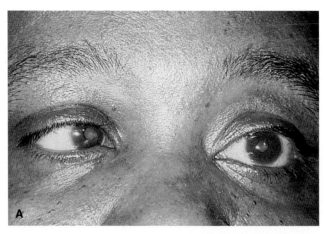

FIGURE 9-3. **Primary and secondary deviation. A.** Patient has a right CN VI palsy with inability to abduct the right eye.

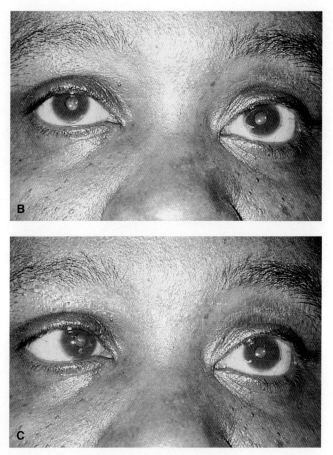

FIGURE 9-3. (*continued*) **B.** The esotropia decreases markedly with the left eye fixing. **C.** There is a marked left esotropia with the right eye fixing (bottom).

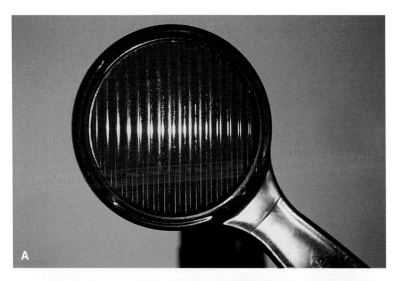

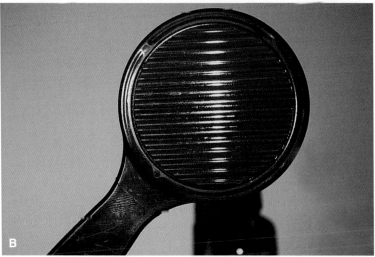

FIGURE 9-4. **Maddox rod test.** A vertical red line is appreciated when the Maddox rod is placed horizontally (**A**) and a horizontal line when it is positioned vertically (**B**).

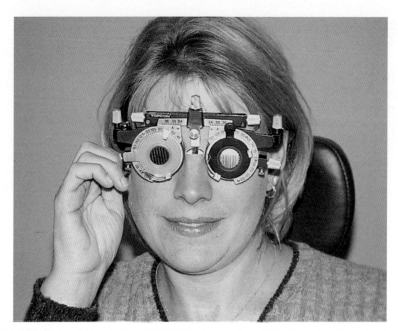

FIGURE 9-5. **Maddox rod test.** Patient with CN IV palsy rotating red Maddox rod to determine the torsional component.

EXAMINE DUCTIONS AND VERSIONS

The patient is asked to follow an object horizontally and then vertically. The ocular excursions are judged to be full or limited in one or more directions of gaze. This is then recorded as the percentage either of ductional deficit or of ductional ability (Fig. 9-6). At times ductional deficits may not be seen, but "overactions" of muscles may be noted. This is often seen in CN IV palsies where the inferior oblique muscle ipsilateral to the paretic superior oblique muscle tends to elevate in adduction. This is a result of Hering's law.

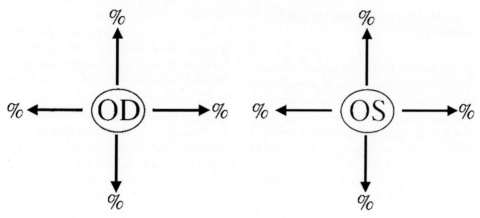

FIGURE 9-6. **Ocular duction chart.** Chart to record ductions in percentages.

EXAMINE SACCADES AND PURSUITS

On saccadic testing, the patient is asked to look quickly from one direction of gaze to the primary position. For example, right gaze to primary position or left gaze to primary position. The speed of the saccade is noted, as well as its extent and stability. Normally, patients make refixational movements quickly and in one movement. Saccades may be slowed or absent, may overshoot the end point, or may occur in a series of smaller movements (hypometric saccades) in order to bring the eye into the required position.

PERFORM FORCED DUCTION TEST (IF APPROPRIATE)

Not all ocular misalignments that produce double vision are due to ocular motor paresis. Restrictive ocular myopathies caused by orbital inflammatory disease (myositis), orbital trauma, or thyroid eye disease are frequent causes of ocular misalignment and double vision. Likewise, myasthenia gravis (MG) may cause a pattern of double vision that can mimic any isolated muscle palsy, isolated CN palsy, combined CN palsies, or supranuclear ocular motility disturbance.

A forced duction test (Fig. 9-7) should be performed if there is any suspicion that a restrictive myopathy is the cause of the patient's diplopia. The examiner grasps the eye with the restricted duction and attempts to move it into the field of ductional deficit as the patient looks in that direction. The ability to easily move the eye in that direction is a *negative* forced duction test and indicates that restriction is not present. Perceived difficulty or inability to passively rotate the eye into the direction of ductional deficit is evidence that a restriction exists. This is a *positive* forced duction test and suggests that the cause of the eye movement abnormality is not a neurologic disorder but is most likely due to local orbital disease.

We prefer to perform the forced duction test by anesthetizing the muscle opposite the direction of ductional deficit. For example, with an elevation deficit, we grasp the inferior rectus muscle. This is done with broad forceps after a cotton-tipped applicator soaked with cocaine 10% has been applied over the inferior rectus muscle for 2 minutes. The patient is asked to look up; the inferior rectus muscle is grasped and the eye is rotated superiorly. The degree of resistance to this passive duction is recorded.

EXAMINE LIDS AND PUPILS

Other clues to the cause of diplopia may be obtained by observing other aspects of the ocular examination. In all patients who present with diplopia, specific attention should be paid to the lid position and the pupillary size. A combination of diplopia and either a lid and/or pupillary abnormality will often provide the examiner with the precise cause of the patient's double vision.

ASSESS OCULAR CEPHALIC MOVEMENTS

In patients who appear to have bilateral ductional deficits, it is important to determine if this is due to an infranuclear or supranuclear lesion. Supranuclear lesions will produce ductional deficits on voluntary gaze, but by performing doll's head maneuvers, the eyes rotate normally into the field of the ductional deficit. This is often seen in patients with dorsal midbrain syndrome and progressive supranuclear palsy (see p. 358).

ASSESS FOR NYSTAGMUS

Part of the examination of the efferent system is to look for abnormal rhythmic eye movements. If nystagmus is present, the direction of the nystagmus is named by the direction of the fast phase (right beating, left beating, etc.) and in what cardinal gazes it is present. The amplitude of nystagmus should also be recorded. Torsional nystagmus is recorded as being clockwise or counterclockwise as the examiner looks at the patient, not as the patient's eyes are moving (e.g., clockwise nystagmus is when the 12- to 6- o'clock axis rotates toward the examiner's right as the examiner faces the patient).

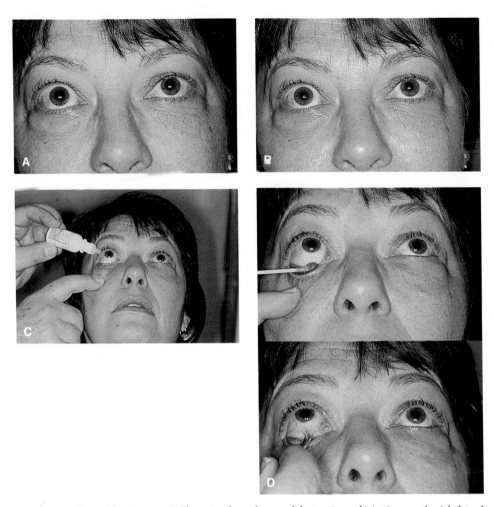

FIGURE 9-7. **Forced duction test. A.** The patient has right upper lid retraction and injection over the right lateral rectus muscle characteristic of thyroid eye disease (TED). **B.** She cannot elevate either eye (bottom). **C.** An ophthetic solution is placed in both eyes. A cotton tip applicator soaked in cocaine 10% is placed over the muscle to be grasped for 2 minutes. **D.** The body of the muscle opposite to the defective duction is grasped with a broad-based forceps and the patient is asked to look in the direction of defective gaze while the examiner attempts to rotate the eye in that direction. Resistance to passive rotation of the eye is a positive test.

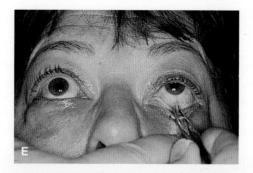

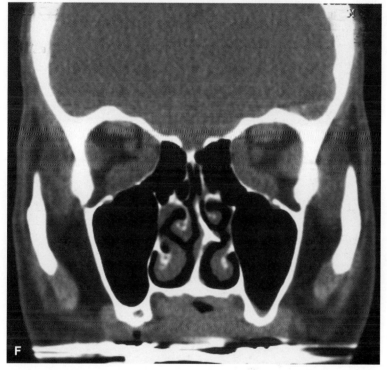

FIGURE 9-7. (*continued*) **E.** The fellow eye is tested in a similar manner. **F.** Coronal CT scan showing enlarged inferior rectus muscles bilaterally consistent with TED.

PERFORM BINOCULAR SINGLE-VISION VISUAL FIELD

When a patient has diplopia, an excellent way to follow progression of the ocular misalignment is by doing binocular single-vision visual fields. The patient is seated in front of a bowl kinetic perimeter with both eyes open. She is then asked to *follow* the III_4e light with her eyes only and to indicate when the light switches from being single to double. The points are plotted so that a diagram of the area in which the patient sees single is created. This diagram may then be used on subsequent visits to determine whether the patient's field of single vision is changing (Fig. 9-8).

Ocular Motility Disturbances without Diplopia

Some patients present with ocular motility disturbances but do not have diplopia. This may be because of poor vision in one or both eyes or because the ocular motility disturbance has not produced an ocular misalignment. In these patients, the examination consists of evaluation of ductions and version, saccades and pursuits, forced ductions, and evaluation for MG.

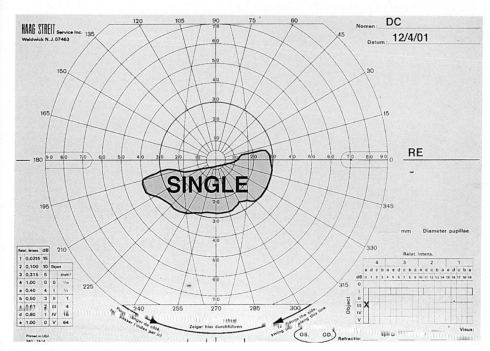

FIGURE 9-8. Binocular single vision visual field. A small area of binocular single vision is present outside of which diplopia occurs.

Ocular Misalignment and Other Ocular Motor Disorders

CRANIAL NERVE III PALSY (OCULOMOTOR NERVE)

Cranial nerve III (CN III) innervates the superior, inferior, medial recti, and the inferior oblique muscles. It also innervates the levator palpebrae superioris and carries with it the parasympathetic innervation to the pupil. Involvement of CN III will produce a symptom complex that involves one or several of these muscles and usually results in double vision.

ANATOMY

The subnuclei that give rise to CN III reside in the midbrain. These subnuclei give rise to the fascicles of each of the extraocular muscles. The superior rectus (SR) subnuclei are crossed so that the fibers from the left SR subnucleus eventually innervate the right SR muscle. Another peculiarity of the nuclear structure of CN III is that the nucleus for the upper lids is a single midline structure innervating the levator muscles of both lids. The pupillary constrictor and accommodation muscles are under the control of an ipsilateral subnucleus.

As CN III leaves the brainstem near the medial aspect of the cerebral peduncle and enters the subarachnoid space, it travels between the superior cerebellar artery and the posterior cerebral artery next to the tip of the basilar artery. It then travels medially along the posterior communicating (PCOM) artery and lateral along the internal carotid artery. When the nerve enters the cavernous sinus, it lies in the lateral wall superior to cranial nerve IV (CN IV) and then goes through the superior orbital fissure dividing into a superior and an inferior division. The superior division contains the SR and levator innervation, whereas the inferior division contains the rest of the innervation for CN III including the parasympathetic pupillary fibers. There is convincing evidence that the functional organization into a superior and an inferior division occurs before anatomic division occurs in the cavernous sinus.

ETIOLOGY AND PATHOPHYSIOLOGY

Cranial III neuropathy may be caused by a variety of processes, but the most frequent causes are either microvascular infarction of the nerve itself or compression. Microvascular infarction occurs in older patients (over 50 years of age) and is due to occlusion of the vasa nervorum. This infarction involves the axial portion of CN III. Because the pupillary fibers are on the periphery of the nerve, the pupil is not usually involved by the axial infarction in microvascular disease. These patients often have identifiable risk factors such as diabetes mellitus, hypertension, atherosclerosis, and hyperlipidemia.

Compressive CN III palsies may be produced by tumors or aneurysms. The clinical syndrome of aneurysmal CN III palsy is an important one because it is a medical emergency. The patient will usually present with a painful (usually, but not always present) isolated CN III palsy. This is usually due to a PCOM artery aneurysm. The aneurysm exerts pressure from the outside; thus, the pupillary fibers are often involved early, and the CN III palsy is characterized by ptosis, ocular misalignment, and, usually, a dilated pupil.

CLINICAL CHARACTERISTICS

- See **Figure 10-1**.

Symptoms

- Pain may be present with CN III palsies because of microvascular infarction or compression. It *does not* distinguish between the two causes.

- Ptosis may be complete or incomplete.
- Diplopia is usually oblique in nature.

Signs

- Ptosis may be complete or incomplete.
- Ophthalmoplegia: There is usually an exotropia in primary position with defective adduction, elevation, and depression of the eye.
- Anisocoria: occurs with compression; otherwise, the pupils are normal.
- The presence of anisocoria with a dilated pupil is critical to the diagnosis of aneurysmal CN III palsy. Thus, any patient diagnosed with a lesion of CN III must have the pupil evaluated. The *rule of the pupil* states that in a *complete* CN III palsy, the pupil will be normal if the cause is microvascular infarction but will be dilated and less reactive to light if the lesion is compressive, especially by a PCOM aneurysm. There are certain caveats to invoking the rule of the pupil.

  - It may be invoked only in the presence of a complete CN III palsy. It would be unwise to invoke this rule in incomplete or partial palsies (**Fig. 10-2**).

  - It has been reported that the pupil may initially be uninvolved with PCOM aneurysms, with anisocoria developing at any time within 5 days of the start of diplopia.

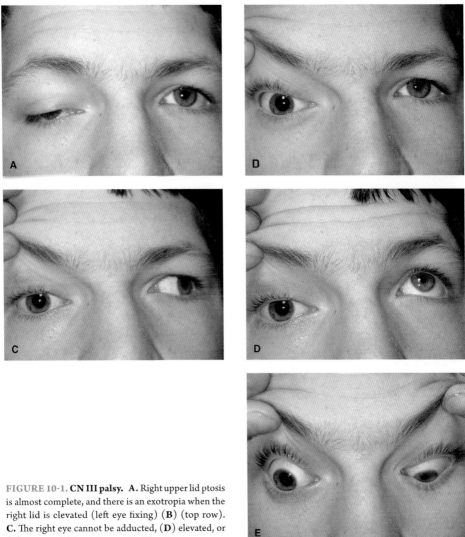

FIGURE 10-1. CN III palsy. A. Right upper lid ptosis is almost complete, and there is an exotropia when the right lid is elevated (left eye fixing) (**B**) (top row). **C.** The right eye cannot be adducted, (**D**) elevated, or (**E**) depressed. The right pupil is dilated.

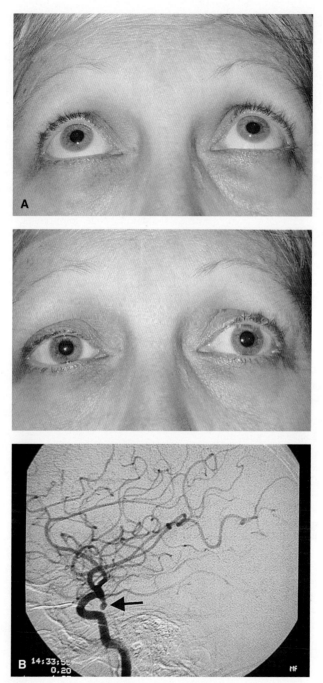

FIGURE 10-2. Incomplete or partial CN III palsy. A. There is small left exotropia and hypertropia in primary gaze with the right eye fixing and slight ptosis of the right upper lid (middle photograph). Upgaze is minimally less OD. The pupils are equal (upper photograph). MRI, MRA, and lumbar puncture were normal, but because of the patient's young age and the presence of headaches, catheter arteriography was done and revealed a right posterior communicating aneurysm (**B**, *arrow*).

SYNDROMES ASSOCIATED WITH CN III PALSY

Nuclear III Nerve Lesions

• Nuclear CN III palsies are extraordinarily infrequent (**Fig. 10-3** and **Table 10-1**).

• Ipsilateral CN III palsy, contralateral SR paresis (because the SR muscle is innervated by contralateral subnuclei), and bilateral ptosis (levators innervated by central midline nuclei)

• Bilateral CN III palsies without ptosis

• Bilateral ptosis alone

• Any isolated palsy of a muscle innervated by CN III

CN III Fascicle Syndromes

• Weber syndrome: Ipsilateral CN III paresis with contralateral hemiparesis (involvement of cerebral peduncle)

• Nothnagel syndrome: Ipsilateral CN III paresis and cerebellar ataxia (involvement of superior cerebellar peduncle)

• Benedikt syndrome: Ipsilateral CN III paresis with contralateral hemitremor (involvement of red nucleus)

Lesions in the Subarachnoid Space

• PCOM artery aneurysm: This is the most common cause of an isolated pupil involving CN III palsy, with the aneurysm occurring at the junction of the PCOM artery and internal carotid artery.

• Uncal herniation: As CN III travels through the subarachnoid space, it rests on the edge of the tentorium cerebelli with the uncal portion of the temporal lobe above it. A supratentorial mass may cause a downward displacement and herniation of the uncus across the tentorial edge, compressing the nerve. The patient usually has an altered mental status.

Cavernous Sinus Syndrome

• CN III paresis inside the cavernous sinus usually occurs in association with paresis of other CNs (IV, V, or VI).

Orbital Syndromes

• Because CN III divides into a superior and an inferior division as it enters the orbit, involvement in the orbit may result in paresis of structures innervated by either of these divisions.

TABLE 10-1. Midbrain Fascicular Third Cranial Nerve Palsies

Syndrome	Signs	Location of Lesion
Weber	CN III palsy	Corticospinal tracts
	Contralateral hemiplegia	Cerebral peduncle
Benedikt	CN III palsy	Red nucleus
	Contralateral ataxia and involuntary movements	
Nothnagel	CN III palsy	Brachium conjunctivum
	Ipsilateral ataxia	

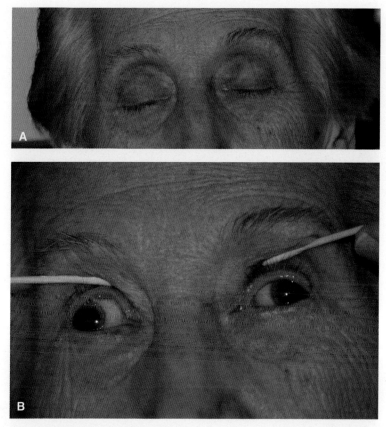

FIGURE 10-3. **Nuclear III palsy with bilateral ptosis.** Nuclear III palsy with bilateral ptosis (**A**), exotropia in primary position (**B**), and

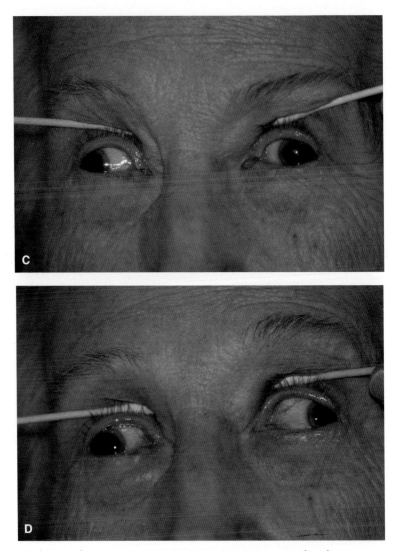

FIGURE 10-3. (*continued*) inability of any eye movement except abduction OU (**C, D**).

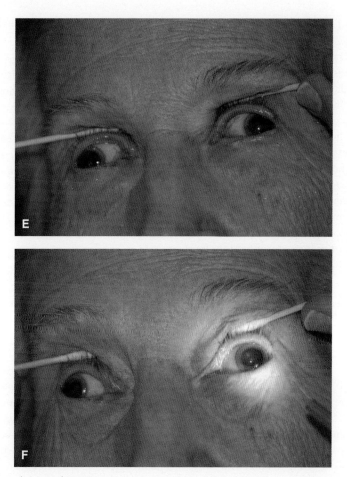

FIGURE 10-3. (*continued*) **E.** There is no vertical movement. **F.** Both pupils are dilated and nonreactive to light.

DIAGNOSTIC EVALUATION

Once CN III palsy has been diagnosed, the next step is to determine whether the palsy is isolated. An associated cranial nerve VI (CN VI) deficit is usually easily identified, but an accompanying CN IV palsy may be less obvious. The primary action of CN IV is depression in adduction; however, in the presence of a complete CN III palsy, the eye cannot be adducted to test for CN IV integrity. The determination is made by looking for the secondary action of CN IV, intorsion of the globe. The patient is instructed to look down while the examiner looks for intorsion. Its absence indicates CN IV paresis (Fig. 10-4).

The investigation of an isolated CN III palsy will depend on the age of the patient, the completeness of the palsy, and the state of the pupil. Guidelines for investigations using these factors are listed in Table 10-2. However, it is becoming the rule for all patients with CN III palsies to undergo MRA or CTA.

• Aneurysms are extraordinarily rare in children under 10 years of age, but ophthalmoplegic migraine is a frequent cause of CN III palsies with pupillary involvement, thus the rationale for subjecting children with CN III palsies to MRI and MRA, but not catheter angiography.

• Patients in the vasculopathic age range with risk factors and no pupillary involvement require investigation to identify those risk factors if none are known to be present, for example, determination of glucose status and blood pressure. In addition, giant cell arteritis may present with any isolated CN palsy; so the patient should specifically be questioned regarding the signs and symptoms associated with giant cell arteritis. Erythrocyte sedimentation rate/C-reactive protein may be helpful if this diagnosis is considered.

• However, if the pupil is involved, the patient should have an urgent MRI/MRA or CT/CTA, and if negative, because the chances of a PCOM aneurysm are still high, we still recommend catheter angiography.

• Patients younger than the vasculopathic age range but older than 10 years require MRI and MRA to rule out tumors or aneurysms even if the pupil is normal. If the pupil is abnormal, however, catheter angiography should be performed even if the neuroimaging is negative. If all imaging tests are unrevealing, then further hematologic and spinal fluid investigations are recommended.

TABLE 10-2. Investigation of Third Cranial Nerve Palsies

	Under 10 Y	11–50 Y	Over 50 Y
Anisocoria less than 2 mm	MRI MRA	MRI, MRA If negative, perform medical workup	Observe without imaging*
Anisocoria greater than 2 mm	MRI MRA†	MRI, MRA If negative, catheter angiography	MRI, MRA If negative, catheter angiography

*Determine the status of the blood pressure, glucose metabolism, and the presence of other medical risk factors.
†Catheter angiography may be justified if these tests are negative.

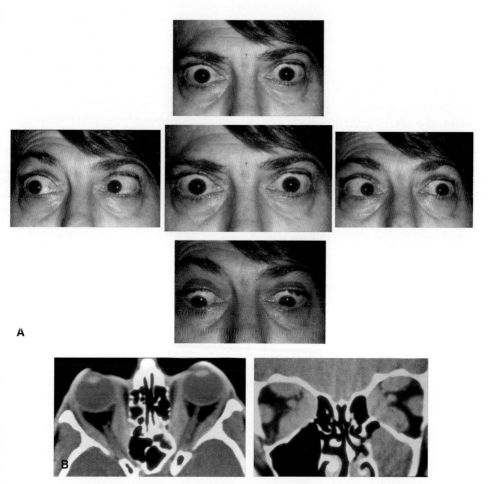

FIGURE 10-4. **Thyroid eye disease.** **A.** Patient with thyroid eye disease with lid retraction in primary gaze and decreased ocular ductions especially in upgaze. **B.** Axial and coronal CT shows enlargement of the extraocular muscles.

DIFFERENTIAL DIAGNOSIS

- A variety of entities produce ocular motor syndromes that can be confused with complete or partial CN III palsies.

  - Thyroid eye disease often produces restriction of the inferior rectus muscles. However, typically, medial rectus restriction is also present producing esotropia and not the exotropia of CN III. Lid retraction, if present, and a positive forced duction test help to establish the correct diagnosis (see Fig. 9-5).

  - Myasthenia gravis (MG) also may simulate any pattern of CN III palsy. The pupil is never involved in MG, and the ptosis and ocular motility disturbances are variable.

  - Orbital trauma can produce an upgaze defect as the result of entrapment of the inferior rectus muscle or as part of a traumatic orbital apex/superior orbital fissure syndrome (Fig. 10-5; see p. 311). Vertical diplopia can also occur following cataract surgery utilizing retrobulbar anesthesia (Fig. 10-6). The cause of the SR "weakness" is actually trauma to the inferior rectus muscle and/or its nerve by the retrobulbar injection. These misalignments may resolve over several months but at times require corrective surgery.

  - Orbital inflammation involving the extraocular muscles may resemble partial CN III palsy. Orbital imaging will reveal the true cause of the ocular misalignment (Fig. 10-7).

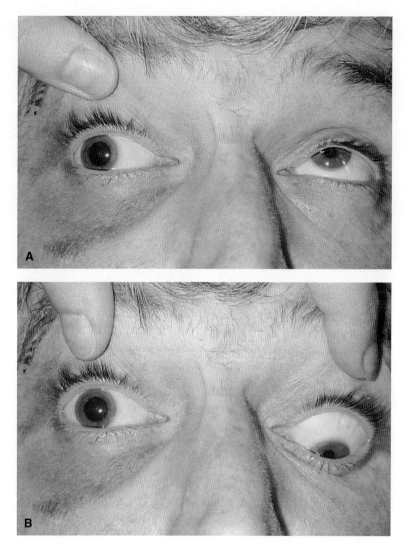

FIGURE 10-5. **Orbital trauma. A, B.** Patient has a right pupil involving CN III following trauma. Note that the conjunctival blood vessel below the right upper lid is in the same position on both up- and downgaze. This lack of intorsion on attempted downgaze indicates a paresis of CN IV.

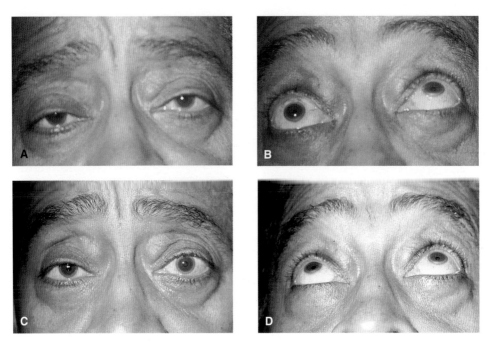

FIGURE 10-6. **Post cataract surgery.** Vertical diplopia appeared after cataract surgery OD with retrobulbar anesthesia. Right upper lid ptosis and poor upgaze (**A**) improved over several months (**B–D**).

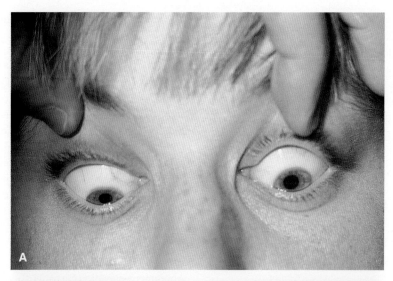

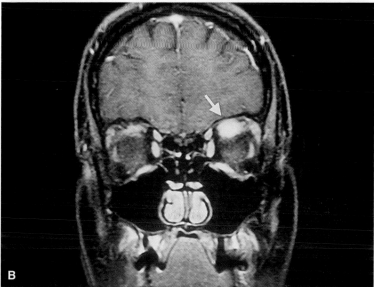

FIGURE 10-7. Orbital inflammation. **A.** Diplopia present on downgaze because of the inability to depress the left eye. **B.** Coronal MRI scan reveals enlargement and increased enhancement of the left superior rectus, levator complex (*arrow*). The forced duction test was positive.

NATURAL HISTORY

- Vasculopathic CN III palsies will resolve spontaneously over a period of 6 to 12 weeks. It is very uncommon for there to be residual diplopia.

- CN palsies because of compression will resolve if the compression is removed or will resolve in a pattern called *aberrant regeneration*.

- The conditions that should prompt investigation of a CN III palsy under observation are listed in **Table 10-3**.

ABERRANT REGENERATION OF CN III

Aberrant regeneration of CN III (**Fig. 10-8**), a stereotypic pattern, most often follows an acute CN III palsy because of a PCOM

TABLE 10-3. When to Investigate a Cranial Nerve III Palsy Under Observation

The pupil dilates
An incomplete CN III palsy progresses after 1 wk
Other neurologic signs or symptoms develop
Aberrant regeneration appears
There is no resolution in 3 mo

aneurysm or pituitary apoplexy. The ptosis resolves completely or is minimally evident. The eye usually will not elevate or depress well, but adduction usually is restored. Aberrant regeneration can be either lid-gaze dyskinesis or pupil-gaze dyskinesis. In pupil-gaze dyskinesis, some of the medial rectus fibers innervate the pupillary sphincter, so that there is more pupil constriction on adduction than to light stimulation (a pseudo-Argyll Robertson pupil). With lid-gaze dyskinesis some of the inferior rectus or medial rectus fibers innervate the levator, so that the upper lid elevates on adduction and downgaze fissure. This widening of the interpalpebral fissure on downgaze is known as the pseudo-Graefe sign.

Aberrant regeneration is a pattern of resolution in compressive or traumatic CN III palsies. It should never be attributed to vasculopathic CN III palsy.

Primary Aberrant Regeneration

Some patients never experience acute CN III palsy but develop a slowly progressive form of CN III aberrant regeneration. Slow growing compressive lesions, usually within the cavernous sinus, produce this syndrome. These lesions are usually meningiomas or cavernous sinus aneurysms, although other causes have been reported.

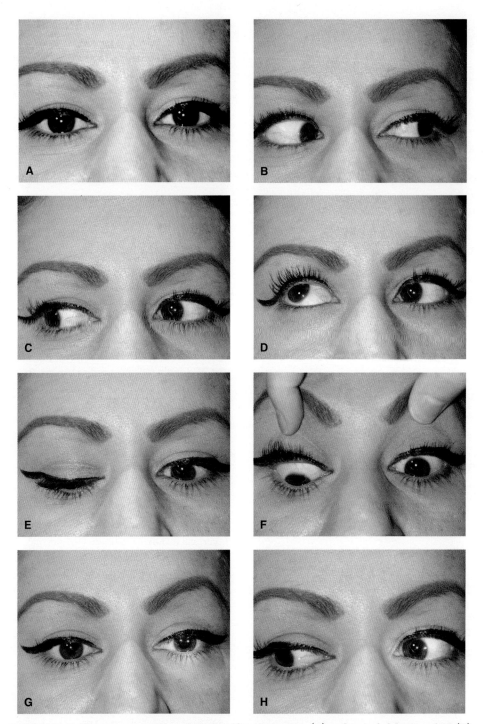

FIGURE 10-8. Abberant regeneration of CN III. There is no ptosis (**A**), and normal abduction of OS (**B**). There is mild limitation in adduction of OS (**C**). There is some limitation of elevation of OS (**D**). The left upper lid elevates on downgaze (**E**) and OS shows some limitation of downgaze. **F.** The left pupil is larger and does not constrict to light (**G**) but does so on adduction (**H**) and depression of OS. The patient had pituitary apoplexy 6 months before with a complete CN III palsy OS.

CRANIAL NERVE IV PALSY

CN IV innervates only the superior oblique muscle, which depresses the eye in adduction and intorts the eye. CN IV is the only CN that exits the brainstem dorsally, and it has the longest intracranial course. It also decussates so that the right nucleus of CN IV will eventually innervate the left superior oblique muscle. CN IV is enveloped in the anterior medullary velum where it is vulnerable to head trauma.

ETIOLOGY

- Head trauma
- Microvascular infarction
- Congenital
- Other causes such as tumors, multiple sclerosis, and inflammation are less frequent

CLINICAL CHARACTERISTICS

Symptoms
- Diplopia is oblique in nature
- Difficulty in reading or walking downstairs

Signs
- Vertical misalignment: The ocular misalignment is usually a hypertropia ipsilateral to the side of the CN involvement. It is worse on gaze to the contralateral side and on ipsilateral head tilt. (For example, a right CN IV palsy produces a right hypertropia worse in left gaze and right head tilt.) The method to most easily detect this misalignment is the Parks Three-Step Test, which determines by using cover–uncover test whether (Fig. 10-9)

  - there is a hypertropia in primary position
  - the hypertropia increases in left or right gaze
  - the hypertropia increases on head tilt (Bielschowsky head-tilt test)

- The head is tilted away from the side of the CN palsy. The chin may be depressed (Fig. 10-10A).

- Elevation in adduction of the ipsilateral inferior oblique muscle, the antagonist of the paretic superior oblique muscle, is demonstrable (Fig. 10-10B).

- Excyclotorsion may be documented using the following:

  - The double Maddox rod or Lancaster red–green glasses (Fig. 10-10C)
  - Ophthalmoscopy: Normally, the fovea is 0.3 mm below imaginary line drawn through the geometric center of the optic disc. With direct ophthalmoscopy, the fovea will appear *lower* if excyclotorsion is present (Fig. 10-11). However, with indirect ophthalmoscopy the fovea appears higher than the optic nerve.

- Vertical fusional amplitude: The normal vertical fusional range is 1 to 3 prism diopters. Patients with a congenital CN IV palsy have an increased range of fusional amplitudes.

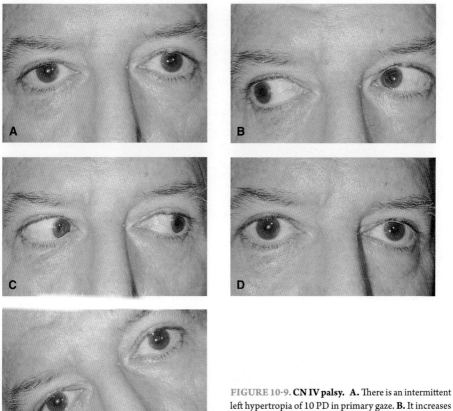

FIGURE 10-9. CN IV palsy. A. There is an intermittent left hypertropia of 10 PD in primary gaze. **B.** It increases dramatically in right gaze because of elevation in adduction of the left inferior oblique muscle. **C.** Left gaze is normal. It is larger on left (**D**) than on right head tilt (**E**).

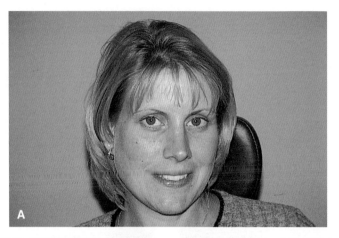

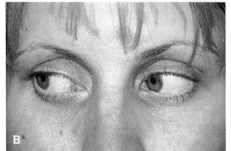 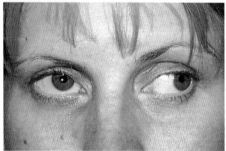

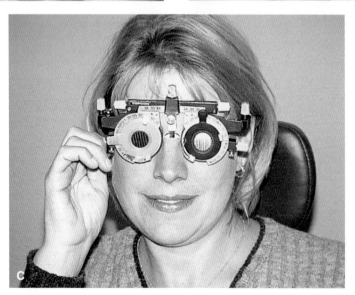

FIGURE 10-10. **CN IV palsy. A.** Patient with right CN IV palsy with a left head tilt and a chin down position.
B. Right gaze is normal but there is marked elevation in adduction of the right inferior oblique muscle in left gaze.
C. Excyclotorsion is measured with the double Maddox rod.

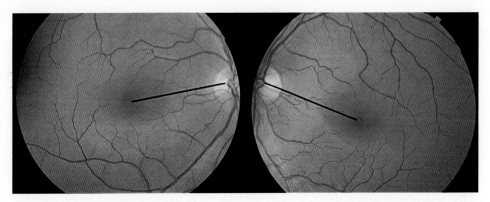

FIGURE 10-11. **Excyclotortion in CN IV palsy.** Fundus photograph shows the normal position of the macula in relation to the optic disc in the right eye (left) and the lower position of the macula in the extorted left eye (right) of a patient with a left CN IV palsy.

SYNDROMES ASSOCIATED WITH CN IV PALSY

- Nuclear-fascicular lesions: CN IV palsy with a contralateral Horner syndrome because the sympathetic pathways descend through the midbrain adjacent to the trochlear fascicles.

- Subarachnoid space lesions: Usually produces an isolated CN IV palsy; bilateral CN IV palsies may occur when the site of injury is at the anterior medullary velum.

- Cavernous sinus lesions: CN IV palsy is seen in combination with CN III palsy. To diagnose CN IV paresis, the patient should be instructed to abduct the eye and then asked to look down. The ability of the eye to intort in this position is an indication of intact CN IV function.

- Orbital lesions: In the orbit, CN IV palsy occurs in conjunction with other CN palsies as well as other features of orbital disease such as proptosis, chemosis, or conjunctival injection.

DIAGNOSTIC EVALUATION

In the presence of isolated CN IV palsy, a history of head trauma should be sought. In the absence of history of head trauma, isolated CN IV palsy in a patient over 50 years of age is assumed to be vasculopathic in nature. Patients younger than the vasculopathic age group should undergo neuroimaging. Patients over the age of 55 years should be investigated for giant cell arteritis. Congenital CN IV palsies may become manifest later in life. These patients complain of intermittent diplopia that becomes more frequent and more prolonged. Examination reveals increased vertical fusional amplitudes, which establish the diagnosis of a congenital process. Examining old family photographs likewise may reveal a long-standing head tilt,

another clue to the congenital nature of the strabismus. In patients with increased vertical fusional amplitudes, no further investigations are required. Vertical fusional amplitudes should be measured in all patients with CN IV palsy.

NATURAL HISTORY

- Patients in the vasculopathic age group with an isolated CN IV palsy and normal vertical fusional amplitudes require investigation for risk factors (e.g., diabetes mellitus and hypertension). These patients may then be observed because most of these palsies will resolve spontaneously within 6 to 12 weeks.

- Patients with traumatic CN IV palsies may also be observed. The misalignment, however, may take longer to resolve.

TREATMENT

- Prisms may be tried, but because of the incomitant and at times the torsional nature of this ocular misalignment, they are often not successful. Surgical realignment of the eyes is often the final solution for these patients.

BILATERAL CN IV PALSIES

Trauma often produces bilateral CN IV palsies. The bilaterality of the process may be masked and patients will sometimes appear to have a unilateral palsy. Clues to bilateral involvement include the following:

- Large cyclorotational misalignment: Patients with an apparent "unilateral" CN IV palsy but with excyclotorsion greater than 10 degrees should be suspected of having bilateral CN IV palsies.

- V-pattern esotropia

- Alternating hypertropia (right hypertropia on left gaze and left hypertropia on right gaze)

SKEW DEVIATION

A skew deviation is a vertical/torsional strabismus caused by a supranuclear lesion that must be differentiated from CN IV palsy. It is usually caused by a lesion in the prenuclear vestibular inputs to the oculomotor nuclei. It may be part of a full ocular tilt reaction (see below). Characteristics of a skew deviation include the following:

- Comitant or incomitant vertical misalignment

- With lower brainstem lesions the ipsilateral eye is usually hypotropic, whereas with pons or midbrain lesions the ipsilateral eye is hypertropic. An alternating skew is characteristic of cerebellar degeneration, with the abducting eye being hypertropic.

- The upright-supine test: A vertical deviation that decreases by 50% from the upright to supine position suggests skew deviation.

- Rarely, it may alternate with eye position so that there is right hypertropia in right gaze and left hypertropia in left gaze.

- Skew deviation may be associated with the ocular tilt reaction, which is the triad of the following:

  - Skew deviation

  - Ocular torsion—such that the upper poles of both eyes rotate in the same direction as that of the head tilt (i.e., the hypotropic eye is excyclotorted and the hypertropic eye incyclotorted). This is the opposite of the physiologic counterroll during which the upper poles of both eyes rotate in the opposite direction to that of the head tilt.

  - Head tilt— the pathologic head tilt is ipsilateral to the hypotropic eye.

CRANIAL NERVE VI PALSY

CN VI has one of the longest intracranial courses. Involvement of this nerve throughout its extranuclear course results in esotropia and ipsilateral abduction deficit.

ANATOMY

The anatomical peculiarity of CN VI is that a lesion in its nucleus will *not* produce an isolated ipsilateral CN VI palsy. The abducens nucleus contains, in addition to cells that give origin to CN VI, interneurons, which give origin to fibers that eventually end in the contralateral medial rectus subnucleus of CN III. This anatomic arrangement ensures conjugate horizontal eye movements; however, it also means that a lesion involving the CN VI nucleus will produce not an ipsilateral abduction deficit but an ipsilateral gaze palsy.

CN VI also lies in proximity to certain other structures throughout its fascicular and peripheral course. It is in close proximity to CN VII in the brainstem and is contained along with CN III, IV, and V within the cavernous sinus. Lesions in these areas are likely to produce combined CN palsies instead of an isolated CN VI palsy.

ETIOLOGY

- The more frequent causes of CN VI palsies are
  - vasculopathic (microvascular) infarction
  - trauma
  - meningitic processes (inflammatory, infectious, and neoplastic)
  - increased intracranial pressure from any cause (**Figure 10-12**)
  - mass lesions (**Figure 10-13**)
  - multiple sclerosis
  - postlumbar puncture or spinal anesthesia (**Figure 10-14**)
  - stroke
  - postflu or vaccination
  - congenital

SYNDROMES ASSOCIATED WITH CN VI PARESIS

Brainstem Lesions Involving CN VI Nucleus or Nerve

- Foville syndrome is due to the involvement of the pontine tegmentum (dorsolateral pons) and consists of
  - ipsilateral CN VI palsy or gaze palsy
  - ipsilateral CN VII palsy
  - ipsilateral Horner syndrome
  - ipsilateral analgesia of the face
  - peripheral deafness
  - loss of taste to anterior two-thirds of the tongue
- Millard-Gubler syndrome is due to the involvement of the ventral paramedian pons and consists of
  - ipsilateral CN VI palsy
  - ipsilateral CN VII palsy
  - contralateral hemiplegia
- Raymond syndrome consists of
  - ipsilateral VI nerve palsy
  - contralateral hemiparesis

Subarachnoid Involvement

CN VI palsy may be a "nonlocalizing" sign as elevated intracranial pressure may result in downward displacement of the brainstem stretching CN VI, which is tethered at its exit from the pons and Dorello canal.

Petrous Apex Syndrome

- CN VI makes contact with the tip of the petrous bone within the Dorello canal. Characteristic neurologic features caused by pathology in this location include
  - CN VI palsy

- ipsilateral facial pain in distribution of the CN V
- ipsilateral facial paresis (CN VII)
- ipsilateral hearing loss (CN VIII)

● The most common causes of abnormalities in this area include localized inflammation/ infection following complicated otitis media (Gradenigo syndrome) and petrous bone fracture. A cerebellopontine angle tumor may result in the above in addition to papilledema and ataxia.

Cavernous Sinus Syndrome

● CN VI may be involved in isolation or associated with involvement of the CN III, IV, and VI, sympathetic plexus, and optic nerve or chiasm (see below).

Orbital Lesions

● CN VI involvement is associated commonly with proptosis or other orbital signs. There may be involvement of the optic nerve.

CLINICAL CHARACTERISTICS

Symptoms

● Double vision

● Pain around the eye at times, depending on the cause

Signs

● Esotropia is usually present in primary gaze and increases in lateral gaze (Fig. 10-14). The esotropia is worse when the paretic eye is fixating [secondary deviation is greater than primary deviation (p. 288, Fig. 9-3)]. This differs from congenital esotropia, in which the measurement of the esotropia is the same with either eye fixating.

● Abduction defect may be partial or total.

● The saccade in the direction of the paresis is usually slowed.

CONGENITAL CN VI PALSY

● Isolated congenital CN VI palsies usually result from birth trauma.

● Several syndromes occur that combine congenital CN VI palsies with other features.

Möbius Syndrome

● Children with Möbius syndrome have mask-like faces because of facial diplegia and mostly bilateral, but at times unilateral, abduction deficits. They may have no esotropia in primary position. Complete absence of horizontal gaze may be a feature of the disorder.

Duane Retraction Syndrome

● Of the three types of Duane retraction syndrome, type I consists of an isolated abduction deficit, which may be unilateral or bilateral. These patients do not usually have esotropia in primary position and do not appreciate diplopia. They may, however, have abnormal eyelid movements, with the lid retracting on ipsilateral adduction (Fig. 10-15).

● Duane retraction syndrome has actually been shown to be due to a prenatal lesion in the CN VI nucleus. The nuclear cells that give rise to the ipsilateral abducens nerve are absent. A portion of CN III, therefore, innervates the lateral rectus muscle, thus producing the cocontracture that results in retraction of the globe that characterizes Duane syndrome.

DIAGNOSTIC EVALUATION

● The type and extent of the investigation will depend on multiple factors including the patient's age, associated ophthalmologic and neurologic findings, and the uni- or bilaterality of the CN VI palsies.

● Patients over 50 years of age who develop unilateral, isolated CN VI palsy will often have the so-called *vasculopathic* cause for their deficit. This is a vascular occlusion to the CN

VI itself. These infarcts in the nerve are usually sudden in onset and painless, although pain at times may be a feature of isolated vasculopathic CN VI palsy. These palsies are usually self-limiting and tend to resolve within 3 months. In a patient in the vasculopathic age range who has an *isolated* CN VI palsy and who has vasculopathic risk factors such as diabetes mellitus, hypertension, hypercholesterolemia, and so forth, a workup may be deferred. If the CN VI palsy resolves in the specified period of time, a vasculopathic etiology may be inferred. It is recommended that investigations, including MRI, be performed if

- the CN VI palsy does not resolve within the 3-month period of time (Fig. 10-16)

- the esotropia progresses after 2 weeks from its onset

- other signs or symptoms develop

- anyone with a previous history of malignancy even if the CN VI is isolated (Fig. 10-17)

• Although vasculopathic CN VI palsies can be recurrent either on the same or opposite side, the bilateral simultaneous occurrence of CN VI palsies should never be considered vasculopathic in origin. In this circumstance, a workup for other causes should be undertaken.

• In all patients with unilateral or bilateral CN VI palsy, ophthalmoscopy with examination of the optic discs looking for papilledema is required. Increased intracranial pressure from any cause can produce unilateral or bilateral CN VI palsies as a nonlocalizing sign of the increased intracranial pressure.

• Patients under the age of 50 years who present with acquired uni- or bilateral CN VI palsies require investigation. If there is no preceding history of trauma or any other obvious cause for the CN VI palsy, a complete medical history and general neurologic examination

should be conducted. MRI is a critical part of the workup in these patients and should be performed on all of them. If the MRI is unrevealing, a lumbar puncture with examination of the cerebrospinal fluid (CSF) should be considered.

TREATMENT

• Treatment of the CN VI palsy obviously depends on its cause. In the isolated vasculopathic scenario, controlling the risk factors might prevent the recurrence of the problem but will not result in a more prompt resolution of the esotropia.

• Treatment of the esotropia itself is similar to that for other forms of ocular misalignment, that is, patching, prisms, or surgery if the ocular misalignment persists.

PSEUDO-CN VI PALSIES

• All abduction defects are not CN VI palsies. A variety of other disorders can produce abduction defects, including

- Duane retraction syndrome (see above)

- Thyroid eye disease (Fig. 10-18)

- Orbital inflammatory disease (myositis, pseudotumor) (Fig. 10-19)

- MG

- Medial rectus muscle entrapment

- Spasm of the near reflex (SNR): Patients with SNR usually have an intermittent esotropia. This is produced by the patient voluntarily activating the near triad of convergence, accommodation, and pupillary miosis. Every time the esotropia and abduction defect occur, the pupils will become miotic (Fig. 10-20). SNR is rarely due to organic disease.

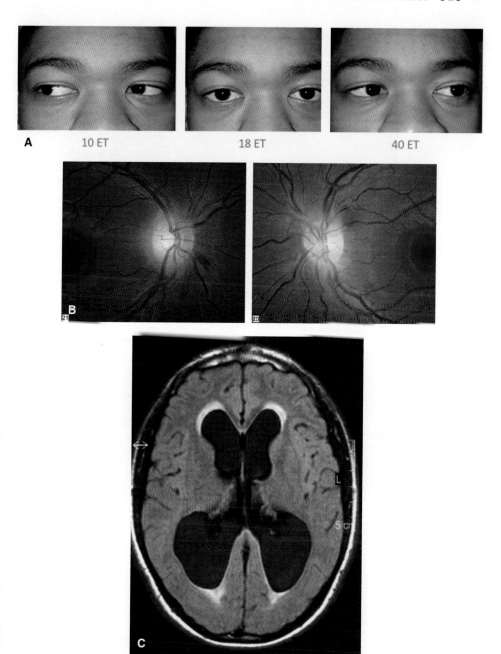

A   10 ET   18 ET   40 ET

FIGURE 10-12. **CN VI palsy.** **A.** Esotropia with bilateral abduction defects in patient with increased intracranial pressure. **B.** Fundus shows bilateral papilledema. **C.** MRI shows hydrocephalus.

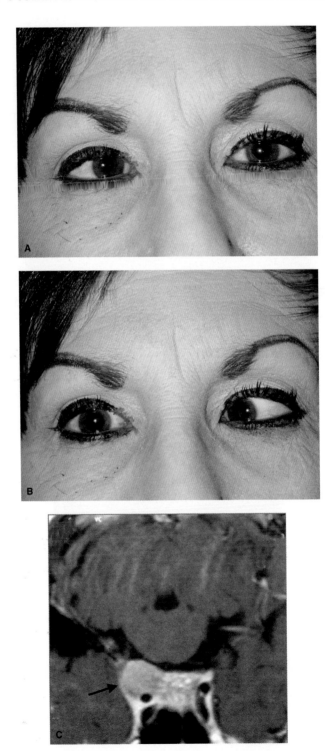

FIGURE 10-13. CN VI palsy. A, B. A 53-year-old woman with esotropia in primary gaze with a right abduction defect. **C.** MRI shows cavernous sinus meningioma (*arrow*).

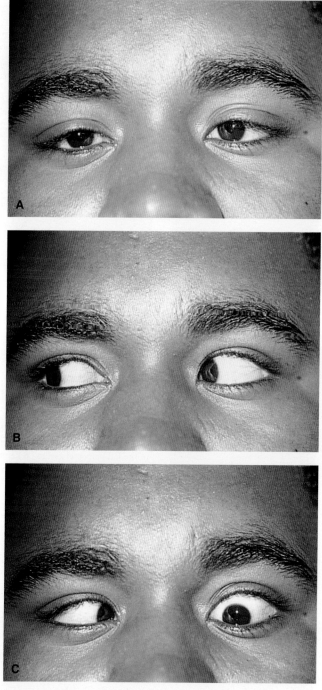

FIGURE 10-14. **CN VI palsy.** **A.** Left esotropia. **B.** There is normal adduction of OS on right gaze but a total left CN VI palsy appeared after lumbar puncture. **C.** The ocular motility returned to normal within 4 months.

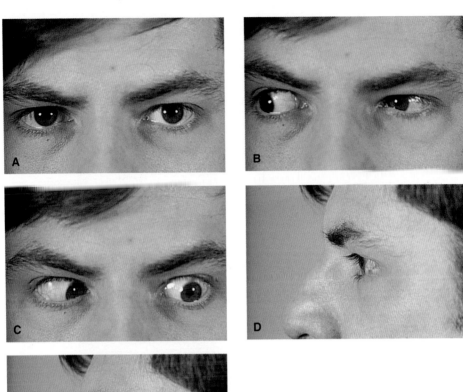

FIGURE 10-15. Duane syndrome: There is an esotropia in primary gaze (**A**); normal right gaze but narrowing of the left palpebral fissure (**B**) and a left abduction deficit (**C**). Side view of OS in primary position (**D**), but it retracts on adduction (**E**).

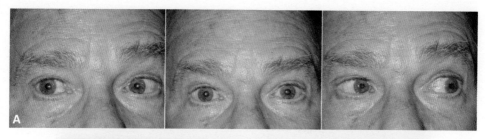

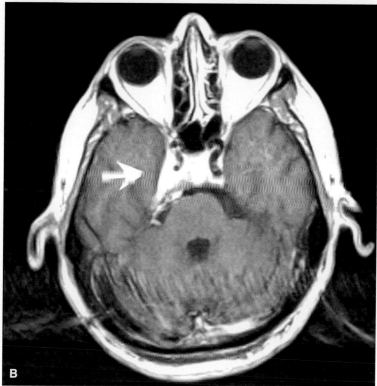

FIGURE 10-16. **CN VI palsy.** **A.** Esotropia and right abduction deficit began 6 months before but has not resolved. **B.** Axial MRI reveals enhancing mass in the right cavernous sinus with a tail characteristic of meningioma (*arrow*).

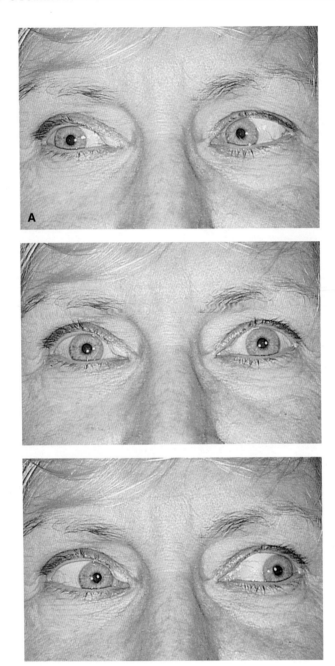

FIGURE 10-17. **CN VI palsy. A.** A 58-year-old woman with an esotropia of 4 PD in her primary gaze (middle) although she appears exotropic, and 14 PD on right gaze with a right abduction deficit (top). Left gaze (bottom) is normal. Her examination was otherwise unremarkable, but because she had breast cancer 10 years before, an MRI was performed (Fig. 10-15).

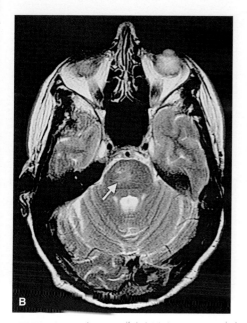
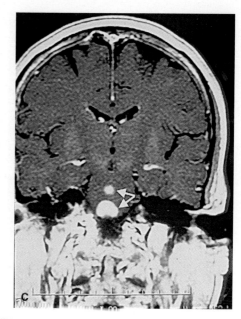

FIGURE 10-17. (*continued*) Axial (**B**) and coronal (**C**) MRIs show two areas of enhancement in the pons (*arrows*). There also were asymptomatic multiple metastatic enhancing lesions in the cerebellum and frontal and temporal lobes

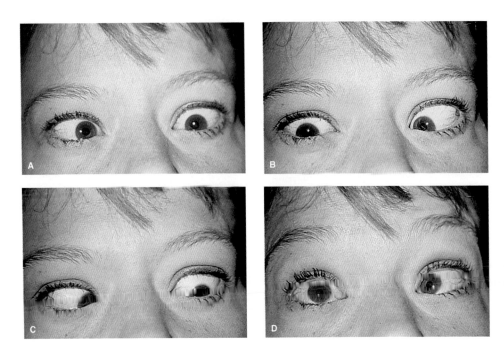

FIGURE 10-18. **Thyroid eye disease.** There is a large esotropia in primary gaze (**A**) with inability to abduct (**B** and **C**) or to elevate (**D**) either eye. The clues to the diagnosis of thyroid eye disease (TED) are lid retraction, the characteristic injection over the lateral rectus muscles, and inability to look up with either eye (bottom).

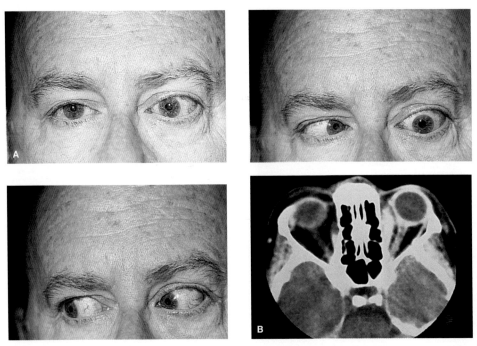

FIGURE 10-19. **Orbital inflammatory disease. A.** Esotropia in primary gaze with absent abduction left eye. Right gaze is normal. The left eye is injected. **B.** Axial CT scan shows an enlarged, enhancing left medial rectus muscle.

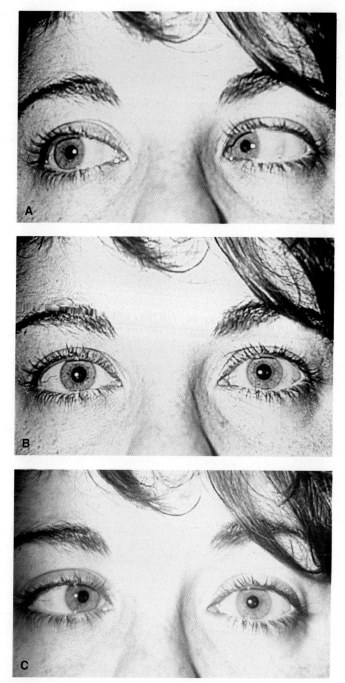

FIGURE 10-20. **Spasm of the near reflex. A–C.** The pupils become markedly miotic when the left abduction defect appears (bottom).

MULTIPLE CN PALSIES

The guidelines for the investigation of CN III, IV, or VI palsies are based largely on their being isolated. The simultaneous presence of more than one CN palsy, or other neurologic signs or symptoms, implies the involvement of different anatomic regions and, by and large, the presence of different disease processes than those that produce isolated CN palsies. Associated neurologic findings that accompany the CN palsy help point to the localization of the disease process. For example, a CN III palsy combined with a contralateral hemiparesis indicates a brainstem lesion.

The simultaneous presence of two or more cranial neuropathies requires the clinician to determine whether one or multiple lesions are causing the clinical signs. Most of the lesions that produce multiple CN palsies involve the peripheral nerves, whereas lesions producing other neurologic problems, for example, hemiparesis or contralateral tremor associated with CN palsies, will be found in the brainstem. CNs III, IV, and VI come together in close proximity in the cavernous sinus, and in this location a single lesion may affect more than one cranial nerve.

CAVERNOUS SINUS SYNDROME

The cavernous sinus is a venous structure on either side of the pituitary gland. The lateral wall of the sinus contains CN III, IV, and V. CN VI traverses the body of the cavernous sinus relatively isolated from the other CNs. The internal carotid artery occupies the central portion of the cavernous sinus (Fig. 10-21). The ocular sympathetic fibers destined for the iris dilator muscle are also contained in this portion of the cavernous sinus. A lesion in the cavernous sinus may produce involvement of any of the CNs or other structures contained therein.

Mass lesions in the cavernous sinus (tumors or aneurysms) may at times produce an isolated CN VI palsy. Because of its location within the body of the cavernous sinus and not within its dural walls, an isolated CN VI palsy may be the first and, at times, the only sign of cavernous sinus disease (Fig. 10-15). More frequently, however, patients with cavernous sinus lesions present with an ocular motility disturbance that is a combination of involvement of CN III, IV, and VI and often with symptoms attributable to CN V.

ETIOLOGY

- Any lesion in the cavernous sinus may produce the so-called *cavernous sinus syndrome*. The most frequent causes are

  - meningiomas
  - intracavernous aneurysms
  - extension of parachiasmal or skull-based mass lesions into the cavernous sinus, for example, pituitary apoplexy
  - metastatic lesions (Fig. 10-22)
  - inflammation or infection: For example, sarcoidosis, syphilis, mucormycosis (Fig. 10-23), herpes zoster, or idiopathic granulomatous inflammation (Tolosa-Hunt syndrome)
  - arteriovenous fistula (carotid-cavernous or dural) (Fig. 10-24)
  - cavernous sinus thrombosis (Fig. 10-25)

CLINICAL CHARACTERISTICS

Symptoms

- Diplopia may be caused by a combination of CN III, IV, and VI or at times isolated CN VI palsy.

- Pain (often severe) or numbness in the distribution of CN V.

- Lid malposition may be secondary to lid edema from venous engorgement produced by a cavernous sinus mass or may be due to a ptosis produced by concomitant Horner syndrome or CN III involvement.

- Anisocoria may be due to CN III palsy, Horner syndrome, or both. If both are present, the pupil may be small or mid dilated and poorly reactive. That combination is virtually pathognomonic of a cavernous sinus lesion.

Signs

- An ocular motility pattern with or without lid and pupillary signs indicating combined involvement of CN III, IV, and VI.

- Decreased sensation over the distribution of CN V_1 and V_2.

- Ocular sympathetic paresis (Horner syndrome). The combination of an isolated CN VI paresis and Horner syndrome may suggest an intracavernous aneurysm or another lesion in the body of the sinus. This is because the sympathetic fibers leave the internal carotid artery within the cavernous sinus and join briefly with CN VI before separating and fusing with the ophthalmic division of CN V.

DIAGNOSTIC EVALUATION

The simultaneous presence of two or more CN palsies requires that an MRI scan of the brain and skull base be performed.

SUPERIOR ORBITAL FISSURE SYNDROME

The anteriormost border of the cavernous sinus is the superior orbital fissure. The clinical signs and symptoms of involvement of this area are identical to the cavernous sinus syndrome with one exception. With lesions of the posterior cavernous sinus, CN V_3 may be involved, whereas this branch is not present in the superior orbital fissure.

ORBITAL APEX SYNDROME

Immediately in front of the superior orbital fissure is the orbital apex. CNs III, IV, V, and VI may be involved here as well. However, because the optic nerve is contained in the orbit, an orbital apex syndrome must be suspected when signs of optic neuropathy accompany CN ocular motility disturbances. Proptosis is another sign of orbital apex syndrome.

Lesions of the orbit may produce ocular motor disturbances that resemble multiple CN palsies. Thyroid eye disease is the most frequent cause, but any orbital lesion can produce a similar clinical picture.

OTHER CAUSES OF MULTIPLE CN PALSIES

The clinical abnormalities found in the cavernous sinus, superior orbital fissure, and orbital apex syndromes are all ipsilateral. However, simultaneous involvement of more than one CN on opposite sides may occur. In this situation, one should suspect a more diffuse disease process that involves the meninges or the CSF. MRI scanning looking for dural enhancement followed by lumbar puncture should be the first investigations performed.

Although it is possible to have the simultaneous involvement of more than one CN on a vasculopathic basis, this is extraordinarily rare and must remain a diagnosis of exclusion.

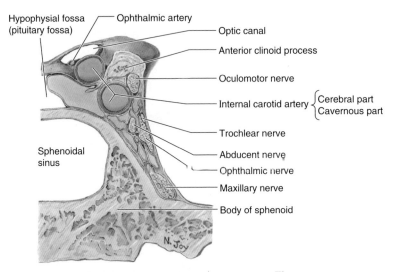

FIGURE 10-21. **Schematic of cavernous sinus anatomy.** (Reprinted from Kline LB. The Tolosa-Hunt Syndrome. *Surv Ophthalmol* 1982;27:79–95, with permission from Elsevier Science.)

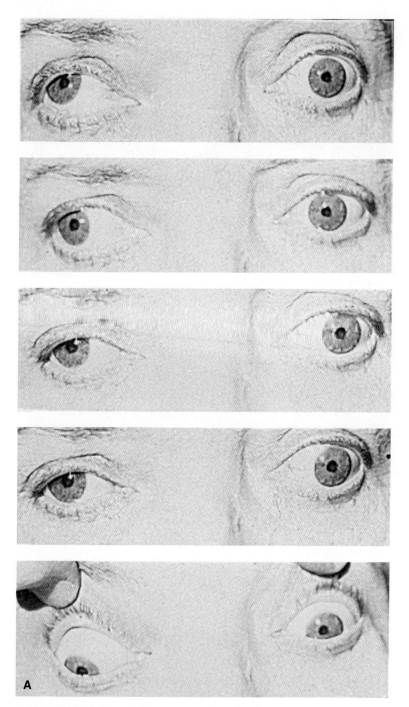

FIGURE 10-22. Metastatic lesions. A. There is exotropia in primary gaze (middle photograph) with globally decreased ductions.

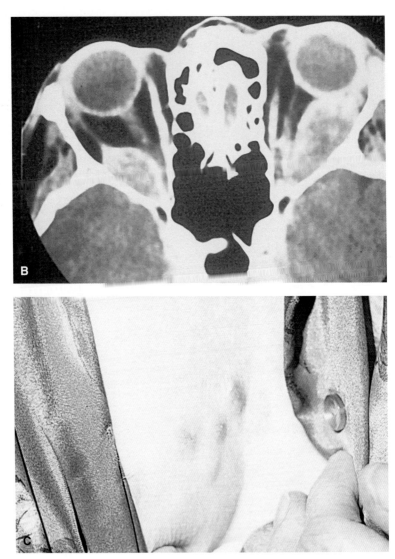

FIGURE 10-22. (*continued*) **B.** CT scan reveals masses in each orbit involving the lateral rectus muscles. **C.** The patient had breast cancer with metastasis to the chest wall as well as the orbits.

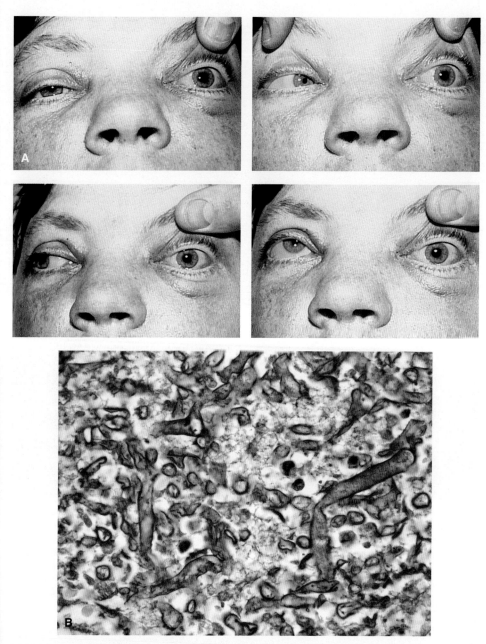

FIGURE 10-23. **Orbital mucormycosis. A.** Left ptosis and total ophthalmoplegia (downgaze not shown). The patient also had a retinal artery occlusion (not shown). **B.** Nonseptate hyphae diagnostic of mucormycosis were identified on orbital biopsy. (Courtesy of Ralph Eagle, MD.)

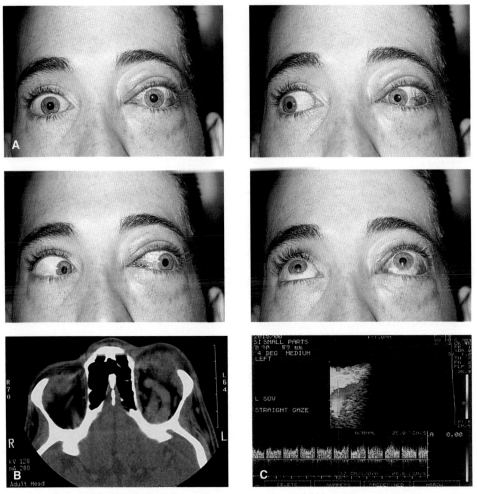

FIGURE 10-24. Arteriovenous fistula. A. The eyes are straight in primary gaze (top), but there is decreased adduction, abduction, depression (not shown), and elevation of the left eye. There are typical arterialized conjunctival blood vessels of a carotid cavernous fistula (CCF). **B.** Axial CT scan shows a greatly enlarged left superior ophthalmic vein (SOV). **C.** Color Doppler reveals reversal of flow in the left SOV (it appears red instead of its normal blue color).

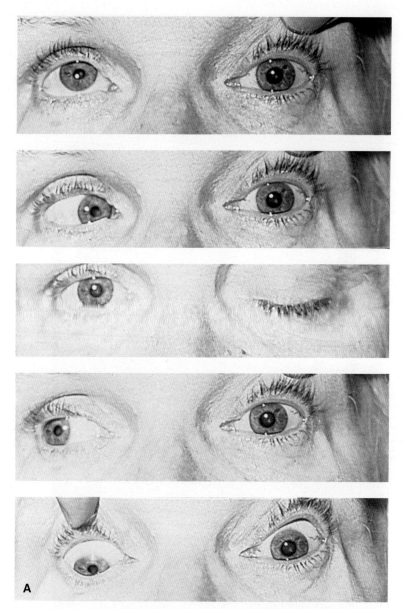

FIGURE 10-25. **Cavernous sinus thrombosis. A.** Total left ophthalmoplegia. The pupil is dilated. CN IV is involved (the conjunctival blood vessel OS does not intort on attempted downgaze).

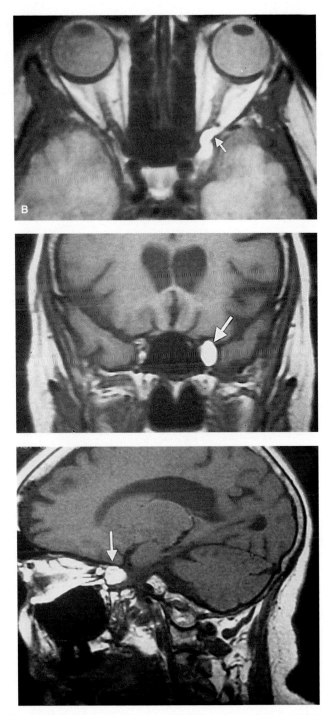

FIGURE 10-25. (*continued*) **B.** Axial, coronal, and sagittal MRI scans reveal a mass with the characteristics of hemorrhage in the cavernous sinus (*arrow*).

INTERNUCLEAR OPHTHALMOPLEGIA

The medial longitudinal fasciculus (MLF), a tract that extends from the pons to the mesencephalon, links the nucleus of CN VI to the contralateral medial rectus subnucleus of CN III to produce conjugate eye movements. The MLF also contains fibers that connect the vestibular nuclei with the ocular motor nuclei. A lesion in the MLF will produce an ocular motility disturbance termed internuclear ophthalmoplegia (INO).

ETIOLOGY

Any disease process that involves the MLF can produce an INO. However, the two most frequent causes of this eye movement abnormality are multiple sclerosis and stroke.

CLINICAL CHARACTERISTICS

Symptoms

• Patients with INOs do not usually appreciate diplopia. They may complain of a vague visual disturbance that is difficult for them to define.

• Patients who do appreciate diplopia have the double vision on the basis of an associated neurologic finding, for example, a skew deviation.

Signs

• Adduction paresis or paralysis and contralateral abducting nystagmus: The typical picture of an INO is an adduction defect in one or both eyes (resembling an isolated medial rectus paresis) associated with disassociated abduction nystagmus in the contralateral eye. If the adduction deficit is complete, this is termed INO (Fig. 10-26); if it is incomplete, it is called internuclear ophthalmo*paresis* (Fig. 10-27). The side of the INO is named for the side of the adduction deficit. Therefore,

a right INO will have a right adduction deficit and nystagmus of the abducting left eye. Rarely, a patient may not have a deficit of adduction but will have only a slowing of the saccadic velocity in the adducting eye, an adduction lag. This is shown by having the patient look from abduction to primary position and noting that there is a marked slowing of the medial rectus saccade. The eye appears to float inward instead of crisply coming to the midline.

• Convergence may be intact or impaired.

• Skew deviation: Commonly occurs with unilateral INO and rarely with a bilateral INO. The hypertropic eye is usually on the side of the lesion.

DIAGNOSTIC EVALUATION

• The presence of an INO indicates a brainstem lesion; therefore, MRI scanning should be performed. It is not unusual for MRI scans to be normal in the presence of an INO. At times, however, the causative lesions may be evident (Fig. 10-28).

TREATMENT

There is no treatment specifically for the INO. Patients are treated depending on the underlying cause of the INO. Multiple sclerosis routinely occurs in younger patients and produces bilateral INOs (Fig. 10-29). These often resolve. Older patients have INOs on the basis of stroke, and these tend to be unilateral. These may also resolve spontaneously.

SPECIAL FORMS OF INO

Wall-eyed bilateral internuclear ophthalmoplegia (WEBINO) is a bilateral INO because of a lesion in the mesencephalon. These patients are exotropic (Fig. 10-30), whereas most patients with an INO (even bilateral INOs) are orthotropic in primary position. The causes of the WEBINO syndrome are identical to those of INO.

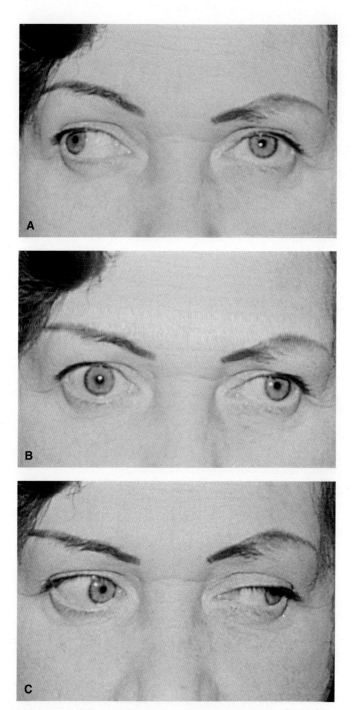

FIGURE 10-26. **Internuclear ophthalmoplegia. A–C.** Unilateral left internuclear ophthalmoplegia with inability to adduct the left eye past the midline. There is exotropia in primary gaze (middle).

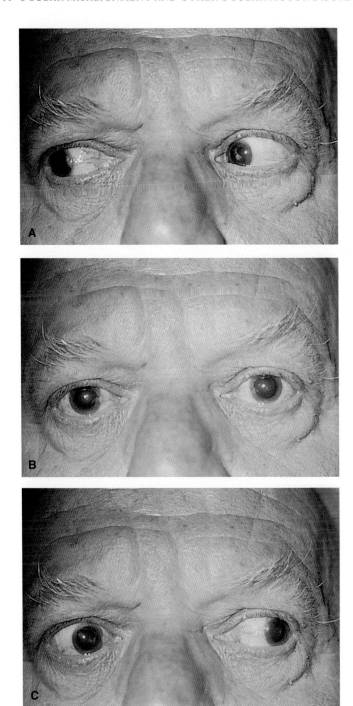

FIGURE 10-27. Internuclear ophthalmoparesis. A–C. No ocular misalignment in primary gaze (middle). Right gaze is full, but there is a small right adduction deficit on left gaze.

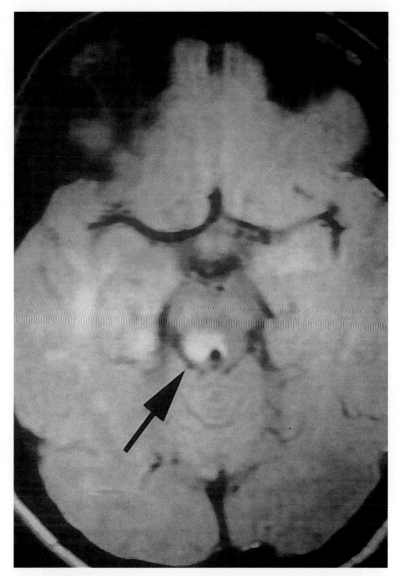

FIGURE 10-28. Internuclear ophthalmoplegia. Axial MRI shows demyelinating lesion (*arrow*) in a patient with internuclear ophthalmoplegia.

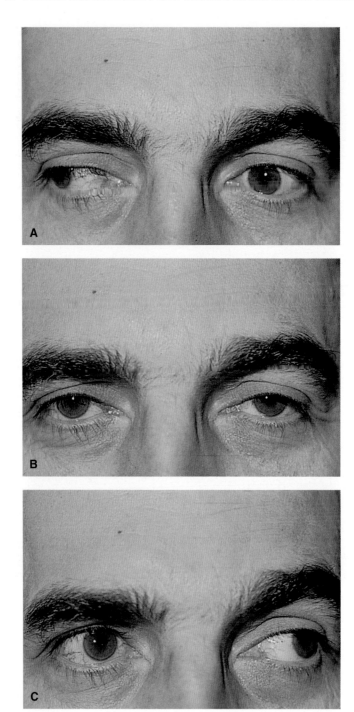

FIGURE 10-29. Bilateral internuclear ophthalmoplegia. A–C. Bilateral internuclear ophthalmoplegia, but the eyes are straight in primary gaze (middle).

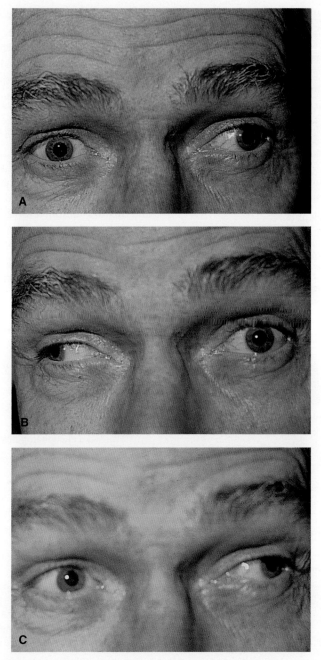

FIGURE 10-30. Wall-eyed bilateral internuclear ophthalmoplegia. There is exotropia in primary position (**A**), with decreased adduction on right (**B**) and left (**C**) gaze.

GAZE PALSIES

Complete inability to move the eyes into right or left gaze is called gaze palsy, whereas incomplete or limited horizontal excursions are termed gaze paresis (**Table 10-4**).

Gaze palsies may be caused by lesions in several sites. The most common are

- frontal lobe,
- pontine paramedian reticular formation (PPRF),
- abducens nucleus.

FRONTAL LOBE

Cortical lesions acutely may produce a gaze deviation toward the side of the involved hemisphere and gaze palsy toward the intact hemisphere. This deviation, unlike those of brainstem origin, may be overcome with oculocephalic movements. The gaze deviation and preference usually resolve within 1 week. Ophthalmologists rarely see these patients because they have neurologic deficits, including alteration of levels of consciousness that require hospitalization often in an ICU.

PONTINE PARAMEDIAN RETICULAR FORMATION

The PPRF is located rostral to the CN VI nucleus within the pons. A lesion in the PPRF will produce ipsilateral conjugate horizontal gaze palsy. The eyes may be deviated to the side opposite the acute lesion. Vestibular stimuli may produce ocular deviation to the side of the palsy if the lesion spares the CN VI nucleus and its vestibular connections.

ABDUCENS NUCLEUS

Lesions of the nucleus of CN VI will also produce gaze palsy because the nucleus contains, in addition to abducens neurons, interneurons destined for the medial rectus subnucleus of the contralateral CN III. Therefore, a lesion in the right CN VI nucleus will produce right gaze palsy and not right CN VI palsy. The causes of gaze palsies are the same as for INO (see p. 344).

ETIOLOGY

- The most frequent causes of gaze palsies are the following:
  - Multiple sclerosis
  - Stroke
  - Wernicke encephalopathy
  - Infectious or inflammatory meningoencephalitis
  - Tumors or other mass lesions
  - Degenerative disorders [see progressive supranuclear palsy (PSP)]

TABLE 10-4. Location of Lesions That Produce Gaze Palsies and Clinical Characteristics

Location of Lesion	Gaze Palsy	Direction of Deviation of Eyes	Response to Oculocephalic Testing
Frontal lobe	Contralateral to lesion	Toward involved hemisphere	Overcome with oculocephalic movements
PPRF	Ipsilateral to lesion	Opposite side of lesion	Overcome with oculocephalic movements
Abducens nucleus	Ipsilateral to lesion	Opposite side of lesion	No change with oculocephalic movement

PPRF, pontine paramedian reticular formation.

CLINICAL CHARACTERISTICS

Symptoms

• Patients with gaze palsies of brainstem origin are asymptomatic unless they have other signs such as a skew deviation, which produces double vision.

Signs

• Decreased or absent conjugate eye movement to either the right or left or both (Fig. 10-31). The gaze palsy is ipsilateral to the side of the lesion, for example, a lesion in the right PPRF produces right gaze palsy. Oculocephalic movements will produce horizontal gaze in patients with lesions of the PPRF but will fail to produce horizontal eye movements in a patient whose gaze palsy is due to a lesion of the CN VI nucleus.

• Ipsilateral CN VII palsies are often associated with lesions in the CN VI nuclear area.

SPECIAL FORMS OF GAZE PALSIES

Lesions in this area may produce a combination of unilateral gaze palsy and an INO. Such a patient will have an inability to look to one side with either eye (gaze palsy) and, on attempted gaze to the opposite side, will have intact abduction, but no adduction (INO). Therefore, of the four possible horizontal eye movements that may be made with the two eyes, only one is possible. Because of this, the syndrome is referred to as the *one-and-a-half* syndrome. This has the same localizing value as an INO or gaze palsy. The causes of this syndrome are likewise identical to those of an INO and gaze palsy.

Some patients with a one-and-a-half syndrome have exotropia. This combination is referred to as a *pontine paralytic exotropia* (Fig. 10-32).

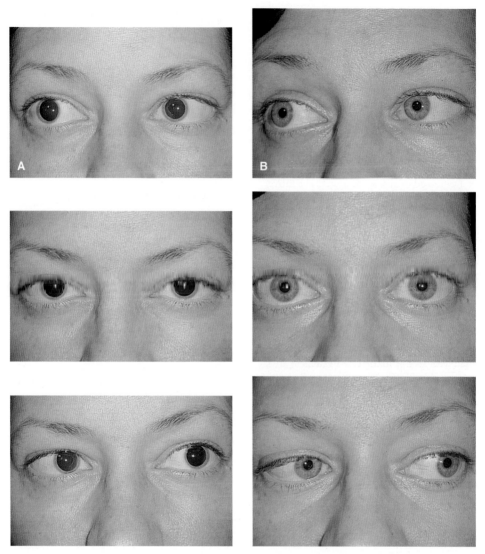

FIGURE 10-31. Gaze palsy. A. (Left row) The patient has no ocular misalignment in primary position. Gaze to right and left is incomplete. The pupils are dilated pharmacologically. **B.** (Right row) Spinal tap was consistent with viral meningoencephalitic process. No treatment was given. Six weeks later, primary gaze is unchanged. Right and left gazes have improved.

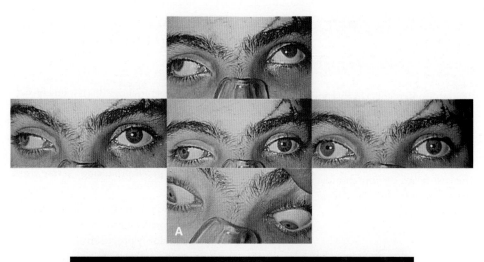

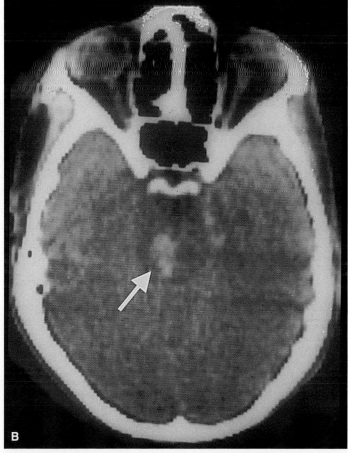

FIGURE 10-32. **Gaze palsy. A.** There is a large exotropia in primary gaze with a left internuclear ophthalmoplegia on right gaze and complete inability to move either eye to the left. **B.** CT scan without contrast shows a brainstem hemorrhage (*arrow*).

CHRONIC PROGRESSIVE EXTERNAL OPHTHALMOPLEGIA

The disorders collectively known as chronic progressive external ophthalmoplegias (CPEO) comprise a group of ocular motility disorders called mitochondrial myopathies or cytopathies.

The two forms of mitochondrial myopathy that are most likely to be encountered by the ophthalmologist are

1. CPEO,
2. Kearns-Sayre syndrome (KSS).

ETIOLOGY

● These disorders are due to mutations in mitochondrial DNA. These mitochondrial abnormalities lead to decreased protein syntheses and structural abnormalities in the muscle, which on skeletal muscle biopsy appear as *ragged red fibers.*

INHERITANCE

● The CPEOs are caused by mutations (usually deletions) in mitochondrial DNA.

● Many instances of CPEO are sporadic, but some are maternally transmitted. This means that the mutation may only be transmitted to future generations through the female line.

CHRONIC PROGRESSIVE EXTERNAL OPHTHALMOPLEGIA

This is the most frequently encountered mitochondrial myopathy.

CLINICAL CHARACTERISTICS

● Droopy upper eyelids: This is a slowly progressive process that is almost always bilateral. The ptosis usually precedes the other ocular manifestations of this disorder. Ptosis may progress to the point where the lids cover the pupils producing a severe visual deficit.

● Double vision: Usually, there is no diplopia (because the ocular motor defects are symmetrical and slowly progressive). Patients are unaware of the problem until it is pointed out to them during their evaluation for ptosis or until their eyes become almost completely immobile causing interference with their peripheral vision. These patients often have to move their heads to see to the left and the right. Downgaze may be better preserved in these patients relative to the other directions of gaze.

● Weakness of other muscles may or may not be present.

Signs

● Ptosis is usually bilateral and symmetrical.

● Ophthalmoplegia is bilateral, symmetrical, and often complete.

● Pupils are normal.

● Weakness of orbicularis oculi or limb and facial muscles (Fig. 10-33).

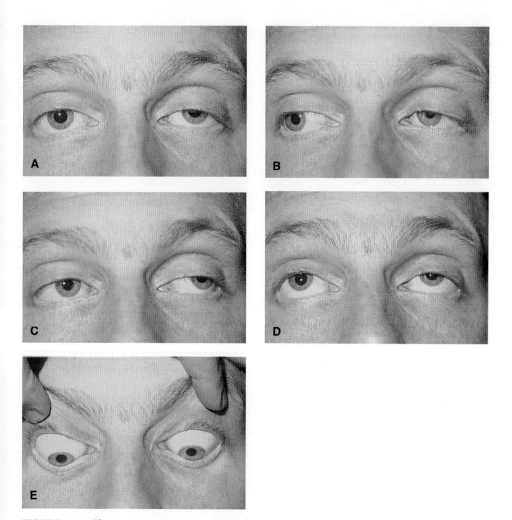

FIGURE 10-33. Chronic progressive external ophthalmoplegia. A–E. Ptosis is prominent, with mildly depressed ductions in all directions. Downgaze is relatively preserved; upgaze is most affected.

KEARNS-SAYRE SYNDROME

- KSS, a special form of CPEO, develops exclusively in young patients (onset before the age of 20 years). KSS is defined by the combination of the following:

  ▪ CPEO (Fig. 10-34A): Development of the eye movement and lid anomalies is similar to those seen in other forms of CPEO except that they develop at a much younger age (usually before 20 years of age).

  ▪ Pigmentary retinopathy: Although originally described as atypical retinitis pigmentosa (RP), this pigment retinopathy has a more salt and pepper appearance and resembles more closely the retinopathy of measles (Fig. 10-34B). Also in contrast to RP, which normally involves the midperipheral and peripheral retina, the pigmentary retinopathy of KSS initially involves the posterior fundus. Furthermore, pallor of the optic disc and attenuation of blood vessels rarely occur in KSS. It does not usually produce severe visual loss, although visual field abnormalities may be plotted. The pigmentary retinopathy may develop before the CPEO.

  ▪ Complete heart block is often the fatal event in these patients. Patients diagnosed with KSS should be under the care of a cardiologist. If heart block is not present, continued monitoring should be performed because heart block may develop at any time during the course of the disease.

- In addition, these patients may develop one or more of the following:

  ▪ Cerebellar ataxia

  ▪ Short stature, with delayed sexual maturity

  ▪ Deafness

  ▪ Dementia

  ▪ Endocrine abnormalities (hypoparathyroidism)

  ▪ CSF protein greater than 1 mg/mL

DIAGNOSTIC EVALUATION AND TREATMENT

- There is no known treatment for CPEO or KSS. However, KSS patients should be investigated with an ECG, and regular cardiac, neurologic, and endocrinologic assessments.

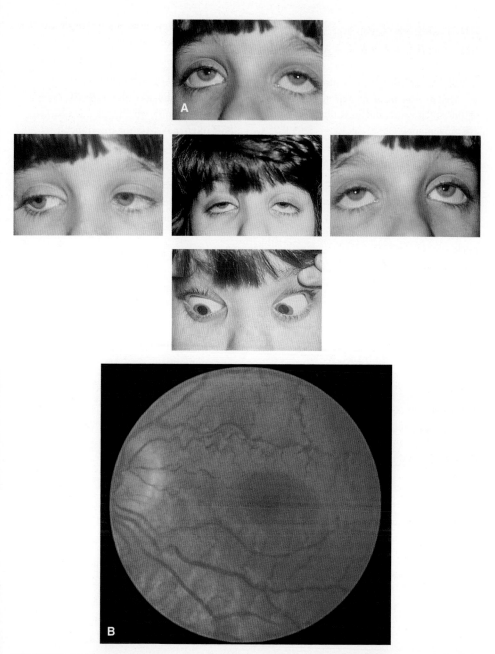

FIGURE 10-34. **Chronic progressive external ophthalmoplegia from Kearns-Sayre syndrome. A.** Ptosis is marked in primary gaze of this 10-year-old girl. Ductions are mildly limited bilaterally. **B.** Posterior pole shows typical pigmentary changes associated with Kearns-Sayre syndrome.

PROGRESSIVE SUPRANUCLEAR PALSY

PSP is a neurodegenerative disease character-ized by slowing of mentation, disturbances of tone and posture, and limitation of voluntary eye movements.

ETIOLOGY

• This is a supranuclear disorder of unknown cause that affects predominantly the brain-stem reticular formation and the ocular motor nuclei.

• It usually occurs later in life and is slowly progressive and is usually fatal within 10 years.

CLINICAL CHARACTERISTICS

Symptoms

• The patient usually has no ocular symp-toms or may complain of difficulties because of poor downward vision, for example, seeing their food, walking off the curb or down the stairs.

Signs

• Slowing of the vertical saccades is the first sign.

• Impairment of vertical gaze. Usually, down-ward gaze is affected earlier and more severely (Fig. 10-35).

• Horizontal eye movements are affected late and usually not to the same extent as vertical gaze.

• Loss of Bell phenomenon.

• Intact vestibular ocular response, except that *axial rigidity*, which is characteristic of PSP, often makes testing this difficult.

• Eyelid disturbances may occur and include apraxia of lid opening or blepharospasm.

• Other neuro-ophthalmic signs including square-wave jerks, impaired vergence eye movements, and abnormal ocular pursuit.

NATURAL HISTORY

• Nonophthalmic signs:
  ▪ Axial and particularly nuchal rigidity
  ▪ Impaired swallowing and speech
  ▪ Terminal event is usually aspiration pneumonia

DIFFERENTIAL DIAGNOSIS

• Parkinson disease
• Whipple disease
• Multiple infarcts
• Hydrocephalus

TREATMENT

• There is no specific therapy for the eye movement disorder of PSP.

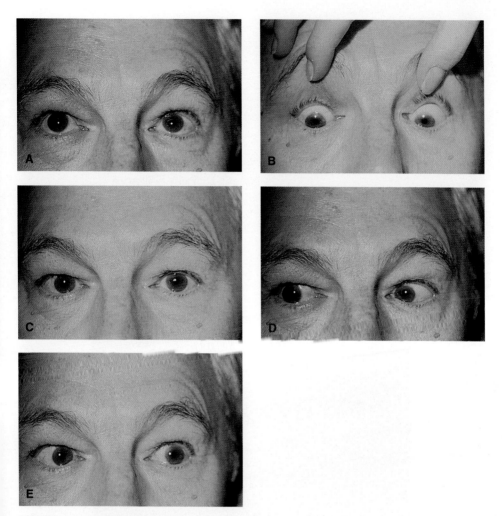

FIGURE 10-35. Progressive supranuclear palsy.   A–E. There is no ocular misalignment but ductions are decreased in all directions, especially upgaze (top row, left).

OCULOPHARYNGEAL MUSCULAR DYSTROPHY

Oculopharyngeal muscular dystrophy (Fig. 10-36) is a genetically inherited disorder usually in an autosomal dominant fashion.

ETIOLOGY

The genetic abnormality is an expansion of 2 to 7 additional base triplets in a repeat sequence in exon 1 of the *PABPN1* (PABP2) gene and results in an increase in length of the polyalanine tract in the PABPN1 protein from 10 to 12–17 residues.

Clinical Characteristics

- Symptoms
  - Ptosis
  - Dysphagia
  - Facial, proximal muscle weakness
- Signs
  - Bilateral ptosis
  - Ophthalmoplegia
  - Difficulty swallowing
  - Dysarthria
  - Proximal muscle weakness
- Diagnosis
  - Genetic testing
  - Muscle biopsy-myocyte nuclei contain discrete PABP2 immunoreactive intranuclear inclusions

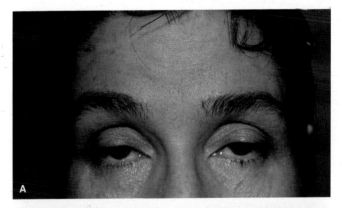

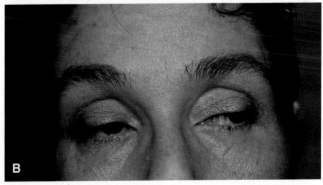

FIGURE 10-36. **Ocular pharyngeal muscular dystrophy. A–E.** Woman with family history and positive genetic testing for oculopharyngeal muscular dystrophy. Bilateral ptosis with decreased eye movements in all directions.

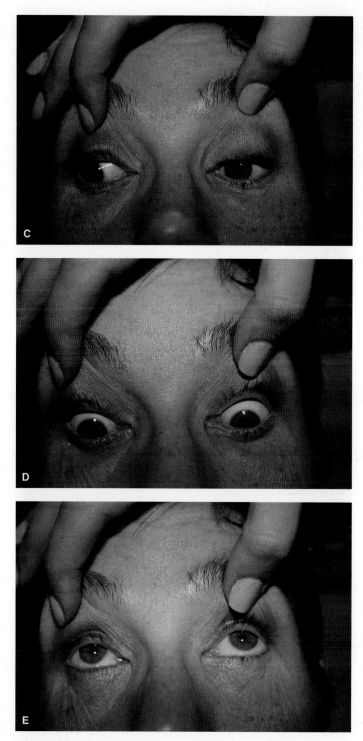

FIGURE 10-36. (*continued*)

GUILLAIN-BARRÉ SYNDROME

The Guillain-Barré syndrome (GBS) is an acute inflammatory demyelinating polyneuropathy that often has neuro-ophthalmologic signs and symptoms.

ETIOLOGY

• This disorder is usually seen after a bacterial or viral infection. The most frequent bacterial agent associated with GBS is *Campylobacter jejuni*.

CLINICAL CHARACTERISTICS

Symptoms

• Patients usually develop symmetrical muscle weakness that progresses relatively rapidly. There is usually a mild respiratory or gastrointestinal illness or a history of vaccinations 1 to 3 weeks prior to the onset of weakness.

• The diagnosis of GBS requires the presence of

▪ progressive motor weakness of more than one limb

▪ areflexia (or hyporeflexia)

Signs

• The ophthalmologic and neuro-ophthalmologic features of the disorder are (Fig. 10-37) as follows:

▪ Ophthalmoplegia: May be partial or total. The most commonly affected nerve is CN VI.

▪ Ptosis: Is usually present when the patient has ophthalmoplegia. It would be unusual for ptosis to occur in the absence of eye movement disorder.

▪ Pupils: GBS may be associated with internal ophthalmoplegia, with the pupils being sluggishly reactive or nonreactive to light.

▪ Optic nerve anomalies in the form of *optic neuritis* or *papilledema* because of increased intracranial pressure.

DIAGNOSTIC EVALUATION

• Most patients have serum antibodies against ganglioside-type GQ1b of which the pathophysiologic relevance is unclear.

• Electrophysiologic testing shows slowing or blocking of nerve conduction.

• Lumbar puncture shows albuminocytologic dissociation, with a high protein and a normal cellular composition in the CSF.

TREATMENT

• The treatment is supportive. This is usually a self-limiting disease, which recovers completely.

• Systemic corticosteroids, plasmapheresis, and the administration of intravenous immune globulin have been advocated by some and may shorten the course of the disorder.

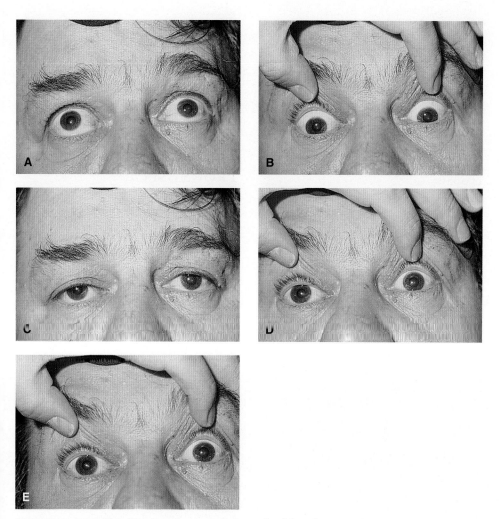

FIGURE 10-37. Guillain-Barré syndrome.   A–E. Patient has bilateral ptosis and mid-dilated, poorly reactive pupils. Gaze is limited bilaterally in all directions. The eye movement and pupillary reactions returned to normal.

MILLER FISHER SYNDROME

- A particular subgroup of patients with GBS may be seen more frequently by the ophthalmologist because of the predominance of signs and symptoms localized to the visual system.
- The triad that characterizes this subgroup of GBS is
  - ophthalmoplegia
  - ataxia
  - areflexia
- The ophthalmoplegia can be identical to that of GBS. In both the GBS and the Miller Fisher syndrome, patients with ophthalmoplegia are found to have an elevated level of anti-GQ1b IgG antibodies.

DIAGNOSTIC EVALUATION

- The CSF findings are usually identical to those of GBS. In addition, MRI scanning is usually normal; however, there may be instances of increased abnormal enhancement of the CNs.

TREATMENT AND PROGNOSIS

- There is no proven treatment for Miller Fisher syndrome, although intravenous immunoglobulins and plasmaphresis are utilized.
- The prognosis for recovery is excellent.

MYASTHENIA GRAVIS

MG is an autoimmune disease that causes weakness in the voluntary muscles.

ETIOLOGY AND PATHOGENESIS

• The acetylcholine receptor at the neuromuscular junction is essential for the transmission of the nerve signal to the muscle. MG results when antibodies bind to these receptor sites, rendering them unavailable. These antiacetylcholine receptor antibodies are the immediate cause of MG.

CLINICAL CHARACTERISTICS

• The basic characteristics of the muscle weakness in MG are variability and fatigability.

Symptoms

• Ophthalmic symptoms include the following:

■ Ptosis is eventually experienced by almost all myasthenic patients. It is the initial symptom in approximately 50% of patients with MG. The ptosis is absent or less upon awakening but progresses as the day goes on and the patient tires. It may involve one or both lids and is usually asymmetric. At times, the lids may be completely ptotic to the point where the patient must manually elevate them to see.

■ Double vision: The diplopia of MG also worsens with prolonged effort or as the day wears on.

• Nonophthalmic complaints include the following:

■ Weakness in one or more muscle group, for example, proximal limb muscles, resulting in difficulty in walking or getting up from a chair.

■ Pharyngeal muscles: Patients may note a change in their voice, which may take on a nasal quality.

■ Difficulty in swallowing or breathing constitutes a medical emergency for any patient with MG.

Signs

• Ptosis. There are several characteristics of the ptosis in MG.

■ The lid droop may be accentuated by having the patient maintain upgaze for 2 minutes (**Fig. 10-38**).

■ Manually elevating the more ptotic lid will result in the other lid becoming noticeably more ptotic (**Fig. 10-39**). This is termed *enhanced ptosis.*

■ When MG patients look from downgaze to primary position, the lids will often overshoot and then come to rest in their customary position. This phenomenon is the *Cogan sign.* However, intermittent lid twitching may be seen in these patients independent of Cogan sign.

• Ocular misalignment and decreased ocular motility: MG may manifest any ocular motility disturbance. Diplopia is usually, but not invariably, present. The more frequently encountered abnormal ocular motility patterns include the following:

■ Upgaze paresis: Difficulty in elevating either eye is often seen, especially when ptosis is present.

■ Pseudo-INO: There is defective adduction of one or both eyes simulating the INO of brainstem disease (**Fig. 10-40**).

■ Ophthalmoplegia: The eyes become virtually immobile in all directions of gaze (**Fig. 10-41**).

■ Simulating CN palsies (**Fig. 10-42**)

- Saccades:
  - May show slow velocity with fatigue.
  - May have abnormal rapid dart-like saccades ("quiver" or lightning eye movements).
- Lid weakness: The eyelids are easily opened during forced lid closure, indicating orbicularis muscle weakness.

DIAGNOSTIC EVALUATION

- Office tests for MG include the following:
  - Tensilon test: The intravenous injection of edrophonium chloride (Tensilon) causes the reversal of lid and ocular motility signs in MG in the majority of patients. The patient will revert to baseline in approximately 2 minutes.
  - Ice test: Ice is placed over the closed ptotic lid for 2 minutes. Myasthenic ptosis will be greatly improved, whereas ptosis from other causes will not (Fig. 10-43). Ocular motility limitations will improve after 5 minutes of ice application.
  - Rest test: The patient keeps his or her eyes closed for 20 minutes and the ptosis improves.

- Laboratory tests include the following:
  - Acetylcholine receptor antibody assay. The detection of an elevated titer of these blocking or binding antibodies is virtually diagnostic of MG. Approximately, 30% to 50% of patients with ocular myasthenia will have an elevated antibody titer.
  - Repetitive nerve stimulation reveals a decremental response to repetitive stimulation of affected muscles. The single-fiber EMG may be diagnostic of MG when the routine EMG is not.
  - Chest imaging to detect thymic enlargement or thymoma is performed in all patients diagnosed with MG.
  - Thyroid function studies are performed because there is an increased incidence of dysthyroidism in patients with MG.

TREATMENT

- The therapy options for MG include cholinesterase inhibitors, corticosteroids or other immunosuppressive therapy, thymectomy, and plasmapheresis.

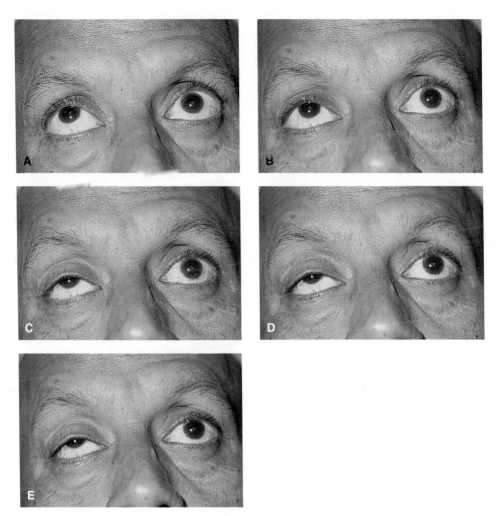

FIGURE 10-38. **Myasthenia gravis.** **A–E.** Right upper lid ptosis gradually worsens with sustained upgaze.

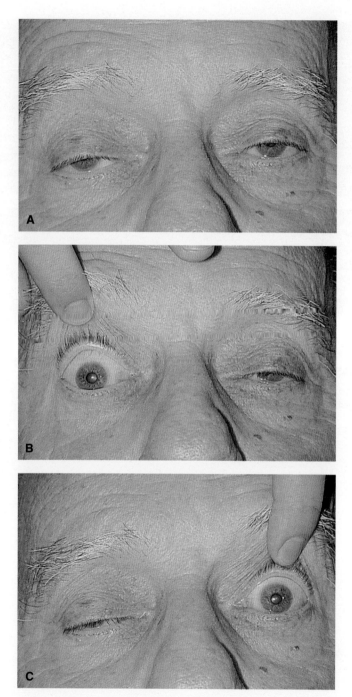

FIGURE 10-39. Myasthenia gravis. A–C. Bilateral ptosis is present in primary position. Note: use of brow to try to open the lids. Manually elevating each lid will cause the other to become more ptotic (enhanced ptosis).

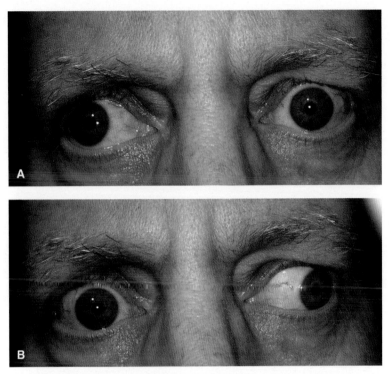

FIGURE 10-40. Myasthenia gravis. Bilateral adduction defects in patient with myasthenia gravis (MG). Ocular motility returned to normal with treatment of MG.

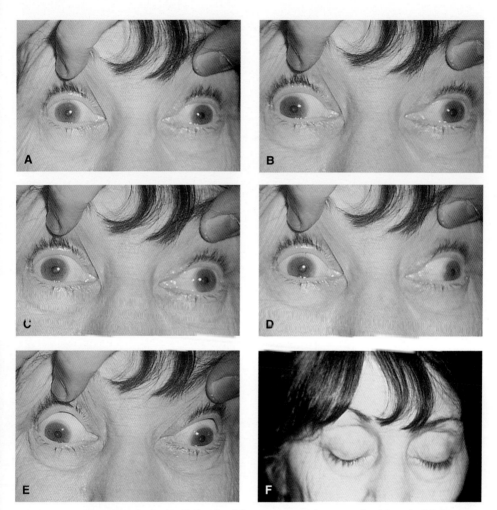

FIGURE 10-41. Myasthenia gravis.   A–F. Complete bilateral ptosis and almost complete bilateral ophthalmoplegia resolved completely with oral Mestinon.

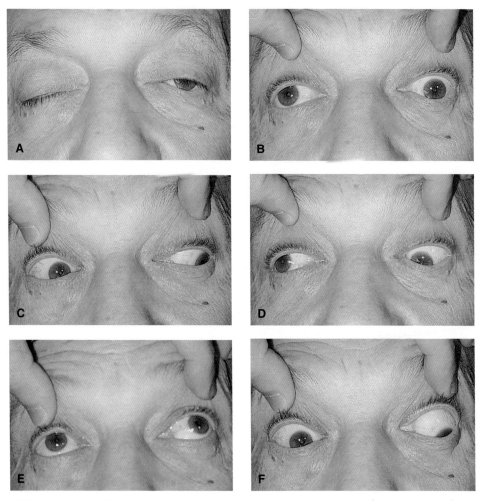

FIGURE 10-42. Myasthenia gravis simulating a CN palsy. **A–F.** Complete left ptosis (right lid also ptotic). The eyes are exotropic in primary position with decreased adduction, elevation, and depression of the left eye. There is a small adduction deficit OD.

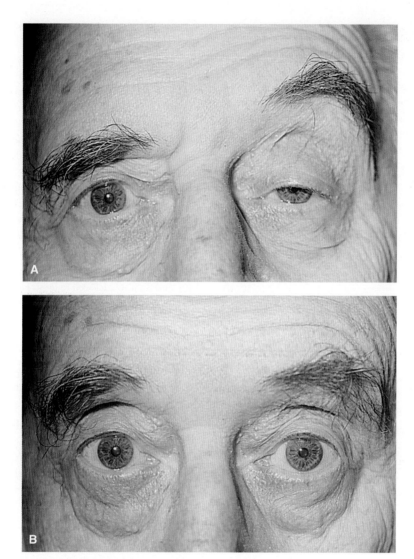

FIGURE 10-43. **Myasthenia gravis.** Ptosis on left upper lid (**A**) improves dramatically following the application of ice to the lid for 2 minutes (**B**).

DORSAL MIDBRAIN (PARINAUD) SYNDROME

Dorsal midbrain (Parinaud) syndrome produces a deficit in upward gaze caused by the involvement of the vertical gaze centers in the dorsal midbrain (Fig. 10-44).

ETIOLOGY

- Lesions in the area of the dorsal midbrain that produce Parinaud syndrome include
  - pineal region tumors
  - hydrocephalus from any cause
  - trauma
  - stroke
  - multiple sclerosis

CLINICAL CHARACTERISTICS

Symptoms

- Diplopia: Patients may experience diplopia, which is due to either an associated skew deviation or unilateral or bilateral CN IV palsies.
- Transient visual obscurations occur when papilledema is present.

Signs

- Lid retraction is usually present in primary position.

- Defective upgaze: Patients cannot voluntarily look up, and when attempting to do so, they will develop convergence and retraction of the eyes into the orbits (*convergence retraction nystagmus*). This phenomenon can be elicited by asking the patient to perform an upward saccade or by utilizing downward moving optokinetic targets. This upward gaze paresis is a supranuclear paresis that can be overcome by performing the doll's head maneuver. Although the patient cannot elevate the eyes voluntarily, the eyes will go into upgaze when the head is moved into a chin down position while fixation is maintained on a distant target.

- Pupillary mydriasis: The pupils are usually large and do not react well to light. However, the reaction to near response is preserved (light-near dissociation). Corectopia is seen in some patients.

- Papilledema: The mass lesions that produce a dorsal midbrain syndrome including hydrocephalus will often produce papilledema

DIAGNOSTIC EVALUATION

- Patients with dorsal midbrain syndrome should have an MRI scan to look for the causative lesion.

TREATMENT

- Treatment depends on the cause of the dorsal midbrain syndrome.

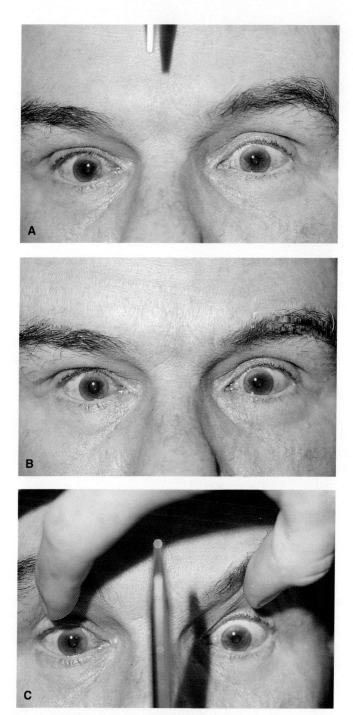

FIGURE 10-44. Dorsal midbrain syndrome.   Bilateral lid retraction is seen in primary gaze (**B**). Upward saccades cannot be performed (**A**). The pupils constrict to near (**C**) but not to light stimulus.

Nystagmus

INTRODUCTION

Nystagmus is a repetitive oscillation of the eyes that is usually rhythmic. Generally, nystagmus is considered as either jerk or pendular. *Jerk* nystagmus refers to rhythmic back-and-forth movements in which there is a fast and a slow phase. By convention, nystagmus is described by the direction of the fast phase. *Pendular* nystagmus refers to rhythmic back-and-forth movements of the eyes in which the velocity is equal in each direction. The nystagmus may be a mixed combination of both jerk and pendular. This chapter is a clinical-based approach to nystagmus, and other texts should be consulted for a detailed pathophysiologic understanding of nystagmus.

Nystagmus may cause visual blurring, but usually does not produce other clinical symptoms or signs. Table 11-1 lists the clinical characteristics of congenital nystagmus that allow its differentiation from acquired nystagmus. Table 11-2 lists specific forms of nystagmus that can be localized to particular portions of the central nervous system. Table 11-3 lists those eye movements that can be confused with nystagmus.

Several questions can be asked to better determine the nature of the nystagmus.

TABLE 11-1. Clinical Characteristics of Congenital Nystagmus

Onset at birth or in the immediate perinatal period

Almost always conjugate and horizontal

Horizontal nystagmus remains horizontal in vertical gaze

It is dampened by convergence and accentuated by fixation

May have a latent component

There is inversion of the optokinetic reflex

There may be head oscillations

Presence of a null point

Absence of oscillopsia

Strabismus is common

Head turns are common

TABLE 11-2. Localization of Nystagmus

Nystagmus	Location	Causes
See-saw	Diencephalon interstitial nucleus of Cajal or its connections	Parasellar masses, brainstem stroke, septo-optic dysplasia, congenital
Convergence–retraction	Mesencephalon (posterior commissure, dorsal midbrain)	Pineal region tumors
Torsional	Central vestibular connections	Demyelination, infarction (Wallenberg syndrome), tumors, syringobulbia, arteriovenous malformations
Bruns	Cerebellopontine angle	Acoustic neuroma
Upbeat	Cerebellum	Cerebellar degeneration, demyelination, infarction
Periodic alternating	Cerebellum	Chiari malformation, demyelination, cerebellar degeneration, infarction, cerebellar mass lesions, congenital
Downbeat	Craniocervical junction Cerebellum	Chiari malformation, basilar invagination, cerebellar degeneration, infarction, demyelination, toxic-metabolic

TABLE 11-3. Conditions That Mimic Nystagmus

Condition	Features	Lesion Location
Ocular flutter	Rapid, conjugate, horizontal oscillations	Probably abnormalities of burst neurons
Opsoclonus	Combined horizontal, vertical, and/or torsional oscillations	Probably abnormalities of burst neurons
Ocular bobbing	Rapid downward deviation with a slow drift up to primary position	Pontine dysfunction
Inverse bobbing (ocular dipping)	Slow downward movement, fast upward movement	Nonlocalizing
Oculopalatal myorhythmia (myoclonus)	Rhythmic oscillations associated with simultaneous contraction of nonocular muscles (palate, tongue)	Interruption of connections in Mollaret triangle: inferior olive, red nucleus, and dentate nucleus

IS THE NYSTAGMUS MONOCULAR OR BILATERAL?

Monocular nystagmus or rhythmic oscillations are most frequently seen in the following settings:

- Internuclear ophthalmoplegia: A dissociated horizontal gaze nystagmus that occurs in the abducting eye contralateral to the side of the medial longitudinal fasciculus (MLF) lesion (see p. 344, Chapter 10).
- Heimann–Bielschowsky phenomenon: Long-standing visual loss (from any cause including optic nerve disease, profound amblyopia, dense cataract) can lead to low-frequency, monocular vertical pendular or jerk nystagmus in the involved eye.
- Spasmus nutans: This consists of the triad of *nystagmus* that is usually vertical, dissociated, rapid, unilateral or bilateral, of small amplitude, and pendular; *head nodding* and *torticollis.* It is of unknown etiology and usually starts at 4 to 12 months of age and disappears by the age of 2 years. These children should undergo an MRI because chiasmal gliomas have been associated with this eye movement anomaly.
- Superior oblique myokymia is a monocular periodic oscillation.
  - Symptoms: Monocular blurring of vision or shimmering of the environment lasting less than 10 seconds but occurring multiple times a day.
  - Cause: Majority have no underlying disease.
  - Looking down or converging may precipitate an attack.
  - Signs: Difficult to elicit during examination, but if attack occurs, these are small-amplitude, irregular, intorsional oscillations in one eye.
  - Course: Usually resolves spontaneously

IS THE BINOCULAR NYSTAGMUS PHYSIOLOGIC OR PATHOLOGIC?

The forms of physiologic nystagmus are as follows:

- End-point: This is a fine-jerk nystagmus seen in extreme gaze.
- Optokinetic: This is a jerk nystagmus elicited by a repetitive stimuli moving across the visual field.
  - Slow phase: In the direction of the target movement
  - Fast phase: In the opposite direction of target movement
- Vestibular nystagmus induced by caloric testing
  - Cold water in ear: Produces nystagmus with the fast phase in opposite direction to the ear that is being tested
  - Warm water: Produces nystagmus with the fast phase in same direction to the ear being tested

IS THE PATHOLOGIC NYSTAGMUS DISSOCIATED?

The frequently encountered dissociated nystagmus patterns are as follows:

- Convergence–retraction nystagmus: Convergence-like movements associated with retraction of the globe into the orbit. Usually seen with pineal region tumors or other midbrain abnormalities (see p. 371, Fig. 10-41).
- See-saw nystagmus: One eye elevates and intorts, whereas the other eye depresses and extorts; the lesion usually involves the optic chiasm or third ventricle, usually in patients with a bitemporal hemianopia.

The forms of nondissociated nystagmus include the following:

• Upbeat: The fast phase is up and the amplitude is greatest in upgaze. The causes include drugs (phenytoin) or lesions of the brainstem, cerebellar vermis, and posterior fossa.

• Downbeat: Fast phase is downward. This is caused by lesions in the craniocervical junction. This is usually present in the primary position, but the amplitude may be so small that it goes unnoticed. It usually obeys Alexander's law (increase in the amplitude when eyes move in the direction of fast phase), that is, nystagmus is greatest in downgaze but often in oblique downgaze.

• Congenital nystagmus

• Rebound: This is a jerk nystagmus in which the fast phase is in the direction of gaze. However, with sustained gaze, the fast phase changes direction. When gaze is returned to the primary position, the fast phase increases in the direction the eye takes in returning to the primary position. This is caused by lesions of the cerebellum.

• Periodic alternating: The direction of the fast phase changes in cycles of 60 to 90 seconds.

• Gaze evoked: Nystagmus is absent in the primary position and is not visually disabling. It is a jerk nystagmus in the direction of gaze.

  ▪ Bruns' nystagmus: Lesions in the cerebellopontine angle may produce a low-frequency, large-amplitude nystagmus when the patient looks to the side of the lesion and a high-frequency, small-amplitude nystagmus when the patient looks in the opposite direction.

  ▪ Drug induced: Anticonvulsants/sedative medication

  ▪ Gaze paretic

• Vestibular: Vestibular nystagmus can be peripheral or central. Peripheral nystagmus is caused by disease of the vestibular organ or nerve, such as labyrinthitis or Ménière disease. Peripheral nystagmus is usually associated with severe vertigo that is aggravated by head movements. There is usually no associated ocular motility disturbance. Fixation tends to inhibit the nystagmus. The nystagmus itself shows an increase in the intensity of the horizontal component when the eyes are turned in the direction of the fast phase. The fast phase is away from the lesion. Central vestibular nystagmus is caused by disorders of the brainstem with its vestibulocerebellar connections. The patient only complains of mild vertigo if any (except Wallenberg syndrome). The nystagmus is neither inhibited by fixation nor induced by head movements. There may be associated saccadic or pursuit defects.

• Latent nystagmus: Jerk nystagmus that is absent when both eyes are viewing but appears when one eye is covered. Both eyes beat toward the fixating eye.

• Acquired pendular nystagmus: This occurs in multiple sclerosis and can be visually disabling because of oscillopsia.

CHAPTER

12

Pupil

BASICS

ANATOMY

The pupil receives both sympathetic and parasympathetic innervation. The sympathetic input dilates the pupil and the parasympathetic input constricts it. Therefore, a sympathetic paresis will produce pupillary miosis, whereas a parasympathetic paresis will cause mydriasis.

SYMPATHETIC SYSTEM

The sympathetic innervation of the pupil is a three-neuron chain that begins in the posterior hypothalamus with the *first-order neuron* that extends down through the brainstem to the spinal cord and synapses at the ciliospinal center of Budge (C8–T2 level) (Fig. 12-1). In the midbrain, the sympathetic pathway runs close to the cranial nerve (CN) IV nucleus. The *second-order neuron* leaves the spinal cord and enters the paravertebral

sympathetic chain ascending in the abdomen and thorax to come into contact with the apex of the lung, and in the neck it is associated with the carotid artery. At the angle of the jaw, it synapses in the superior cervical ganglion from which the *third-order neuron* originates. The first- and second-order neurons are also known as preganglionic; the third-order neuron is termed postganglionic. It ascends within the adventitia of the internal carotid artery to enter the skull. It then travels through the cavernous sinus where it is in close association with CN VI and joins the ophthalmic division of CN V to enter the orbit. The oculosympathetic fibers innervate the iris dilator muscle, Müller muscles, and inferior tarsal muscle. The sympathetic fibers are responsible for facial sweating and vasodilation following the external carotid artery branching off at the superior cervical ganglion.

Any abnormality along this three-neuron chain produces Horner syndrome that consists of relative ipsilateral pupillary miosis, upper lid ptosis, and lower lid elevation (Fig. 12-2).

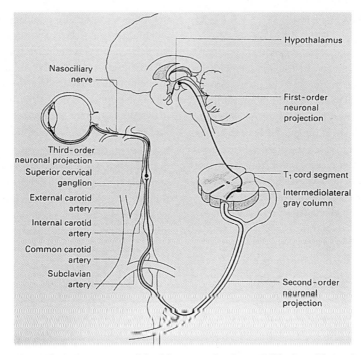

FIGURE 12-1. Sympathetic innervation of the dilator muscle of iris. Cell bodies of first-order sympathetic neurons in hypothalamus project axons through brainstem to intermediolateral gray column of lower cervical and upper thoracic spinal cord. Second-order neurons project via white rami communicantes through paravertebral sympathetic chain to superior cervical ganglion. On the left side, chain in its course splits around subclavian artery. Third-order neurons travel within pericarotid plexus to cavernous sinus, where they join the sixth cranial nerve briefly before entering orbit on first division of trigeminal nerve. These axons enter globe to innervate iris dilator muscle.

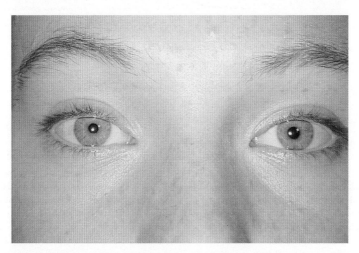

FIGURE 12-2. Horner syndrome. The patient has right upper lid ptosis, with the right pupil being smaller than the left. The right lower lid is elevated compared to the left.

PARASYMPATHETIC SYSTEM

The parasympathetic system (Fig. 12-3) begins at the retinal ganglion cells with the fibers destined to innervate the pupil coursing with the visual fibers. The pupillomotor fibers leave this pathway before the lateral geniculate body is reached via the brachium of the superior colliculus to reach the pretectal area. Both pretectal nuclei receive input from both eyes via intercalated neurons. Each pretectal nucleus sends axons to both Edinger–Westphal nuclei. Parasympathetic efferent fibers leave the Edinger–Westphal nucleus and are incorporated into CN III to the ipsilateral ciliary ganglion within the orbit. The postganglionic fibers innervate the iris sphincter muscle for pupillary constriction and the ciliary muscle for accommodation. The proportion of fibers to the iris sphincter to the ciliary muscle is 30:1. Acetylcholine released at the neuromuscular junction of the iris sphincter results in pupillary constriction, and an abnormality of the efferent parasympathetic input to the iris results in pupillary mydriasis.

Pupillary constriction to a near stimulus (near-reflex) bypasses the pretectal nuclei in the dorsal midbrain and descends directly to the area of the Edinger–Westphal nuclei from higher cortical centers. Hence, in light–near dissociation, the dorsal midbrain and pretectum are damaged, but the near-reflex pathway and Edinger–Westphal nuclei are not damaged.

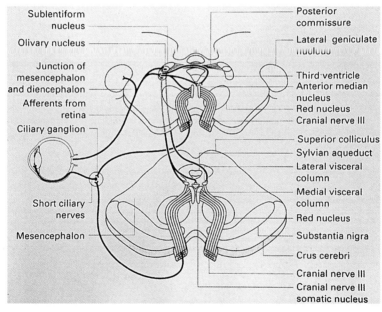

FIGURE 12-3. Parasympathetic innervation: pupillary light reflex. Afferents arising in retina project to lateral geniculate nucleus and pretectal (sublentiform and olivary) nuclei. Fiber arising from pretectal nuclei project above and below third ventricle and sylvian aqueduct to anterior median nucleus and to medial and lateral visceral columns of Edinger–Westphal complex. These nuclei send axons through fascicles of CN III to synapse in ciliary ganglion. Fibers arising from this ganglion project to eye via short ciliary nerves.

EXAMINATION TECHNIQUES

Examination of the pupil is an integral part of the ophthalmologic examination.

The technique of pupillary examination is as follows:

1. The *pupillary size* of each eye is determined first in a dimly lit room with the patient fixating a distant target. The pupils are diffusely illuminated from below (Fig. 12-4A). The pupillary size is examined in bright light by turning on the examination room lights (Fig. 12-4B) or by using either a halogen muscle light or indirect ophthalmoscope turned up to its highest brightness level.

2. *Reactivity* of each pupil is tested in a dimly lit room with the patient fixing on a distance target. A bright light is shone in each eye and the briskness of the pupillary reactions is recorded (Fig. 12-4C and D).

3. The swinging light test is then performed looking for the presence of a relative afferent pupillary defect (RAPD) (see Chapter 1).

4. The pupillary *near response* is tested by having the patient fix on a target at near (approximately 12 inches or 30 cm) while the pupils are diffusely illuminated (Fig. 12-4E). Effort is an important aspect of this test, so if convergence does not occur, it is difficult to tell whether the problem is pathologic or effort related.

5. Slit lamp assessment of iris and pharmacologic testing is carried out in specific instances (see sections "Adie (Tonic) Pupil," "Mydriasis," "Horner Syndrome") (Chart 1).

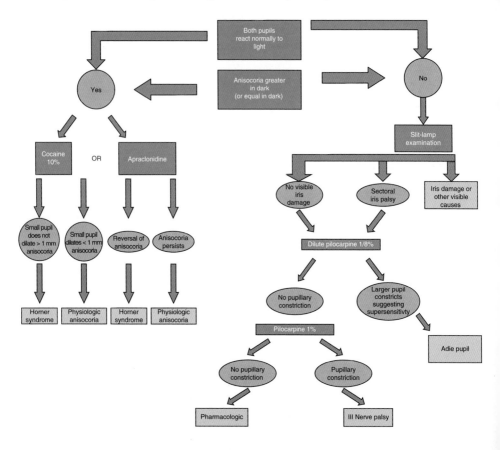

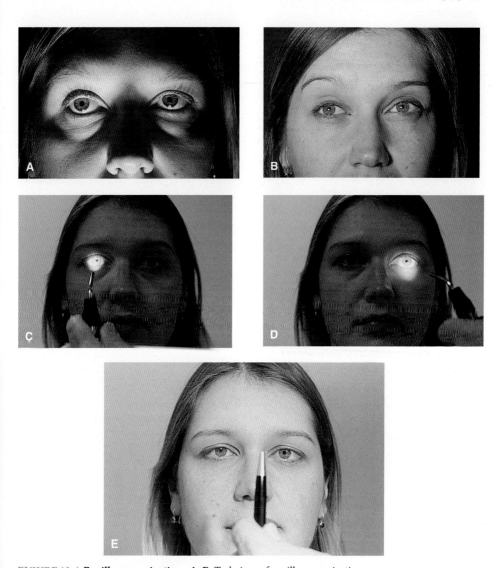

FIGURE 12-4. **Pupillary examination.   A–E.** Technique of pupillary examination.

PUPILLARY SIZE

Under normal circumstances, the pupils are equal in size, although some people have smaller pupils (particularly older patients) and some have larger pupils (particularly younger, anxious patients). Therefore, anisocoria, that is, a difference in size between the two pupils, must always be suspected of being potentially a pathologic finding. Not all anisocoria, however, is pathologic. *Physiologic anisocoria* (Fig. 12-5) is seen in approximately 10% to 20% of the patients. To determine if anisocoria is physiologic, as opposed to being due to a pathologic process, the pupillary size is determined as just described in both bright and dim illumination. In physiologic anisocoria, the degree of anisocoria between the pupils is relatively the same in both illumination levels. For example, if there is a 30% difference in pupillary size in dim light, a 30% difference will also be present in bright light. Any change in the degree of the anisocoria in bright and dim light indicates pathologic anisocoria.

Pathologic anisocoria can be due to an abnormality of either the sympathetic or the parasympathetic pathway. If the anisocoria is greater in dim light, the abnormal pupil is the smaller one and a sympathetic paresis should be suspected. The most likely manifestation of this sympathetic paresis is Horner syndrome, which is usually accompanied by ptosis (Fig. 12-6).

If the anisocoria is greater in bright light, the abnormal pupil is the larger one, which does not constrict normally. There are a number of causes for this, including abnormalities in the pupillary parasympathetic innervation system. Adie pupil and a parasympathetic paresis due to CN III palsy are the most likely causes of a parasympathetic abnormality. Likewise, pharmacologic blockade of one pupil will produce anisocoria that is greater in bright light (Fig. 12-7). In this condition, the larger pupil is of greater diameter than produced in other neuro-ophthalmic causes of anisocoria.

In any patient who has anisocoria, it is critical to examine

- the lids and
- ocular motility

This will enable the physician to identify the more important causes of anisocoria, that is, Horner syndrome and CN III palsy.

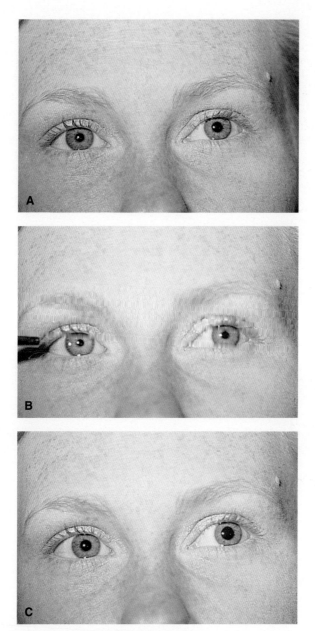

FIGURE 12-5. Physiologic anisocoria. The left pupil is larger than the right in ambient light (**A**). The degree of anisocoria is the same in bright (**B**) and dim illumination (**C**).

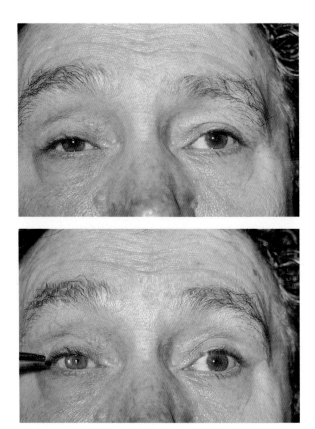

FIGURE 12-6. **Horner syndrome.** Anisocoria is more prominent in dim illumination (top photo), indicating the smaller pupil is abnormal.

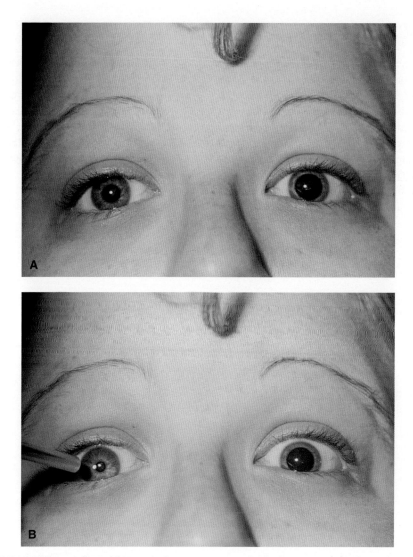

FIGURE 12-7. **Pharmacologic dilation. A.** Greater anisocoria in bright illumination (**B**) indicates that the larger pupil is abnormal (left). The large diameter of the left pupil indicates pharmacodilation.

REACTIVITY OF THE PUPIL

Even in the presence of isocoria (pupils of equal size), pupillary reactivity should be assessed. The pupils may be abnormal in reactivity and yet be of equal size. Such abnormalities are usually due to parasympathetic disorders and may be seen in Guillain–Barré syndrome, dorsal midbrain syndrome, or botulism. Adie pupil, which has a tendency to become bilateral, may also produce bilateral poorly reactive pupils that at times may be isochoric.

RELATIVE AFFERENT PUPILLARY DEFECT

At this point, the patient is examined for the presence of an RAPD. The method of examination and its significance is outlined in Chapter 1.

NEAR RESPONSE

Testing for near response is not performed routinely but is important to document in specific clinical situations, usually to detect light–near dissociation. This pupillary disconnect, where the pupil does not react to light but does to near, is seen in Adie pupil, Argyll Robertson (AR) pupils, and the dorsal midbrain syndrome, among others.

HORNER SYNDROME

Horner syndrome is caused by a decrease in the sympathetic innervation to the eye. The defining signs of the syndrome are *ptosis* and *miosis*.

ETIOLOGY

● Any lesion occurring at any point along the three-neuron sympathetic chain will produce the clinical signs of Horner syndrome.

CLINICAL CHARACTERISTICS

Symptoms

● Often, the patient is asymptomatic or may notice a slight ptosis. Initially, increased accommodation might cause fluctuation of vision.

● Discomfort in the ipsilateral eye or supraorbital area is highly suggestive of carotid

dissection. The presence of associated signs or symptoms may assist in localizing the level of the lesion (**Table 12-1**).

Signs

● Ptosis of the upper eyelid combined with elevation of the lower lid produces narrowing of the interpalpebral fissure and apparent enophthalmos (**Fig. 12-8A**).

● Anisocoria, with the pupil on the affected side being smaller due to decreased innervation to the iris dilator muscle. The anisocoria is greater in dim light because the pupil with the sympathetic paresis does not dilate normally, but the anisocoria is less or disappears completely in bright light. Several factors affect the degree of anisocoria:

  ▪ Alertness of the patient: In an alert patient, the normal pupil is dilated, whereas the pupil of Horner syndrome is less so.

  ▪ Resting size of pupils

TABLE 12-1. Horner Syndrome

Level	Associated Signs and Symptoms	Causes	Pharmacologic Test
I	Contralateral hemiparesis Contralateral hemianesthesia Hemihypohydrosis Wallenberg syndrome Contralateral CN IV palsy Ipsilateral CN VI palsy	Stroke Multiple sclerosis Vertebral artery dissection	Nondiagnostic
II	Hoarseness Cough Pain in scapula region	Tumors of the lung, breast, and schwannomas Trauma (including surgery) Epidural anesthetic	Hydroxyamphetamine negative
III	Orbital and neck pain Decreased taste Dysphagia Palatal hemianesthesia Headache Involvement of CN III, IV, V, and VI	Carotid artery dissection Neck trauma Tumors and inflammation of neck Cluster headache Raeder's paratrigeminal neuralgia Cavernous sinus masses and inflammation	Hydroxyamphetamine positive

- Completeness of the injury and extent of reinnervation

- Degree of supersensitivity and concentration of circulating adrenergic substance in the blood

- Anhidrosis: Depending on the site of the lesion, sweat fibers to the ipsilateral face may be involved so that some patients may demonstrate lack of sweating of the forehead. As the postganglionic sudomotor fibers in the face follow the external carotid artery after synapsing in the superior cervical ganglion, a postganglionic lesion may only produce minimal sweat disturbance of the skin of the forehead.

- Iris heterochromia: If the Horner syndrome is congenital, iris heterochromia is present, with the iris on the affected side being a lighter color than on the nonaffected side.

- Paradoxical pupillary dilation: Denervation supersensitivity leads to a widely dilated pupil with adrenergic stimulation. The pupil on the side of the sympathetic lesion may become the larger pupil as a result of the release of endogenous catecholamines that occur with intense emotional excitement.

- Dilation lag: The Horner pupil initially dilates more slowly in the dark. The anisocoria is more prominent after 5 seconds and decreases at 15 seconds. This effect can be exaggerated by interposing a sudden noise (which increases sympathetic discharge).

- Skin changes: Acutely following sympathetic denervation, the skin temperature on the side of the lesion increases because of loss of sudomotor control and dilation of blood vessels. Hence, there may be conjunctival hyperemia, skin flushing, epiphora, and nasal stuffiness. In the long term, the skin on the affected side may actually be paler. This is because denervation sensitivity of blood vessels results in vasoconstriction.

DIAGNOSTIC EVALUATION

In any pharmacologic testing of the pupil, the testing agent being used should be instilled in both cul-de-sacs so that the "normal" pupil is used as a control.

Apraclonidine 0.5% or 1% (Iopidine; Allergan) is increasingly recognized as the first-line pharmacologic test for evaluating a suspected Horner syndrome, appears to have the same specificity and sensitivity as cocaine, and is more readily available. Apraclonidine is a direct alpha-receptor agonist. It does not cause pupillary dilation in eyes with intact sympathetic innervations but will cause mild pupillary dilation in eyes with sympathetic denervation regardless of the lesion location. After 30 to 45 minutes, apraclonidine will produce dilation of the miotic (Horner) pupil but not a normal pupil, thus resulting in reversal of the anisocoria. It will also elevate the ptotic lid. Some reports indicate that it may constrict the normal pupil. The end point, however, is reversal of the anisocoria (Fig. 12-9).

Cocaine 10% can also be used in the investigation of Horner syndrome. Cocaine dilates a normal pupil by blocking the reuptake of norepinephrine into the sympathetic nerve endings, thus allowing its prolonged presence to produce mydriasis. Under normal circumstances, there is sufficient norepinephrine constantly present to cause the pupil to dilate. When there is sympathetic denervation, an insufficient quantity of norepinephrine is present at the sympathetic effector cells. Therefore, blocking the reuptake does not result in pupillary dilation. Cocaine dilates a normal pupil but not the pupil with sympathetic paresis. The presence of 0.8 mm of postcocaine anisocoria establishes the diagnosis (Fig. 12-10). The larger the amount of anisocoria 45 minutes after cocaine instillation, the more secure is the diagnosis of Horner syndrome. It is important to inform the patient that after this test, their urine will test positive for cocaine for approximately 48 hours.

Hydroxyamphetamine actively releases norepi-nephrine from the stores in the adrenergic nerve endings, thus dilating a normal pupil. It also will dilate first- and second-order Horner pupils, where the norepinephrine is present in the nerve ending of the third-order neuron but is not being released because of the preganglionic sympathetic paresis. With a third-order (postganglionic) lesion, the nerve endings are damaged, and there are insufficient stores of norepinephrine to release. Therefore, a Horner pupil due to a third-order (postganglionic) lesion will not dilate.

The combination of these pharmacologic tests has been used as a basis of deciding which pa-tients with Horner pupil should undergo further investigation. Because postganglionic lesions tend to be caused by more benign processes, such as migraine, it has been recommended that patients with preganglionic Horner pupil be investigated, whereas those with an isolated postganglionic Horner pupil need not be.

However, pharmacologic testing will err in de-termining the localization of the Horner lesion about 10% of the time. Therefore, we recommend that all patients with Horner syndrome undergo MRI of the head, MR angiography (MRA)/ CT angiography (CTA) of the neck, and CT of the thorax.

TREATMENT

• Treatment is directed at the underlying etiology if one is found.

SPECIAL FORM: CAROTID ARTERY DISSECTION

This cause of Horner syndrome also pro-duces pain in the neck, ipsilateral face, or the periorbital area; decreased taste is present in approximately 10% of the patients. The dis-section may be spontaneous, caused by minor trauma or by an inherent structural defect of the arterial wall. It may be associated with an underlying connective tissue disorder such as Ehlers–Danlos syndrome type IV, Marfan syndrome, osteogenesis imperfecta type I, and autosomal dominant polycystic kidney disease.

A subintimal dissection usually results in carotid stenosis or occlusion. A subadventitial dissection may cause aneurysmal dilation of the carotid artery. The diagnosis of carotid dissection may be made on MRI scan alone, where a crescent or circular area of bright signal (blood) is seen within the luminal wall of the carotid artery (Fig. 12-8B). An MRA or CTA will show the dissection, usually with marked stenosis or occlusion of the carotid artery (Fig. 12-8C). This testing is sufficient. Catheter angiography need not be performed.

Treatment is aimed at preventing stroke or retinal ischemia and consists of intravenous heparin followed by oral warfarin. The dissections usually heal spontaneously in several months. Repeat MRA/CTA will reveal when arterial patency has been restored and the anticoagulation therapy may be discontinued.

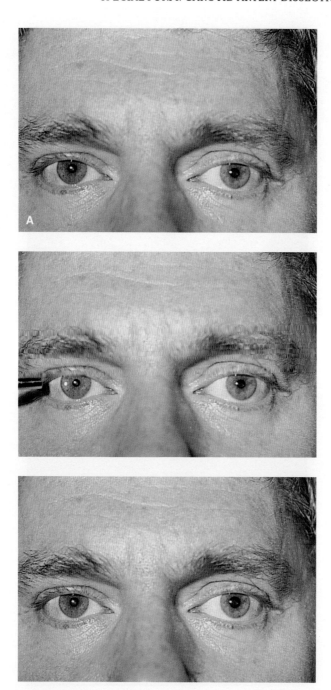

FIGURE 12-8. Horner syndrome. A. A patient with right Horner pupil. The anisocoria is greater in dim light (lower photo). Note that the right lower lid is elevated.

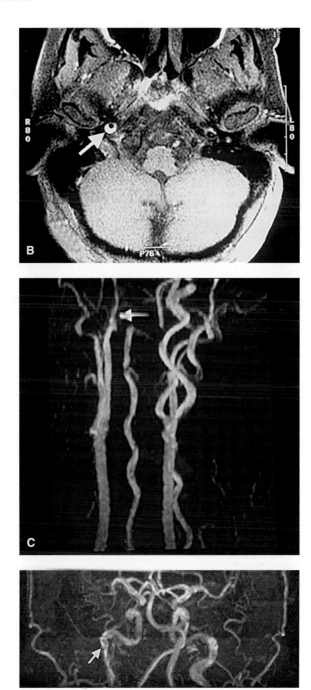

FIGURE 12-8. (*continued*) **B.** MRI reveals the characteristic hyperintense halo of blood in the wall of the carotid artery (*arrow*). **C.** MRA (upper photo) shows narrowing and an irregular contour of the internal carotid artery in the neck (*arrow*). The intracranial artery regains its normal caliber and regular contour above the dissection (*arrow*) (lower photo).

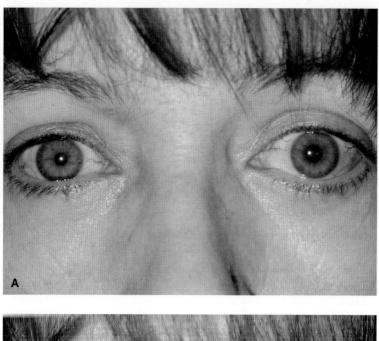

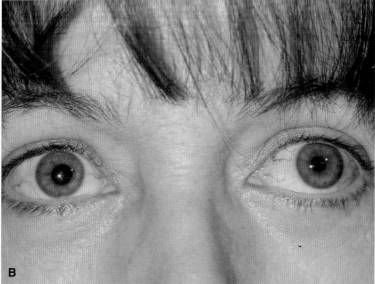

FIGURE 12-9. **Horner syndrome. A.** Left Horner syndrome. **B.** Following instillation of 1% apraclonidine, there is reversal of the anisocoria and the right, previously ptotic lid is elevated. (Courtesy of Jurij Bilyk, MD.)

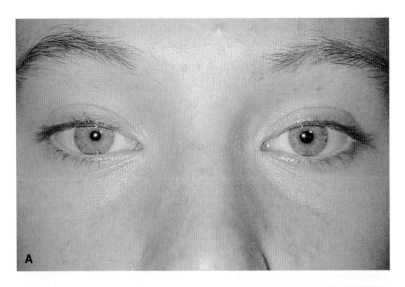

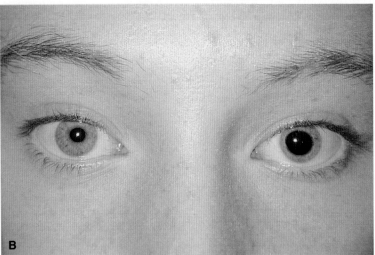

FIGURE 12-10. **Horner syndrome.** There is ptosis and miosis on the right (**A**). After the instillation of cocaine 10% the left pupil dilates (**B**), but the right does not, indicating a right Horner syndrome.

MYDRIASIS

Mydriasis is defined as a dilated pupil. It can be unilateral or bilateral. It also can be isolated or associated with other lid or extraocular muscle findings. Isolated pupillary mydriasis occurs in only a few conditions such as trauma, pharmacologic mydriasis, and cranial nerve III palsy.

TRAUMA

A dilated pupil can be the result of trauma to the globe. The dilated pupil is usually irregular and pupillary constriction to light is decreased or absent, even in the presence of preserved vision. Both the direct and consensual reaction to light and near stimuli are usually decreased.

Slit-lamp examination often reveals rupture of the pupillary sphincter or loss of the sphincter, as evidenced by flattening out of the pupillary collarette. Other anterior segment findings consistent with trauma (e.g., a subluxated lens, hyphema) may also be seen (Fig. 12-11).

PHARMACOLOGIC MYDRIASIS

Certain pharmaceuticals produce mydriasis. At times, systemic medications will produce bilateral dilated pupils with reactivity that is usually decreased.

The most frequently encountered clinical condition, however, is that of unilateral mydriasis with a minimally to nonreactive pupil without any lid or ocular motor abnormalities that may suggest a CN III palsy. Topical instillation of a pupillary dilating agent must be considered in this scenario. This may occur accidentally, with the patient being unaware that a pupillary dilating agent has been introduced into the eye. At times, however, the introduction of the mydriatic agent is purposeful and is done for secondary gain.

The extent of pupillary dilation with the instillation of mydriatic agents is much greater than the pupil dilation encountered in neurologic conditions, for example, CN III palsy. The pharmacologically dilated pupil is usually dilated to approximately 9 mm and does not react to light or near stimulation.

The diagnosis of a pharmacologically dilated pupil is established by obtaining a history, if available, of the instillation of a dilating agent (e.g., contamination of the fingers when helping a family member instill mydriatic eye drops or touching the eye after applying a scopolamine patch). If no such history is obtained, proof of the pharmacologic cause of the mydriasis is obtained by instilling pilocarpine 1% into both eyes. This drug will constrict a normal pupil as well as the dilated pupil due to CN III palsy but will not constrict the pupil that is pharmacologically dilated (Fig. 12-12). Failure of the dilated pupil to constrict is prima facie evidence of pharmacologic instillation if the pupillary sphincter is intact. Once this has been demonstrated, no further testing to detect another cause is indicated.

CRANIAL NERVE III PALSY

It is often suspected that an isolated nonreactive, widely dilated pupil with no other signs of CN III involvement may be due to an aneurysm or mass compressing the interpeduncular portion of the oculomotor nerve. There are few case reports that have documented this association; however, the majority of these patients did not have a truly isolated mydriasis or developed other signs of a CN III palsy within 2 weeks. Therefore, it is far more likely that the cause of a widely dilated nonreactive pupil is direct pharmacologic blockade or an Adie tonic pupil and not CN III palsy.

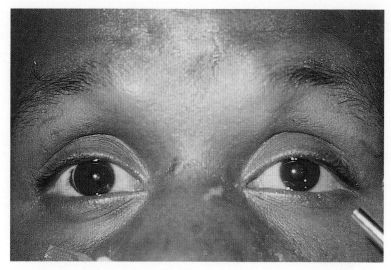

FIGURE 12-11. **Traumatic mydriasis.** The left pupil is dilated, slightly irregular, and does not react to direct light. Note the subconjunctival hemorrhage in the right eye.

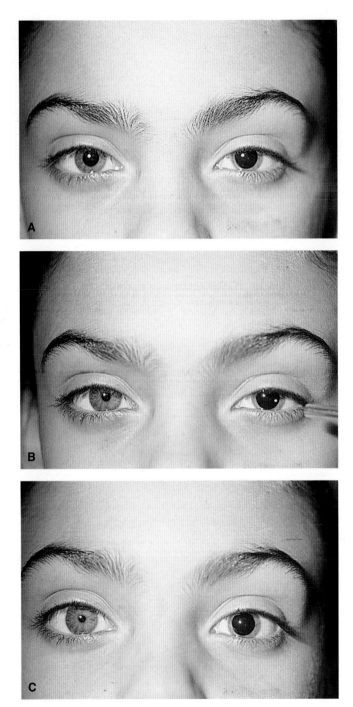

FIGURE 12-12. Pharmacologically dilated left pupil. The left pupil is markedly dilated (**A**) and does not react to direct light (**B**). Note consensual constriction of the right pupil. After the institution of pilocarpine 1% (**C**), the right pupil is miotic, the left unchanged.

ADIE (TONIC) PUPIL

This benign pupillary anomaly is characterized by the sudden onset of parasympathetic paralysis resulting in pupillary mydriasis.

ETIOLOGY AND EPIDEMIOLOGY

This is a disorder predominantly of young women, which appears to occur spontaneously. Patients often notice the anomaly when they look in the mirror and notice that one pupil is larger than the other. Alternatively, it may be noted by coworkers or relatives, who mention it to the patient. Although Adie tonic pupil occurs in both genders, it is more common in women, with 70% of cases occurring in women and 30% in men. Adie pupil is unilateral in 80% of the cases, with the second eye becoming involved at a rate of approximately 4% per year.

It is thought that this represents a viral infection in the ciliary ganglion. The acute event causes the parasympathetic paresis. The regrowth of the fibers occurs, with misdirection of the accommodative fibers that, because they outnumber the pupillary motor fibers, usurp the latter's actions. Most cases of Adie tonic pupil are idiopathic. However, Adie tonic pupil has been associated with herpes zoster, diabetes mellitus, Guillain–Barré syndrome, autonomic neuropathies, orbital trauma (including surgery), and orbital infection.

CLINICAL CHARACTERISTICS

Symptoms

- Patients may be asymptomatic or may experience
  - blurred near vision
  - a cramping sensation in the eye, which is not usually severe or terribly troublesome

  - headache
  - photophobia

Signs

- Pupillary mydriasis (**Fig. 12-13**)
- Initially, the pupil does not react to light or accommodation.
- Subsequently, the pupil does not react well or at all to light, but reacts slowly and tonically to a near stimulus, then redilates slowly and tonically on refixation at a distance.
- There is evidence of sectoral pupillary paralysis with partial or total loss of the iris collarette (**Fig. 12-14**). There is abnormal movement of the iris to a light stimulus. The portion of the iris with preserved collarette will constrict but the portion where it is absent will not, resulting in a purse string–type movement of the pupil instead of the normally seen concentric constriction. This is often referred to as vermiform movements.
- Deep tendon hypo- or areflexia (Adie syndrome).
- Certain features of Adie tonic pupil may change over time:
  - The pupils remain large, but over the years will become progressively smaller. They continue to react poorly to light and tonically to a near target.
  - Some patients may recover a limited amount of accommodation but still experience a noticeable lag period when shifting fixation between distance and near.
  - Deep tendon reflexes become increasingly hyporeflexic.
  - The other eye becomes involved in approximately 20% of the patients.

DIAGNOSTIC EVALUATION

- Pharmacologic testing: Topical pilocarpine 1/8% or 1/10% may be instilled into each eye. These diluted concentrations of pilocarpine will not constrict a normal pupil but will constrict an Adie pupil because of the presence of denervation hypersensitivity. It should be cautioned that early in the development of Adie pupil, pilocarpine 1/10% may not cause the Adie pupil to constrict and will not do so until denervation hypersensitivity occurs (Fig. 12-13D).

● Aside from pharmacologic documentation of the unilateral Adie pupil, no investigations need be conducted because this is a benign condition. Bilateral Adie pupils have been associated with syphilis and sarcoidosis, so the bilateral simultaneous occurrence of Adie pupil should be investigated for these disorders.

DIFFERENTIAL DIAGNOSIS

● Pharmacologically induced mydriasis
● CN III palsy
● Traumatic mydriasis
● Dorsal midbrain (Parinaud) syndrome (see p. 374)

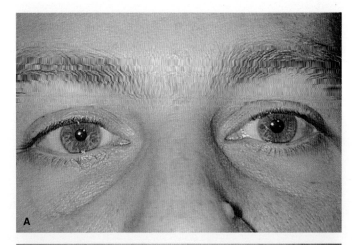

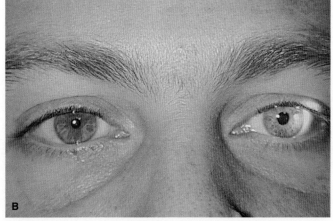

FIGURE 12-13. **Adie pupil. A.** The left pupil is larger than the right in ambient light. **B.** The anisocoria increases in bright illuminations because of poor constriction of left pupil.

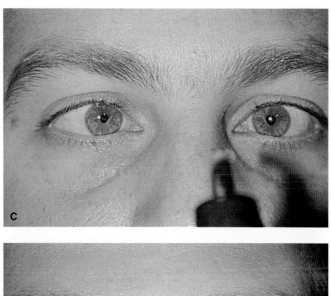

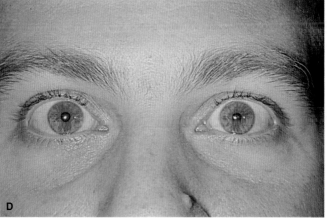

FIGURE 12-13. (*continued*) **C.** Near constriction is slow and tonic, as is redilation where the Adie pupil may momentarily be smaller than the normal side. **D.** After instillation of 1/10% pilocarpine, the left pupil constricts, whereas the right does not.

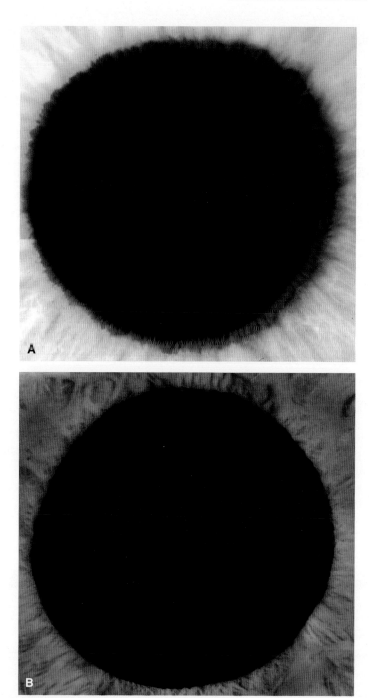

FIGURE 12-14. **Adie pupil. A.** The iris collarette is visible at the pupil margin 360 degrees. **B.** Adie pupil with no reaction to light, where no collarette is visible.

ARGYLL ROBERTSON PUPIL

The Argyll Robertson (AR) pupil is a classic example of the so-called pupillary light–near dissociation. Other causes of light–near dissociation are in **Table 12-2**.

ETIOLOGY AND PATHOGENESIS

- A variety of disorders have been implicated in causing AR pupils. However, most clinicians apply this term only when syphilis is the obvious cause. The exact mechanism by which these patients with syphilis develop AR pupils is unknown.
- AR pupils are almost always bilateral.

CLINICAL CHARACTERISTICS

Symptoms
- The pupil abnormality does not produce any direct symptoms.

Signs
- The following criteria must be met before the diagnosis of AR pupils may be made (**Fig. 12-15**).

- Vision must be present. Nonspecific light–near dissociation will occur with visual loss from any anterior visual pathway cause.
- Miotic pupils are essential. In particular, in darkness, both pupils are smaller than age-matched controls. During the later stages of syphilis, the pupils may be large and still manifest light–near dissociation. These are referred to as *taboparetic pupils.*
- The pupils show a larger reaction to a near stimulus than to light. In fact, they show almost no reaction to light.

- The pupils may also show any of the following characteristics:
  - The abnormality is usually bilateral but at times asymmetric.
  - They may be irregular.
  - Iris atrophy or transillumination defects may develop late.
  - The pupils dilate normally to mydriatics until iris atrophy occurs.
- Associated findings include the following:
  - Slit-lamp examination: interstitial keratitis
  - Dilated fundus examination: chorioretinitis, papillitis, uveitis

TABLE 12-2. Light–Near Dissociation

Cause	Lesion Location
Adie pupil	Ciliary ganglion
Optic neuropathy or severe retinopathy	Anterior visual pathway
Argyll Robertson pupils	Lesion in tectum of midbrain
Parinaud syndrome (dorsal midbrain syndrome)	Lesion in tectum of midbrain
Aberrant regeneration of III nerve	Aberrant innervations of papillary fibers
Peripheral neuropathy (diabetes, Charcot–Marie–Tooth)	Short posterior ciliary nerves

DIAGNOSTIC EVALUATION

• Tests for syphilis: Fluorescent treponemal antigen (FTA-ABS) and venereal disease research laboratory (VDRL)

• Consider lumbar puncture if central nervous system involvement is suspected.

TREATMENT

• The only treatment is directed at the underlying infection if it has not been adequately treated before. The AR pupil remains even after antibiotic therapy is completed.

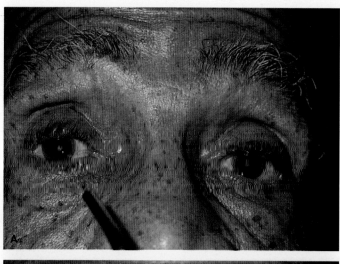

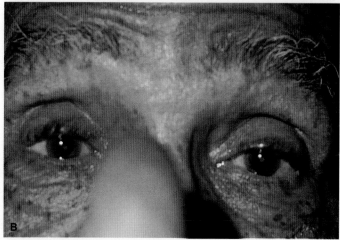

FIGURE 12-15. Argyll Robertson pupils. The pupils react poorly to direct light (**A**) but become more miotic on near testing (**B**).

Orbital Disease of Neuro-ophthalmic Significance

Jurlj R. Bllyk

THYROID EYE DISEASE

Graves' disease is defined as the triad of hyperthyroidism (diffuse thyroid enlargement), orbitopathy, and pretibial myxedema.

ETIOLOGY AND EPIDEMIOLOGY

● Thyroid eye disease (TED) is an autoimmune process. However, the exact mechanism by which the changes in the orbit take place remains elusive.

● TED is associated with other autoimmune disorders, such as myasthenia gravis, which is present in 1% to 2% of the patients with TED.

● Orbital findings are likely due to chronic inflammation and glycosaminoglycan deposition in the soft tissues (extraocular muscles, fat, lacrimal gland) that in turn causes edema and eventual fibrosis. Secondary orbital congestion from decreased venous outflow potentiates the clinical findings.

INCIDENCE

● Thyroid disease is common, occurring in about 2% of the general population, with a female preponderance of 6 to 10:1. TED is seen to some degree in 30% to 70% of patients with thyroid dysfunction, with the female-to-male ratio narrowing to 4:1.

● Although periocular findings usually manifest within 18 months of the thyroid disease, they can either precede or follow the thyroid diagnosis by several years or even decades. Patients are typically hyperthyroid, but a minority of cases are hypo- or euthyroid. The presence of the characteristic eye disease without any thyroid abnormalities is termed euthyroid TED. About 25% of these patients will develop thyroid dysfunction in 1 year and about 50% over 5 years. Approximately 5% to 25% of patients will present initially to the ophthalmologist without evidence of systemic disease.

CLINICAL CHARACTERISTICS

- Systemic: Depending on the specific type of thyroid dysfunction (hyper-, hypo-, eu-), initial symptoms include:
  - Weight loss or gain
  - Increased appetite
  - Sweating
  - Heat/cold intolerance
  - Fatigue
  - Tremors
  - Heart palpitations
  - The thyroid gland may be enlarged
  - Up to 50% may have a family history of thyroid dysfunction

- Periocular and orbital: Many patients experience two distinct phases of the disease. Early in the course, the patient presents with symptomatic, inflammatory signs called "active" (Fig. 13-1). During this phase, patients have a variety of nonspecific complaints, often misdiagnosed as allergy or dry eye syndrome. As additional orbital inflammation develops, the clinical diagnosis becomes more obvious.
  - Six months to 3 years later (mean 12 months), the progressive changes either arrest or abate, and the patient enters a long-term "inactive" or "burnt-out" phase. At this point, the chance of reentering an inflammatory phase is about 5%. TED may present either unilaterally or bilaterally and may be asymmetric.

- Symptoms
  - Eyelid: A variety of lid abnormalities occur, including upper lid retraction in primary gaze ("thyroid stare"), edema ("puffy eyelid"), and lagophthalmos (inability to close the eyelids completely).

  - A foreign body sensation, which may be asymmetric, and is due to corneal exposure from proptosis, lid retraction or both.

  - Double vision is due to infiltration of the extraocular muscles, which become inflamed and subsequently become fibrotic.

- Loss of vision can occur secondary to anterior segment disease (corneal exposure, drying, infection, or perforation) or a compressive optic neuropathy.

- Signs
  - Upper eyelid retraction is a typical and highly sensitive sign of TED and is seen mostly in the hyperthyroid state (Fig. 13-2A). Upper scleral show should always be considered abnormal and should prompt thyroid function testing. Lid edema may occur in the hyper- or hypothyroid state. The upper lid may lag behind the movement of the globe in downgaze (von Graefe sign) (Fig. 13-2B).

  - Proptosis may be unilateral or bilateral. The most frequent cause of proptosis in adults is TED.

  - Increased resistance to attempted retropulsion of the globes is found in some patients. Patients with little or no proptosis and increased resistance to retropulsion are at greater risk of developing optic neuropathy.

  - Exposure keratopathy because of lagophthalmos.

  - Ocular injection. Conjunctival injection is most prominent over the horizontal rectus muscles. Conjunctival chemosis is commonly noted inferolaterally (Fig. 13-3).

  - Superior limbic keratitis may be present.

  - Ocular misalignment in any form may occur. However, the muscles most commonly involved are the medial and inferior rectus muscles. Therefore, esotropias and hypotropias are most frequently encountered (Fig. 13-4). Exotropias are atypical of TED and should prompt a search for another etiology.

▪ Increased intraocular pressure, especially in upgaze; this is usually due to restrictive inferior rectus myopathy or a congested orbit (Fig. 13-5A). Because this is a mechanical form of increased intraocular pressure, topical antiglaucomatous therapy is often ineffective.

▪ Optic neuropathy occurs in approximately 5% of patients with TED and is due to compression of the optic nerve by large indurated muscles at the orbital apex. The clinical risk factors for the development of thyroid-related optic neuropathy are:

  ▸ Lack of proptosis

  ▸ Increased resistance to ocular retropulsion

  ▸ Enlargement of the medial rectus muscles with complaints of diplopia and evidence of restrictive strabismus

DIAGNOSTIC EVALUATION

• The clinical appearance of a patient with lid retraction is sufficient to establish the diagnosis of TED (Fig. 13-5A). In a typical clinical setting, imaging of the orbit is not required but may reveal enlarged extraocular muscles with sparing of the tendinous insertions. The medial and inferior rectus muscles are most frequently involved (Fig. 13-5B). The orbital fat may appear inflamed on MRI and have a diffuse reticular pattern ("dirty fat") on CT.

• Endocrinologic investigation to detect any thyroid dysfunction should be carried out in patients without a history of thyroid disease. Although a battery of tests are available, in general a selective (sensitive, third-generation) TSH is the only screening test needed. This test is especially helpful in patients who are systemically asymptomatic because it is

effective in detecting subtle degrees of hyperthyroidism. In cases where the patient is euthyroid, thyroid-stimulating (TSI) and thyroid peroxidase (TPO) antibodies tests may reveal a markedly elevated titer. Although the predictive utility of TSI and TPO is unclear, a high titer supports the diagnosis of TED in an euthyroid patient.

• Imaging of the orbit should be performed if the diagnosis is in doubt (e.g., absence of upper eyelid retraction, isolated unilateral proptosis, etc.) or in preparation for surgical intervention (see the following discussion).

• Follow-up schedules depend on the clinical setting. Patients with risk factors for optic neuropathy (see previous discussion) should be examined every 2 to 3 months initially to detect decreasing vision or color perception, and the patient should be instructed on how to monitor for red desaturation on a weekly basis between examinations. Patients with no ocular misalignment and normal retropulsion may be seen every 6 to 12 months.

DIFFERENTIAL DIAGNOSIS

• A detailed description is found in **Table 13-1**.

TREATMENT

• General
  ▪ Control the dysthyroid state. Note that control of thyroid function has little effect on the progression of TED.

  ▪ There is controversial evidence that patients treated for hyperthyroidism with radioactive iodine rather than medically or surgically may develop TED more frequently and to a more severe degree. Pretreatment with corticosteroid has been suggested to decrease this problem, but

TABLE 13-1. Etiology of Orbital Inflammation

Infectious Inflammation	Noninfectious Inflammation*
By anatomic site of involvement	Thyroid eye disease
Preseptal cellulitis	Idiopathic orbital inflammatory syndrome (orbital pseudotumor)
Orbital cellulitis	Lymphoid hyperplasia
Subperiosteal abscess	Granulomatous (sarcoidosis)
Intraorbital abscess	Vasculitic (granulomatosis with polyangiitis)
Cavernous sinus thrombosis	Eosinophilic granulomatosis with polyangiitis (Churg-Strauss syndrome)
	Metastatic disease
By infectious agent	Relapsing polychondritis
Bacterial	Polyarteritis nodosa, dermatomyositis
Fungal	Rheumatologic (Sjögren syndrome)
Viral	Other (hypersensitivity angiitis, amyloidosis)
Parasitic	

*An example of each type of noninfectious inflammation is included in parentheses.

remains unproven and may overtreat a significant number of patients. More recent data have concluded that progression of TED may occur more frequently following either thyroidectomy or radioactive iodine therapy if the patient has very high levels of serum T3/T4 before treatment, and these levels drop precipitously and remain low immediately after treatment.

■ Cigarette smoking adversely affects the progression and severity of TED. All patients with Graves' disease should be advised strongly to stop smoking. The patient should be reminded in no uncertain terms that cessation of tobacco use is important in the management of their disease; these conversations should be clearly documented in the medical record.

● Specific

■ Systemic corticosteroids: TED often responds to the systemic administration of corticosteroids. Treatment may improve orbital congestion, acute ocular misalignment, and optic neuropathy. Some patients will respond to this treatment, others will not. Prolonged steroid therapy is not indicated because of the risks of long-term steroid use. In most patients, cessation of corticosteroids will result in a recurrence of inflammation. Recent studies from Europe suggest that the use of high-dose pulsed intravenous corticosteroids may lead to an arrest of progressive orbitopathy with fewer systemic side effects than oral corticosteroids. Whether this therapy is effective in long-term disease control is controversial.

■ Oral selenium: Selenium has known antioxidant effects. A large study from Europe concluded that oral selenium supplementation in patients with mild to moderate TED resulted in less ocular involvement and slowed progression of TED when compared with placebo. It is difficult to directly apply these data to patients in the United States because some parts of Europe suffer from a lack of dietary selenium, whereas no such deficiency has been shown in the American diet. Furthermore, there is some controversy as to whether excess selenium increases the risk of type II diabetes and prostate cancer. We typically offer selenium supplementation to women with mild to moderate active TED at a dose of 100 µg twice daily for 6 months; some clinicians recommend a daily diet of Brazil nuts, which have a high selenium content.

■ Orbital radiation: There is controversy about the efficacy of orbital radiation. Many reports indicate that it is effective in the treatment of the inflammatory phase of TED. Other studies as well as a recent meta-analysis of available data indicate that it may not be effective except in the stabilization of progressive external ophthalmoplegia. However, some criticism about the patient selection and duration of the ocular disease keeps the controversy regarding radiation therapy alive. We still employ radiation therapy in select patients with TED. Orbital radiation is usually given over 10 to 12 sessions (200 cGy each session) for a total dose of 2,000 cGy. It should not be repeated because of the risk of additive radiation, and many experts avoid radiation in patients who smoke or have other vasculopathic risk factors (e.g., diabetes mellitus). It is only indicated in patients who are in the inflammatory phase. Of note, orbital radiation is advocated by some experts in the management of TED compressive optic neuropathy. Although the authors certainly utilize this treatment modality in patients who present with early optic neuropathy, the treating physician should also be aware that radiation therapy frequently has a significant lag of several weeks before any anti-inflammatory effect is seen. The optic neuropathy may progress significantly in the interim. Therefore, advanced or rapidly progressive compressive optic neuropathy is best treated with timely orbital decompression. Patients with early optic neuropathy who undergo orbital radiation therapy should be monitored closely for any progressive visual loss.

■ Surgery usually progresses in a staged, sequential fashion. Orbital abnormalities are addressed first, followed by strabismus and eyelid repair. Not all patients require each step, but the order is important to maximize predictability of the final result.

▶ Orbital decompression is indicated when proptosis must be reduced or when optic neuropathy occurs. For the relief of proptosis, an anterior decompression may suffice; for optic neuropathy, a posterior orbital decompression that involves the deep medial wall of the orbit is usually required. Some experts have reported reversal of optic neuropathy with bony decompression of the deep lateral orbital wall. During the inflammatory phase, surgery is reserved for emergent cases of compressive optic neuropathy. Once the inflammation has subsided, surgery is typically safer and more predictable.

▶ Extraocular muscle surgery: surgical attempts to realign the eyes should be performed only after the ocular misalignment has been stable for several months (we use 3 months as a minimum). Recessions (typically with adjustable suture technique) are recommended rather than muscle resection.

▶ Eyelid surgery is aimed at first correcting upper and lower eyelid retraction and then debulking edematous skin and fat. A variety of techniques are employed, including levator recession, full-thickness blepharotomy, Müllerectomy, and eyelid spacers.

■ Biologics: Limited data on the use of biologic agents in the management of refractory TED have appeared recently in the literature. The physician must be cautioned at this juncture about recommending such therapy to patients with typical TED, given the limited power of these studies (limited patient numbers); the lack of a clear understanding as to the specific biologic agent (i.e., tumor necrosis factor antibody vs. CD20 antibody), dosage, and duration of treatment; the cost of the agents; the off-label use of biologic agents in TED; and the potential systemic side effects. That said, biologic agents present an intriguing potential therapy for TED in the future.

■ Injected corticosteroids: Some experts advocate the use of depot corticosteroid agents in the management of TED. There are several limitations of this modality that must be considered. First, no study shows that orbital injection is superior to the use of systemic corticosteroids, although admittedly fewer systemic side effects occur with injection. Second, some clinicians question the logic of injecting a volume of medication into an already congested orbit. Third, corticosteroid injections carry the risk of glaucoma, globe perforation, optic nerve injury, and extraocular muscle injury. Finally, a recent "black box" warning by the manufacturer of triamcinolone suspension specifically warns against periocular injection because of the risk of arterial occlusion from particulate embolization. This leaves the clinician with few options for long-acting depot injections into the orbit.

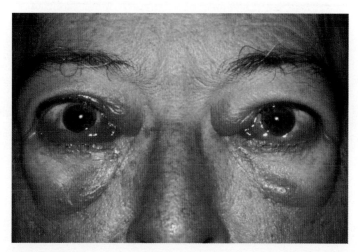

FIGURE 13-1. **Thyroid eye disease.** Acute inflammatory thyroid eye disease with lid retraction, boggy eyelid edema, conjunctival chemosis, and proptosis.

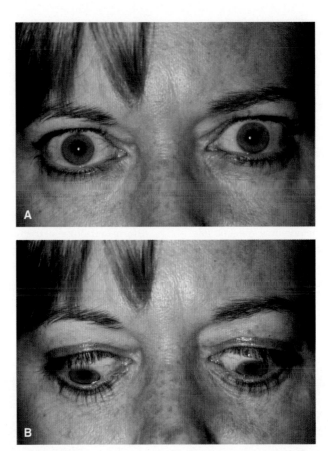

FIGURE 13-2. Thyroid eye disease. A. Upper eyelid retraction ("thyroid stare"). **B.** Lid lag in downgaze. The patient is in the quiescent "burnt-out" phase of TED.

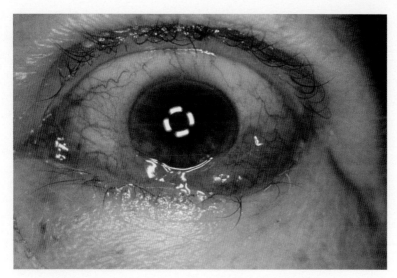

FIGURE 13-3. Thyroid eye disease. Conjunctival chemosis and upper eyelid retraction.

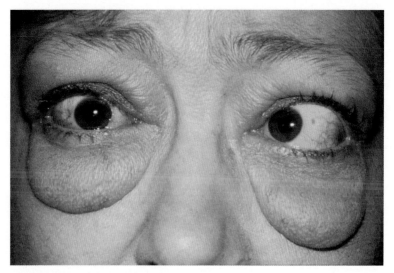

FIGURE 13-4. Thyroid eye disease: Strabismus.

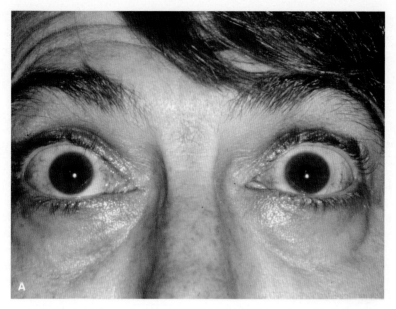

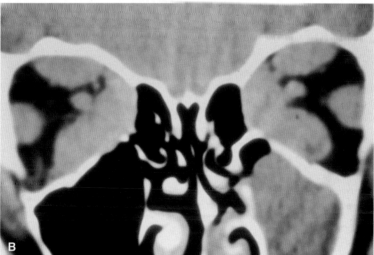

FIGURE 13-5. **Thyroid eye disease. A.** Patient on attempted upgaze. **B.** Coronal CT image demonstrates extraocular muscle enlargement.

IDIOPATHIC ORBITAL INFLAMMATORY SYNDROME (ORBITAL PSEUDOTUMOR)

Idiopathic orbital inflammatory syndrome (IOIS) is an acute inflammation affecting any tissue within the orbit.

ETIOLOGY

● The etiology is unknown. In the vast majority of cases, there is no associated systemic disease. On occasion, patients with other autoimmune or inflammatory conditions (lupus erythematosus, ulcerative colitis) may present with orbital inflammation. IOIS has no clear predilection for a certain age, gender, or race. No clear seasonal pattern has been proven.

● Histopathologically, a mixed, paucicellular inflammatory response is the rule, including neutrophils, lymphocytes, and monocytes, although in some cases (especially children), a preponderance of eosinophils may be seen. Limited recent data suggest that IOIS may be a T-cell–mediated process.

CLINICAL CHARACTERISTICS

● Classically the presentation is acute, with a sudden onset of

  ▪ pain,

  ▪ swelling, and

  ▪ double vision.

● IOIS can affect any soft-tissue component within the orbit and may manifest signs of

  ▪ dacryoadenitis (Fig. 13-6),

  ▪ myositis (Fig. 13-7),

  ▪ optic neuritis,

  ▪ tenonitis (Fig. 13-8),

  ▪ posterior scleritis,

  ▪ orbital apex syndrome, when the disease affects the posterior orbit, and

  ▪ in children, IOIS presenting with systemic symptoms, including fever, which is more often bilateral than in adults.

DIFFERENTIAL DIAGNOSIS

● A more complete differential diagnostic list for IOIS is found in Table 13-1. The main entities to consider include the following:

  ▪ Orbital cellulitis: In some patients, the clinical presentation may be difficult to distinguish from orbital cellulitis. Several findings may be helpful in this regard (Table 13-2). First, IOIS tends to present explosively over several hours. Orbital cellulitis typically has prodromal symptoms lasting several days. In orbital cellulitis, the eyelids tend to be tense and deeply erythematous. Conversely, in IOIS, there is a softer, pinker swelling of the eyelids referred to as a "boggy edema" (Fig. 13-9). Conjunctival edema (chemosis) mirrors this tendency; cases of IOIS have a quieter (less injected) chemosis than cases of infectious orbital cellulitis. Furthermore, in most cases of orbital cellulitis, the adjacent paranasal sinuses will be affected with complaints of nasal congestion and purulent rhinorrhea, in contradistinction to IOIS, where the sinuses will be clear.

  ▪ Lymphoproliferative disease: The spectrum proceeds from polyclonal lymphoid hyperplasia to monoclonal lymphoma. IOIS should *not* be considered part of this spectrum because, unlike lymphoid hyperplasia, there is no evidence that IOIS progresses to lymphoma. Lymphoproliferative disease commonly presents in an indolent, painless fashion over weeks to months, although in a minority of cases, orbital lymphoma may mimic the inflammatory findings of IOIS. Additional distinguishing features are found in Table 13-3.

TABLE 13-2. Features Distinguishing IOIS from Cellulitis

Features	IOIS	Orbital Cellulitis
Onset	Abrupt over several hours	Several days
Eyelid	Soft pink coloration, "boggy edema"	Tense, erythematous
CT	Paranasal sinuses uninvolved	Paranasal sinuses involved
Conjunctiva	Variable	Chemosis, injection
Systemic signs	Usually none	Fever, elevated white count

IOIS, idiopathic orbital inflammatory syndrome.

■ TED (Graves' disease): A detailed discussion is found in a separate section. Distinguishing features are found in **Table 13-4.**

■ Adenoviral conjunctivitis presents with preseptal findings. Although initially a unilateral process, autoinoculation of the contralateral eye almost invariably leads to bilateral complaints. Presence of a follicular conjunctivitis along with a tender preauricular lymphadenopathy is diagnostic.

■ Granulomatosis with polyangiitis (GPA, Granulomatosis with polyangiitis (Wegener granulomatosis)) is a necrotizing vasculitis that may present in either an indolent or explosive fashion. Most patients with GPA are male and between 20 and 40 years. Ocular involvement occurs in 50% of patients. Two variants are seen:

▶ Generalized, with the involvement of the lungs and kidneys. These patients present with significant, fulminant systemic complaints. A positive cytoplasmic antineutrophil cytoplasmic antibodies (c-ANCA) serology is the rule and is diagnostic.

▶ Localized, with the involvement limited to the paranasal sinuses and orbit. Symptoms are reminiscent of chronic sinusitis. Bone destruction on CT is the rule. Biopsy is necessary for definitive diagnosis because c-ANCA serology is negative in a significant percentage of patients.

■ Sarcoidosis: Periocular or intraocular sarcoidosis may present in either an indolent or a fulminant fashion. Involvement of the

TABLE 13-3. Features Distinguishing IOIS from Orbital Lymphoproliferative Disease

Features	IOIS	Orbital Lymphocytic Lesions
Onset	Abrupt	Insidious
Examination	Mimics cellulitis	"Salmon patch" conjunctival mass or orbital mass
CT	Diffuse, poorly defined borders	Molding to orbital structures
Pathology	Polymorphic (mixed cells)	Monomorphic (mostly lymphocytes)
	Hypocellular	Hypercellular
	Occasional fibrosis	Rare fibrosis
Systemic association	Usually none	Lymphoma

IOIS, idiopathic orbital inflammatory syndrome.

TABLE 13-4. Features Distinguishing IOIS from TED

Features	IOIS	TED
Gender	M = F	F > M
Onset	Usually sudden	Usually gradual
Laterality	Usually unilateral	Usually bilateral
Pain	Yes	Variable
Response to steroids	Rapid	Variable
Imaging (myositis variant):		
Number muscles	~1 (50%)	>1
Muscles	SR, MR	IR > MR > SR > LR
Muscle border	Irregular	Regular
Tendon	Involved (Fig. 13-7B)	Spared
Orbital fat	Involved	Relatively clear

Extraocular muscles: IR, inferior rectus; IOIS, idiopathic orbital inflammatory syndrome; LR, lateral rectus; MR, medial rectus; SR, superior rectus; TED, thyroid eye disease.

lacrimal glands is common. History may reveal constitutional symptoms as well as complaints of shortness of breath or a misdiagnosis of asthma. Ocular examination may reveal eyelid and conjunctival nodules, evidence of previous uveitis (keratic precipitates), iris nodules, vitreous debris, and cotton wool spots. Optic neuritis may occur. Angiotensin-converting enzyme and chest X-ray may be helpful but can prove negative in a localized variant known as "orbital sarcoid" or orbital granulomatous inflammation.

■ Orbital metastasis: Metastatic disease to the orbit typically occurs in a more indolent and less inflammatory fashion than classic IOIS. However, inflammatory signs may certainly accompany orbital metastasis. The empiric diagnosis of IOIS should be used with great caution in any patient with a known history of cancer, with a low threshold for attempted orbital biopsy.

• Special forms: One rare variant of orbital inflammation, known as sclerosing pseudotumor, is more chronic and causes significant tissue destruction from secondary fibrosis. This form of orbital inflammation is poorly responsive to corticosteroid therapy and may require more drastic measures, including chemotherapeutic agents, biologics, repeated surgical debulking, and, on occasion, exenteration. The clinical and histopathologic picture is so atypical of classic IOIS that some experts have appropriately questioned whether this diagnosis even belongs within the rubric of orbital inflammation. IgG4-related orbitopathy is a recently described entity in the orbit and may represent either a unique subtype of inflammatory orbitopathy or a variant of other entities (GPA, sarcoidosis). IgG4-related orbitopathy may be associated with fibrosis of other viscera and a higher risk of eventual lymphoma development.

DIAGNOSTIC EVALUATION

• CT or MRI will reveal a poorly circumscribed, infiltrating enhancement of orbital tissue and may be limited to specific tissue (muscle, lacrimal gland). Bone destruction is very atypical and necessitates tissue biopsy.

- On occasion, B-scan ultrasonography is helpful in cases of posterior scleritis, which may not be visible on CT or MRI.

- Systemic workup is rarely helpful and is usually not indicated. In patients where differentiation from infection is difficult, a complete blood count (CBC) with differential may be obtained. An elevated white count and left shift may be seen in both infectious and noninfectious orbital inflammation. Bacterial infection will usually result in neutrophilia with left shift, whereas in some cases of IOIS, eosinophilia may be present. As already noted, a careful history of previous cancer must be sought in all cases of presumed IOIS. Atypical cases of IOIS warrant further investigation, including serologies for sarcoidosis, CRP and IgG/IgG4 levels, and workup for potential malignant sources (prostate-specific antigen, mammography, chest imaging, etc.).

- The need for initial orbital biopsy to either confirm IOIS or refute other confounding diagnoses is controversial. There is no "typical" histopathology that conclusively proves the diagnosis of IOIS; rather, biopsy is usually done to rule out other distinct pathologies. Certainly, biopsy should be considered in atypical cases of IOIS or in patients with a known history of malignancy. Because of the low morbidity of lacrimal gland biopsy, some experts also recommend biopsy of all cases of suspected inflammatory dacryoadenitis. Biopsy may not be feasible if the affected tissue is not readily accessible (e.g., orbital apex) or if surgery carries a significant morbidity (e.g., biopsy of an extraocular muscle). Two additional points must also be considered by the clinician. First, treatment of IOIS with systemic corticosteroids before attempted biopsy may mask the true histopathology of the process. Second, a "negative" biopsy does not necessarily rule out

a potentially dangerous diagnosis: the biopsy may simply have been inadequate. This is a distinct possibility in biopsy of the orbital apex and extraocular muscles, where an attempt to obtain more tissue also increases the risk of permanent morbidity from the procedure.

- In cases that present atypically (subacute/chronic, bilaterally in adults) or respond poorly to corticosteroid treatment (recalcitrant or recurrent cases), a lower threshold for a complete systemic workup and tissue biopsy in search of another cause should be aggressively pursued.

TREATMENT

- Corticosteroids. In adults, prednisone 80 to 100 mg daily usually results in rapid and dramatic clinical improvement, often after only one dose; pediatric doses should be calculated by body weight (1 mg/kg/day). This dramatic response to appropriate doses of corticosteroids bolsters the presumptive diagnosis of IOIS, but is not conclusive: other pathologies, most notably lymphoproliferative disease, may manifest similar dramatic responses. Relapses are common and are usually related to a rapid taper of corticosteroids.

- Nonsteroidal anti-inflammatory medications (NSAIDs). In patients who are intolerant of corticosteroids, the initial corticosteroid dose may be tapered more rapidly, whereas a steady dose of NSAIDs is maintained as a therapeutic bridge, followed by a slow NSAID taper.

- Radiation therapy. A course of low-dose (2,000 cGy) orbital radiotherapy may be considered. Many experts mandate tissue biopsy before proceeding with radiotherapy.

- If any doubt is present between IOIS and orbital cellulitis, as occurs more often in children than in adults, it is prudent to first begin a trial of intravenous antibiotics with close clinical follow-up. If symptoms fail to improve after 48 hours, a "test dose" of corticosteroids may be given while still maintaining antibiotic coverage. A rapid response to corticosteroids is indicative of a noninfectious inflammation.

• Rare cases of IOIS may not respond to corticosteroids and NSAIDs, and in such cases antimetabolite or biologic therapy may be considered, but biopsy should be performed first when feasible.

• The use of corticosteroid injection into orbital tissue for IOIS mirrors the discussion of this modality in TED (see previous section). A recent study noted more rapid resolution of inflammatory dacryoadenitis with surgical debulking and intraoperative injection of corticosteroid.

• All patients with IOIS, even those with classic presentations and rapid, sustained response to systemic corticosteroids, must be warned about the limitations of empiric diagnosis and followed over the long term to assure that no confounding diagnosis manifests.

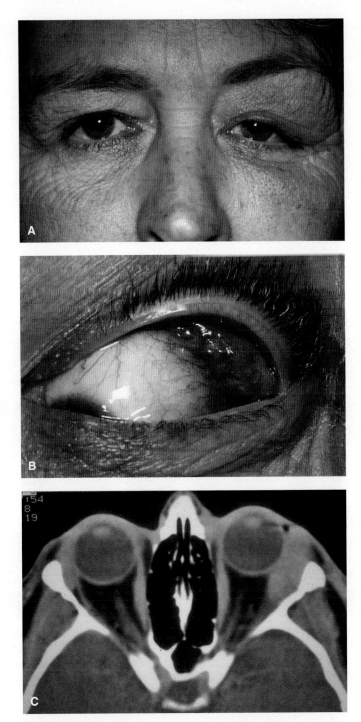

FIGURE 13-6. **Inflammatory dacryoadenitis. A** and **B.** Diffuse injection of the lacrimal gland without purulent discharge. **C.** Axial CT shows diffuse enlargement of the lacrimal gland without bone erosion.

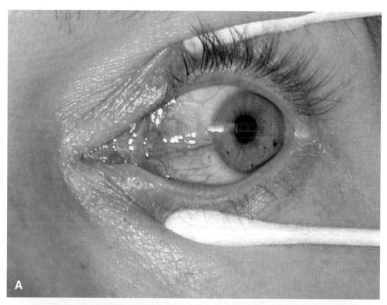

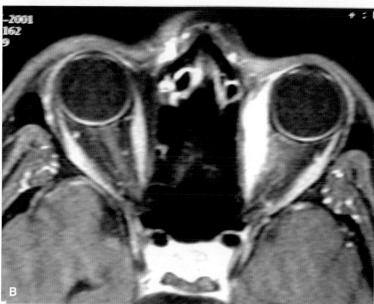

FIGURE 13-7. **Myositis. A.** Thickening of the medial rectus muscle insertion with overlying conjunctival injection. **B.** Axial MRI (T1, gadolinium, fat suppression) reveals diffuse enlargement of the muscle, including the insertion.

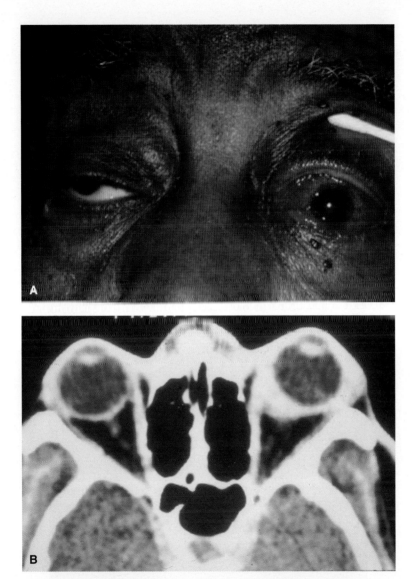

FIGURE 13-8. **Tenonitis.** **A.** Clinical signs of proptosis, external ophthalmoplegia, and conjunctival injection. **B.** On CT, diffuse thickening and enhancement of Tenon's capsule are obvious.

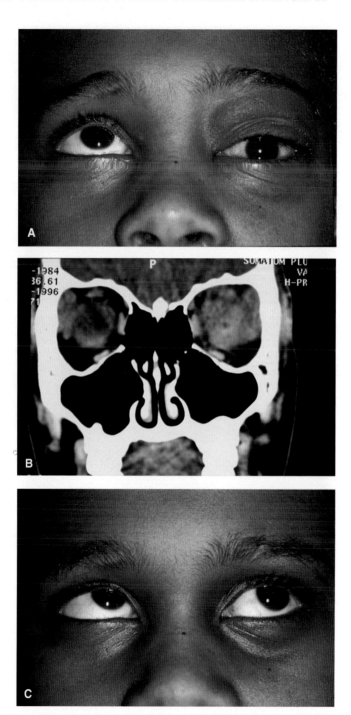

FIGURE 13-9. Idiopathic orbital inflammatory syndrome (IOIS). **A.** Typical pink, boggy eyelids of IOIS. Note limitation in upgaze. **B.** Coronal CT shows diffuse intraconal enhancement. Note that the paranasal sinuses are clear. **C.** Complete clinical resolution 1 week after oral corticosteroids.

CAVERNOUS SINUS FISTULAS

Acquired arteriovenous (AV) communications (fistulas) affecting the orbit most commonly occur in the cavernous sinus.

ETIOLOGY

- In simple terms, AV fistulas within the cavernous sinus generally fall into two categories:
  - *High-flow* fistulas are usually the result of trauma, occur in younger patients, and involve an abnormal connection between the carotid siphon and the cavernous sinus venous plexus (Barrow type A). The term carotid-cavernous fistula (CCF) is used interchangeably with high-flow fistula.
  - *Low-flow* fistulas typically occur spontaneously in older patients. The abnormality occurs between one of the small arterial branches of the internal carotid, external carotid, or both (Barrow type B, C, D) and the venous plexus of the cavernous sinus. This type of fistula is often called a "dural-sinus fistula," or simply subsumed into the more generalized CCF.

- Although practical for the ophthalmologists, this rubric is an oversimplification of the stratification of CCFs used by our neurosurgical colleagues. Other critical parameters that usually require angiography to elucidate include the source (internal vs. external carotid artery), laterality (ipsilateral, contralateral, or both), and, most importantly, the presence or absence of posterior cortical venous outflow. It is impossible for an ophthalmologist to assess this last feature on a clinical basis, yet it remains a critical concept because significant posterior cortical venous outflow by the fistula markedly increases the risk of hemorrhagic stroke. Fortunately, most low-flow fistulas that drain anterior toward the orbit do not drain posteriorly.

CLINICAL CHARACTERISTICS

- Symptoms
  - Visual acuity varies from normal to poor
  - Diplopia
  - Red eye
  - Headache may be present
  - A "whooshing" or "rushing" sound in the head
- Signs
  - Proptosis
  - External ophthalmoplegia at times with ocular misalignment (Fig. 13-10A)
  - Auscultation over the superior orbital rim may reveal a bruit, although this is an admittedly uncommon finding.
  - The conjunctival vessels associated with fistulae are diffusely engorged and tortuous (arterialization, corkscrewing). The vascular engorgement often extends to the limbus (Fig. 13-10B).
  - Intraocular pressure may be elevated. Applanation tonometry often shows a significant pulsatility in the biprism.
  - Iris neovascularization may occur from chronic ocular ischemia.
  - A relative afferent pupillary defect (RAPD) and dyschromatopsia are present if optic neuropathy develops.
  - Venous engorgement or central retinal vein occlusion may be seen on funduscopic examination (Fig. 13-10C). Exudative retinal or choroidal detachments are less common.
  - Ocular or macular ischemia.
  - Because the cavernous sinuses are connected by the circular (intercavernous) sinus around the pituitary stalk, a unilateral CCF may present with unilateral, bilateral, or, rarely, contralateral orbital findings.

DIAGNOSTIC EVALUATION

• Orbital color Doppler ultrasonography (CDU) shows engorgement of the superior ophthalmic vein (SOV), reversal of flow, and an arterial waveform within the SOV (Fig. 13-11). Based on a recent publication, CDU appears to be more sensitive in ruling out CCF than specific in ruling it in. However, given the lack of morbidity of CDU compared with cerebral arteriography, CDU should be used as a screening test if available.

• An enlarged, S-shaped SOV in the superior orbit, just beneath the superior rectus/ levator complex on CT or MRI (Fig. 13-12). Both SOVs may be enlarged with asymmetric clinical findings, depending on flow characteristics. The extraocular muscles too may also be enlarged because of decreased venous outflow and resultant orbital congestion. Note that extraocular muscle and SOV enlargement may be seen in other congestive orbitopathies, most notably TED.

• When suspected, patients with cavernous sinus fistulas should undergo six-vessel cerebral arteriography to better characterize the abnormality, assess for posterior cortical venous outflow, and allow for transarterial or transvenous closure of the abnormality (Fig. 13-13A). Note that some experts will follow suspected low-flow CCFs that are minimally symptomatic, hoping that the fistula will spontaneously thrombose, thereby skirting the low but possible morbidity of cerebral arteriography.

TREATMENT

• In high-flow fistulas that present with severe orbital signs, including progressive optic neuropathy, treatment is indicated.

Treatment is performed by neuroradiologic interventionalists. The location of the abnormal connection is delineated using conventional arteriography, and preferably at the same time, the fistula is closed with a variety of techniques, including glue, balloons, or thrombogenic coils (Fig. 13-13B). On occasion, the fistula cannot be approached using conventional femoral transarterial or transvenous routes. In such cases, the fistula may be closed through a transorbital SOV approach using a lid crease incision. The patient is always warned about the potential complications of arteriography, including stroke and death, as well as the risks of fistula closure, including visual loss, worsening of orbital congestion, marked intraocular pressure rise and orbital compartment syndrome from sudden closure of orbital venous egress, central retinal vein/artery occlusion, and neovascularization because of ocular ischemia.

• Because low-flow fistulas often close spontaneously, they may be followed over time unless the intraocular pressure is uncontrolled, posterior cortical venous outflow is present, the findings persist over months without improvement, or progressive ocular findings develop.

• A paradoxical worsening of symptoms may be seen in low-flow fistulas. As thrombosis forms in the SOV, the patient may present with a marked increase in signs and symptoms. If possible, conservative management is indicated for 48 to 72 hours, at which time the symptoms should begin to abate as alternate orbital venous drainage forms. If no improvement occurs after this time, the patient should undergo repeat workup to assure that a low-flow state has not converted into a high-flow abnormality.

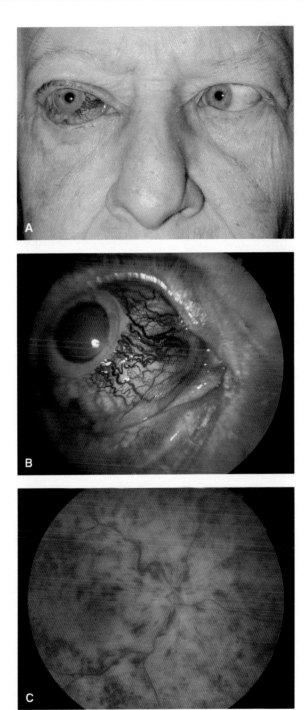

FIGURE 13-10. Clinical signs in cavernous sinus fistulas.   A. Mild proptosis and an abduction deficit are noted on the right. **B.** Arterialization of conjunctival vessels. **C.** Central retinal vein occlusion.

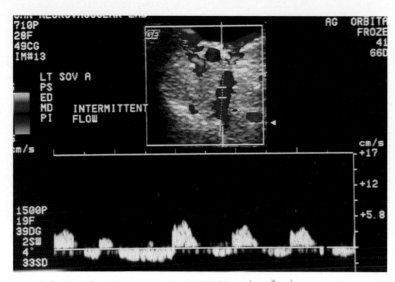

FIGURE 13-11. **Color Doppler ultrasonography in a cavernous sinus fistula.** Reversal of flow (red instead of the usual blue) is noted in the superior ophthalmic vein. Also note the presence of an arterial waveform.

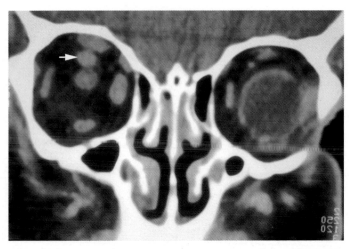

FIGURE 13-12. **Cavernous sinus fistula.** Coronal CT imaging reveals an engorged SOV (*arrow*) along with diffuse enlargement of the extraocular muscles on the affected side.

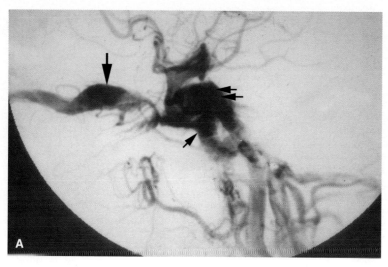

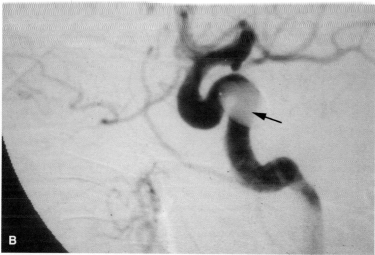

FIGURE 13-13. **Arteriography of a cavernous sinus fistula. A.** An abnormal connection is noted between the carotid siphon (*small arrow*) and the cavernous sinus (*double arrow*), with secondary engorgement of the superior ophthalmic vein (SOV, *large arrow*). **B.** Flow into the SOV ceases after placement of a detachable balloon (*arrow*) into the cavernous sinus.

Index

Note: Page number followed by *f* and *t* indicates figure and table respectively.